Felix Unger (Ed.)

Coronary Artery Surgery in the Nineties

With 92 Figures and 104 Tables

Springer-Verlag Berlin Heidelberg New York
London Paris Tokyo

Universitäts-Professor
Dr. med. FELIX UNGER
Landeskrankenanstalten Salzburg
Herzchirurgie
Müllner Hauptstr. 48
A-5020 Salzburg

ISBN-13: 978-3-642-45624-4 e-ISBN-13: 978-3-642-45622-0
DOI: 10.1007/978-3-642-45622-0

Library of Congress Cataloging-in-Publication Data.
Coronary artery surgery in the nineties.
Based on a workshop held Nov. 22–23, 1985 in Salzburg, Austria under the patronage of the European Society of Cardiology. Includes bibliographies and index.
1. Coronary arteries—Surgery—Congresses. I. Unger, Felix, 1946– . II. European Society of Cardiology. [DNLM: 1. Coronary Vessels—surgery—congresses.
WG 300 C8198 1985]
RD598.C6678 1987 617'.412 87-9511
ISBN-13: 978-3-642-45624-4

Softcover reprint of the hardcover 1st edition 1987

2127/3145-543210

Preface

It was a great pleasure to organize a workshop on Coronary Artery Surgery for the Nineties – Prognosis after Revascularization, held November 22–23, 1985, in Salzburg, Austria. This workshop was under the patrogene of the European Society for Cardiovascular Surgery, of the European Society of Cardiology and of the WHO-Regional Office Europe. It was a continuation of the first workshop, which was held in Innsbruck, Austria, on the topic Coronary Artery Surgery: Controversies and New Trends in 1983.

Within the last few years the surgical treatment of angina has changed the therapeutic possibilities dramatically. Due to the high effectiveness of coronary artery surgery, there is a tremendous demand to cure patients suffering from severe angina. The demand is not met at all. Within the last few years there has been an increase in the number of surgical procedures performed, and it seems that 700 operations on the coronary arteries must be our target if we are to meet the demand in Europe. A specific aim of the workshop was to provide an overview on the present incidence of cardiac surgery. The current mean for Europe and the USA is 235 cases of coronary artery bypass graft surgery per million population, whereby up to 870 procedures in 700 centers are performed in the USA. In 1984 there were 146685 cases of coronary artery surgery for a population of 635 million people. In total, cardiac surgery was performed at 950 centers. In Europe, Switzerland, The Netherlands and Belgium had the highest incidence of 500 operations per million population.

Prevalence studies show that approximately 30000 people per million population have an asymptomatic coronary lesion. Of this group, 5000 have a myocardial infarction whereby 2000 die, and 8000 become symptomatic. Of these last 13000, 3000 need a cardioangiographic evaluation; this standard is met in the USA and in consequence the death rate has dropped to 1900 per million. In Europe there is a dramatically low incidence of diagnostic procedures and, in consequence, a low rate in operations. It is very ferently to be hoped that this will change in the near future, and that it will soon be possible to report 3000 diagnoses per million, 700 coronary procedures per million, and 250 cases of percutaneous transluminal coronary angioplasty per million.

During the preparation for this workshop, the nestor of Austrian cardiology, our beloved Professor Kurt Polzer, Vienna, died in September at the age of 75. He was a great stimulus for the development of cardiology in Austria. This book is dedicated to him as a sign of our great respect for him.

I am very grateful to Springer-Verlag, especially to Jürgen Wieczorek, for making it possible to publish the proceedings of this workshop.

Salzburg, September 1986 FELIX UNGER

Table of Contents

II. Percutaneous Transluminal Coronary Angioplasty

III. Surgical Techniques

IV. Coronary Artery Surgery in Acute Myocardial Infarction

V. Reoperation

List of Authors

ÅBERG T.
Department of Thoracic Surgery, University Hospital,
751 86 Uppsala, Sweden

ACCARDI R.
Centro Cardiopneumologico – Clinica Medica-Policlinico, Via delle Menegone, 37134 Verona, Italy

ALBER G.
Department of Cardiology, Hospital Traunstein, Cuno-Niggl-Straße 3, 8220 Traunstein, FRG

ALFIERI O.
St. Antonius Hospital, Dept. Cardiopulmonary Surgery, Koekoekslaan 1, 3435 Utrecht/Nieuwegein, The Netherlands

ALTIMIRAS J.
Farmacia Hospital de La Sta. Creu, Sant Pau/Av. S. Ant. M. Claret 167, Barcelona 08025, Spain

AMSEL B. J.
Universitair Ziekenhuis Antwerpen, Dept. of Cardiovascular Surgery, Wilrijkstraat 10, 2520 Edegem, Belgium

ARBUSTINI E.
Instituto di Anatomia Patologica, Universita degli Studi di Pavia, 27100 Pavia, Italy

ARÍS A.
Hospital de la Santa Creu i Sant Pau, Hemodinamica i Cardiologia Invasiva, Avda. S. Antoni M. Claret 167, 08026 Barcelona, Spain

ASTORRI, E.
Instituto de Patologia Medica, Via Gramsci 14, 43100 Parma, Italy

AUGÉ J. M.
Hospital de La Sta. Creu, Sant Pau/Av. S. Ant. M. Claret 167, Barcelona 08025, Spain

BASSONS T.
Farmacia Hospital de La Sta. Creu, Sant Pau/Av. S. Ant. M. Claret 167, Barcelona 08025, Spain

BEENISCH J.
Department of Cardiac Surgery, University Hospital of Munich, Klinikum Großhadern, Marchioninistraße 15, 8000 Munich 70, FRG

BENINI A.
Centro Cardiopneumologico – Clinica Medica-Policlinico, Via delle Menegone, 37134 Verona, Italy

BENUSSI P.
Centro Cardiopneumologico – Clinica Medica-Policlinico, Via delle Menegone, 37134 Verona, Italy

BERREKLOUW E.
St. Antonius Hospital, Koekoeslaan 1, 3435 CM Utrecht/ Nieuwegein, The Netherlands

BESA G.
Divisione de chirurgia Thoracico e Cardiovasculare, Ospedale Civile Maggiore Borgo Trento, 37200 Verona, Italy

BETTENDORFF PH.
Clinique Medico-Chirurgicale de Genolier, 1261 Genolier, Switzerland

BIANCHI T.
St. Antonius Hospital, Koekoeslaan 1, 3435 CM Utrecht/ Nieuwegein, The Netherlands

BOS E.
Thoraxcentre, University Hospital Dijkzigt, Dr. Molewaterplein 40, Rotterdam 3015 GD, The Netherlands

BOSSE O.
Department of Cardiology, Hospital Traunstein, Cuno-Niggl-Straße 3, 8220 Traunstein, FRG

BRANDT D.
University Hospital, Department for Surgery, Auenbruggerplatz, 8036 Graz, Austria

BRENNER W.
Kaiser Foundation Hospital, Dept. of Cardiac Surgery and Division of Cardiology, 1526 – N. Edgemont, Los Angeles CA 90027, USA

BRONZWAER J.
St. Antonius Hospital, Dept. Cardiopulmonary Surgery, Koekoeslaan 1, 3435 CM Utrecht/Nieuwegein, The Netherlands

Brower R. W.
Thoraxcentre, University Hospital Dijkzigt,
Dr. Molewaterplein 40, Rotterdam 3015 GD, The Netherlands

Brücke P.
Department of Surgery, Allgemeines Krankenhaus Linz,
Krankenhausstraße 9, 4020 Linz/Donau, Austria

Brugger P.
Rehabilitation Center for Rheumatic and Cardiovascular
Disease of the PVA-Arbeiter, 5760 Saalfelden, Austria

Brunnkvist S.
Department of Thoracic Surgery, University Hospital,
751 86 Uppsala, Sweden

Brutel de la Riviere A.
St. Antonius Hospital, Koekoeslaan 2, 3435 CM Utrecht/
Nieuwegein, The Netherlands

Bücherl E. S.
Chirurgische Univ. Klinik + Poliklinik im Klinikum
Charlottenburg, Freie Universität Berlin, Spandauer Damm 130,
1000 Berlin 19, FRG

Busi M.
Cattetra di Chirurgia del Cuore e dei Grossi Vasi, Universitá
Parmà, Via Gramsci 14, 43100 Parma, Italy

Cameron C.
R. C. Dickson Centre, Victoria General Hospital, Halifax,
Nova Scotia, Canada B3H 2Y9

Caralps J. M.
Hospital de la Santa Creu i Sant Pau, Hemodinamica
i Cardiologia Invasiva, Avda. S. Antoni M. Claret 167,
08025 Barcelona, Spain

Casarotto D.
Cattedra di Chirurgia Cardiovascolare – Universitá di Verona,
37124 Verona, Italy

Chapelle J.-P.
Department of Clinical Chemistry, Anesthesiology and Surgery,
Univ. Liège, Belgium

Chello M.
Department of Naples/Department of Cardiovascular Surgery,
Riviera di Chiaia 168, 80121 Naples, Italy

Conti F.
Divisione di chirurgica Thoracico e Cardiovasculare, Ospedale
Civile Maggiore Borgo Trento, 37100 Verona, Italy

CONTINI A.
Cattedra di Chirurgia del Cuore e dei Grossi Vasi, Universitá
Parma, Via Gramsci 14, 43100 Parma, Italy

CREXELLS C.
Hospital de la Santa Creu i Sant Pau, Hemodinamica
i Cardiologia Invasiva, Avda. S. Antoni M. Claret 167,
08025 Barcelona, Spain

CULLHED I.
Department of Thoracic Surgery, University Hospital,
751 86 Uppsala, Sweden

DAJEE H.
Kaiser Foundation Hospital, Dept. of Cardiac Surgery
and Division of Cardiology, 1526 N. Edgemont,
Los Angeles CA 90027, USA

DE AMICIS V.
University of Naples/Department of Cardiovascular Surgery,
Riviera di Chiaia 168, 80121 Naples, Italy

DEFAUW J.
St. Antonius Hospital, Koekoeslaan 1, 3435 CM Utrecht/
Nieuwegein, The Netherlands

DE GEEST R.
St. Antonius Hospital, Koekoeslaan 2, 3435 CM Utrecht/
Nieuwegein, The Netherlands

DEKEYZER L.
Medical Informatics Department/Gasthuisberg University
Hospital, 3000 Leuven, Belgium

DESEINS L.
St. Antonius Hospital, Dept. Cardiopulmonary Surgery,
Koekoeslaan 1, 3435 CM Utrecht/Nieuwegein, The Netherlands

DEUTSCH M.
2. Chirugische Universitätsklinik Wien, Spitalgasse 23,
1090 Vienna, Austria

DI LELLO F.
Centro Cardiopneumologico – Clinica Medica-Policlinico,
Via delle Menegone, 37134 Verona, Italy

DI TOMMASO L.
University of Naples/Department of Cardiovascular Surgery,
Riviera di Chiaia 168, 80121 Naples, Italy

DIMITRI W. R.
Cardiothoracic Unit, St. Thomas Hospital, London SE1 7EH,
UK

DION R. A. E.
Universitair Ziekenhuis Antwerpen, Dept. of Cardiovascular Surgery, Wilrijkstraat 10, 2520 Edegem, Belgium

ECKEL L.
Clinic for Thoracic and Cardiovascular Surgery, Klinikum der Johann-Wolfgang-Goethe-Universität, Theodor-Stern-Kai 7, 6000 Frankfurt/Main, FRG

EL ALLAF M.
Department of Clinical Chemistry, Anesthesiology and Surgery, University Liège, Belgium

ENGHOFF E.
Department of Thoracic Surgery, University Hospital, 751 86 Uppsala, Sweden

ESTRIN J. A.
Departments of Surgery and Anesthesiology, University of Minnesota, Minneapolis/Minnesota, 55455, USA

FERRETTI P. P.
Servicio di Medicina Nucleare, Ospedale Maggiore Parma, Via Gramsci 14, 43100 Parma, Italy

FLAMENG W.
Cardiovascular Surgery Department/Gasthuisberg, University Hospital, 3000 Leuven, Belgium

FLETCHER A.
Kaiser Foundation Hospital, Dept. of Cardiac Surgery and Division of Cardiology, 1526 N Edgemont St., Los Angeles, California, USA

GAGLIARDI C.
University of Naples/Department of Cardiovascular Surgery, Riviera di Chiaia 168, 80121 Naples, Italy

GAMBA G.
Divisione di Chirurgia Thoracico e Cardiovasculare, Ospedale Civile Maggiore Borgo Trento, 37100 Verona, Italy

GAVARUZZI G.
Servicio di Medicina Nucleare, Ospedale Maggiore Parma, Via Gramsci 14, 43100 Parma, Italy

GEHA A. S.
Yale University School of Medicine, Department of Surgery, 121 FMB/333 Cedar Street New Haven, Connecticut 06510, USA

GOENEN M.
Cliniques universitaires Saint-Luc avenue Hippocrate 10, 1200 Bruxelles, Belgium

GÖRLACH G.
Klinik für Herz- und Gefäßchirurgie, Justus-Liebig-Universität, Klinikstraße 29, 6300 Gießen, FRG

GOGGI C.
Divisione di Cardiochirurgica Policlinico S. Matteo, 27100 Pavia, Italy

GOMBOTZ H.
University Hospital, Department of Surgery, Auenbruggerplatz, 8036 Graz, Austria

GRAFFIGNA A.
Divisione di Cardiochirurgica, Policlinico S. Matteo, 27100 Pavia, Italy

GUITERAS P.
Hospital de la Santa Creu i Sant Pau, Hemodinamica i Cardiologia Invasiva, Avda. S. Antoni M. Claret 167, 08025 Barcelona, Spain

HAALEBOS M. M. P.
Thoraxcenter, Erasmus University Rotterdam, Postbus 1738, 3000 DR Rotterdam, The Netherlands

HABICHT J.
Mèdico-Chirurgicale de Genolier, 1261 Genolier, Switzerland

HALLÉN A.
Department of Thoracic Surgery, University Hospital, 751 86 Uppsala, Sweden

HARTL P.
Department of Surgery, Allgemeines Krankenhaus Linz, Krankenhausstraße 9, 4020 Linz/Donau, Austria

HAUENSTEIN K. H.
Department of Radiology, University Freiburg, Hugstetterstraße 55, 7800 Freiburg, FRG

HAUF E.
Mèdico-Chirurgicale de Genolier, 1261 Genolier, Switzerland

HEHRLEIN F. W.
Klinik für Herz- und Gefäßchirurgie, Justus-Liebig-Universität, Klinikstraße 29, 6300 Gießen, FRG

HELMIUS G.
Department of Thoracic Surgery, University Hospital, 751 86 Uppsala, Sweden

HEMMER, W.
Department of Cardiac Surgery, University Hospital of Munich, Klinikum Großhadern, Marchioninistraße 15, 8000 Munich 70, FRG

HEMPEL B.
Chirurgische Univ. Klinik + Poliklinik im Klinikum Charlottenburg, Freie Universität Berlin, Spandauer Damm 130, 1000 Berlin 19, FRG

HEUSGHEM C.
Department of Clinical Chemistry, Anesthesiology and Surgery, Univ. Liège, Belgium

HILL J. D.
Pacific Presbyterian Medical Center, P.O. Box 7999, San Francisco, California 94594, USA

HITCHCOCK J. F.
University Hospital/Department of Cardio-thoracic Surgery, P.O. Box 16250, 3500 CG Utrecht, The Netherlands

HÖGE R.
Klinik für Herz- und Gefäßchirurgie, Justus-Liebig-Universität, Klinikstraße 29, 6300 Gießen, FRG

HUGENHOLTZ P. G.
Thoraxcenter, Erasmus University, Rotterdam, Postbus 1738, 3000 DR Rotterdam, The Netherlands

IATRIDIS A.
Pacific Presbyterian Medical Center, P.O. Box 7999, San Francisco, California 94594, USA

IVIC N.
Divisione de Chirurgia Thoracico e Cardiovascular, Ospedale Civile Maggiore Borgo Trento, 37100 Verona, Italy

JAMBROES B.
University Hospital/Department of Cardio-thoracic Surgery, P.O. Box 16250, 3500 CG Utrecht, The Netherlands

JAMBROES G.
University Hospital/Department of Cardio-thoracic Surgery, P.O. Box 16250, 3500 CG Utrecht, The Netherlands

JANNELLI G.
University of Naples/Department of Cardiovascular Surgery, Riviera di Chaiai 168, 80121 Naples, Italy

JOHN A.
Chirurgische Universitätsklinik + Poliklinik im Klinikum Charlottenburg, Freie Universität Berlin, Spandauer-Damm 130, 1000 Berlin 19, FRG

KAUL T. K.
Regional Adult Cardio-Thoracic Unit, Broadgreen, Hospital Thomas Drive, Liverpool L14 3LB, Merseyside, UK

KEMKES B. M.
Department of Cardiac Surgery, University Hospital of Munich, Klinikum Großhadern, Marchioninistraße 15, 8000 Munich 70, FRG

KENNEDY J. H.
Physiological Flow Studies Unit, Imperial College of Science and Technology, Prince Consort Road, London SW7, UK

KHADIMI R. A.
Regional Adult Cardio-Thoracic Unit, Broadgreen Hospital, Thomas Drive, Liverpool L14 3LB, Merseyside, UK

KHONSARI S.
Kaiser Foundation Hospital, Dept. of Cardiac Surgery and Division of Cardiology, 1526 – N. Edgemont, Los Angeles CA 90027, USA

KHURI S.
Clinic for Thoracic and Cardiovascular Surgery, Klinikum der Johann-Wolfgang-Goethe-Universität, Theodor-Stern-Kai 7, 6000 Frankfurt/Main, FRG.

KLEIN G.
Rehabilitation Center for Rheumatic and Cardiovascular Disease of the OV Arbeiter, 5760 Saalfelden, Austria

KLEIN W.
University Hospital, Department of Surgery, Auenbruggerplatz, 8036 Graz, Austria

KNAEPEN P.
St. Antonius Hospital, Koekoeslaan 1, 3435 CM Utrecht/ Nieuwegein, The Netherlands

KOBINIA G. S.
Allgemeines öffentliches Krankenhaus des Landes Kärnten in Klagenfurt, Abt. für Herzchirurgie, St. Veiter Str. 47, Klagenfurt, Austria

KRAFT-KINZ J.
University Hospital, Department of Surgery, Auenbruggerplatz, 8036 Graz, Austria

KRAUSE E.
Clinic for Thoracic and Cardiovascular Surgery, Klinikum der Johann-Wolfgang-Goethe-Universität, Theodor-Stern-Kai 7, 6000 Frankfurt/Main, FRG

Kreuzer E.
Department of Cardiac Surgery, University Hospital of Munich, Klinikum Großhadern, Marchioninistraße 15, 8000 Munich 70, FRG

Laird-Meeter K.
University Hospital Dijkzigt, Dr. Molewaterplein 40, Rotterdam 3015 GD, The Netherlands

Lamy M.
Department of Clinical Chemistry, Anesthesiology, and Surgery, University Liège, Belgium

Landymore R. W.
Dept. Cardiac and Vascular Surgery, R. C. Dickson Center, Viktoria General Hospital, Halifax, Nova Scotia, Canada B3H 2Y9

Larbuisson R.
Department of Clinical Chemistry, Anesthesiology, and Surgery, University Liège, Belgium

Laufer G.
II. Chirurgische Universitätsklinik Wien, Spitalgasse 23, 1090 Vienna, Austria

Limet R.
Department of Clinical Chemistry, Anesthesiology and Surgery, Univ. Liège, Belgium

Livermore J.
Kaiser Foundation Hospital, Dept. of Cardiac Surgery and Division of Cardiology, 1526 N Edgemont St., Los Angeles, California, USA

Llewellyn M.
Regional Adult Cardio-Thoracic Unit, Broadgreen Hospital Thomas Drive, Liverpool L14 3LB, Merseyside, United Kingdom

Ludwig K.
Rehabilitationscenter for Rheumatic and Cardiovascular disease of the PV Arbeiter, 5760 Saalfelden, Austria

MacAulay M. A.
Department of Cardiac and Vascular Surgery, R. C. Dickson Center, Viktoria General Hospital, Halifax, Nova Scotia, Canada B3H 2Y9

Macedo M. E. M.
Director de Service Hospitale Santa Cruz, Rua Prof. Dr. Reynaldo Dos Santos, 2795 Carnaxide, Portugal

MARCHESE A. R.
University of Naples/Department of Cardiovascular Surgery, Riviera di Chiaia 168, 80121 Naples, Italy

MARCO J.
Service d'Hemodynamique, Hopital Purpan, Toulouse, France

MARINI A.
Centro Cardiopneumologico – Clinica Medica, Universitá di Verona, 37123 Verona, Italy

MARKEWITZ A.
Department of Cardiac Surgery, University Hospital of Munich, Klinikum Großhadern, Marchioninistraße 15, 8000 Munich 70, FRG

MASOTTI M.
Hospital de la Santa Creu i Sant Pau, Hemodinamica i Cardiologia Invasiva, Avda. S. Antoni M. Claret, 167, 08025 Barcelona, Spain

MASTROROBERTO P.
Corso Vittorio Emanuele 58, 84100 Salerno, Italy

MEADE J. B.
Regional Adult Cardio-Thoracic Unit, Broadgreene Hospital, Thomas Drive, Liverpool L14 3LB, Merseyside, UK

MINZIONI G.
Divisione di Cardiochirurgia, Policlinico, S. Matteo, 27100 Pavia, Italy

MOCHTAR B.
University Hospital Dijkzigt, Dr. Molewaterplein 40, Rotterdam 3015 GD, The Netherlands

MOLINA J. E.
Departments of Surgery and Anesthesiology, University of Minnesota, Minneapolis/Minnesota 55455, USA

MONACO M.
University of Naples/Department of Cardiovascular Surgery, Riviera di Chiaia 168, 80121 Naples, Italy

MOTTA A.
Cattedra di Chirurgia Cardiovascolare – Universitá di Verona, 37124 Verona, Italy

MULCH J.
Klinik für Herz- und Gefäßchirurgie, Justus-Liebig-Universität, Klinikstraße 29, 6300 Gießen, FRG

MUSUMECI A.
University of Naples/Department of Cardiovascular Surgery, Riviera di Chiaia 168, 80121 Naples, Italy

NICHOLAIDES A.
Cardiothoracic Unit, St. Thomas Hospital, SE 7EH, UK

NÖLDGE G.
Department of Radiology, University of Freiburg, Hugstetterstraße 55, 7800 Freiburg, FRG

NORDGREN L.
Department of Thoracic Surgery, University Hospital, 751 86 Uppsala, Sweden

NYSTRÖM S.-O.
Department of Thoracic Surgery, University Hospital, 751 86 Uppsala, Sweden

ORIOL A.
Hospital de la Sante Creu i Sant Pau, Hemodinamica i Cardiologia Invasiva, Avda. S. Antoni M. Claret, 167, 08025 Barcelona

OSTERHOLZER G.
Department of Cardiac Surgery, University Hospital of Munich, Klinikum Großhadern, Marchioninistraße 15, 8000 München 70, FRG

OULHACI M.
Clinique Medico-Chirurgicale de Genolier, 1261 Genolier, Switzerland

PADRÓ J. M.
Hospital de la Santa Creu i Sant Pau, Hemodinamica i Cardiologia Invasiva, Avda. S. Antoni M. Claret, 167, 08025 Barcelona, Spain

PALENKER J.
Chirurgische Univ.-Klinik + Poliklinik im Klinikum Charlottenburg, Freie Universität Berlin, Spandauer-Damm 130, 1000 Berlin 19, FRG

PANTALEO D.
University of Naples/Department of Cardiovascular Surgery, Riviera di Chiaia 168, 80121 Naples, Italy

PEPINO P.
University of Naples/Department of Cardiovascular Surgery, Rivier di Chiaia 168, 80121 Naples, Italy

PERANZONI F.
Divisione di Chirurgia Thoracico e Cardiovasculare, Ospediale Civile Maggiore Borgo Trento, 37100 Verona, Italy

PERAZA C.
Hospital de la Santa Creu i Sant Pau, Hemodinamica i Cardiologia Invasiva, Avda. S. Antoni M. Claret, 167, 08025 Barcelona, Spain

PUGLIESE G.
Cattedra di Chirurgia Cardiovascolare – Universitá di Verona, 37123 Verona, Italy

RAGNI T.
Divisione di Cardiochirurgica, Policlinico, S. Matteo, 27100 Pavia, Italy

RAGUSA R.
Divisione di Chirurgia Thoracico + Cardiovascolare, Ospedale Civile Maggiore Borgo Trento, 37100 Verona, Italy

RAMSDALE D.
Regional Adult Cardio-Thoracic Unit, Broadgreene, Hospital Thomas Drive, Liverpool L14 3LB, Merseyside, UK

RAMSTRÖM J.
Department of Thoracic Surgery, University Hospital, 751 86 Uppsala, Sweden

REBLE B.
Department of Cardiac Surgery, University Hospital of Munich, Klinikum Großhadern, Marchioninistraße 15, 8000 München 70, FRG

REICHART B.
Department of Cardiac Surgery, University Hospital of Munich, Klinikum Großhadern, Marchioninistraße 15, 8000 Munich 70, FRG

REICHENSPURNER H.
Department of Surgery, University Hospital of Munich, Klinikum Großhadern, Hospital of Munich, Klinikum Großhadern, Marchioninistraße 15, 8000 Munich 70, FRG

RICCIARDI G.
University of Naples/Department of Cardiovascular Surgery, Riviera di Chiaia 168, 80121 Naples, Italy

RIGLER B.
University Hospital, Department of Surgery, Auenbruggerplatz, 8036 Graz, Austria

RIZZOTTI R.
Divisione di Chirurgia Thoracico + Cardiovascolare, Ospedale Civile Maggiore Borgo Trento, 37100 Verona, Italy

SATTER P.
Clinic for Thoracic and Cardiovascular Surgery, Klinikum der Johann-Wolfgang-Goethe-Universität, Theodor-Stern-Kai 7, 6000 Frankfurt/Main, FRG

SAPSFORD R.
Cardiothoracic Unit, St. Thomas Hospital, SE1 7EH London, UK

SCHAD N.
City Hospital Passau, 8390 Passau, FRG

SCHELD H. H.
Klinik für Herz- und Gefäßchirurgie, Justus-Liebig-Universität, Klinikstraße 29, 6300 Gießen, FRG

SCHETZ M.
Cardiovascular Surgery Dept./Gasthuisberg, University Hospital, 3000 Leuven, Belgium

SCHIESSLER A.
Chirurg. Universitätsklinik + Poliklinik im Klinikum Charlottenburg, Freie Universität Berlin, Spandauer-Damm 130, 1000 Berlin 19, FRG

SCHLOSSER V.
Department of Cardio-Vascular Surgery, University of Freiburg, Hugstetterstraße 55, 7800 Freiburg, FRG

SCHMUZIGER M.
Hôpital de la Tour, 1, Av. J-D. Maillard, 1217 Meyrin (Geneva), Switzerland

SCHÜTZ A.
Department of Cardiac Surgery, University Hospital of Munich, Klinikum Großhadern, Marchioninistraße 15, 8000 Munich 70, FRG

SCURO A.
Centro Cardiopneumologico – Clinica Medica, Universita di Verona, 37124 Verona, Italy

SERGEANT P.
Cardiovascular Surgery Dept./Gasthuisberg, University Hospital, 3000 Leuven, Belgium

SERRUYS P. W.
University Hospital Dijkzigt, Dr. Molewaterplein 40, Rotterdam 3015 GD, The Netherlands

SHEIBAN I.
Centro Cardiopneumologico – Clinica Medica Universita di Verona, 38124 Verona, Italy

SHERIDAN B.
Dept. Cardiac and Vascular Surgery, R. C. Dickson Center, Viktoria General Hospital, Halifax, Nova Scotia, Canada B3H 2Y9

SIDHU P.
Kaiser Foundation Hospital, Dept. of Cardiac Surgery and Division of Cardiology, 1526 – N. Edgemont, Los Angeles, CA 90027, USA

SINGH M.
Kaiser Foundation Hospital, Dept. of Cardiac Surgery and Division of Cardiology, 1526 – N. Edgemont, Los Angeles, CA 90027, USA

SPAMPINATO N.
University of Naples/Department of Cardiovascular Surgery, Riviera di Chiaia 168, 80121 Naples, Italy

SPILLNER G.
Department of Cardio-Vascular Surgery, University of Freiburg, Hugstetterstraße 55, 7800 Freiburg, FRG

SPREAFICO P.
Divisione di Cardiochirurgica, Policlinico S. Matteo, 27100 Pavia, Italy

STANBRIDGE R.
Cardiothoracic Unit, St. Thomas Hospital, SE1 7EH, UK

STANGL G.
II. Chirurgische Universitätsklinik Wien, Spitalgasse 23, 1090 Vienna, Austria

STASSANO P.
University of Naples/Department of Cardiovascular Surgery, Riviera di Chiaia 168, 80121 Naples, Italy

SUY R.
Cardiovascular Surgery Department/Gasthuisberg, University Hospital, 3000 Leuven, Belgium

TAPPAINER E.
Divisione de Chirurgica Thoracico e Cardiovasculare, Ospedale Civile Maggiore Borgo Trento, 37100 Verona, Italy

TREVI G. P.
Cattedra di Cardiologia, Universita di Verona, 37124 Verona, Italy

UNGER F.
Department of Cardiac Surgery, Landeskrankenanstalten Salzburg, Müllner-Hauptstraße 48, 5020 Salzburg, Austria

URBANYI B.
Department of Cardio-Vascular Surgery, University of Freiburg, Hugstetterstraße 55, 7800 Freiburg, FRG

VALENTI P.
Clinique Medico-Chirurgicale de Genolier, 1261 Genolier, Switzerland

VD BRAND M. J. B. M.
Thoraxcentre University Hospital Dijkzigt, Dr. Molewaterplein 40, Rotterdam 3015 GD, The Netherlands

VAN DOMBURG R.
University Hospital Dijkzigt, Thoraxcenter, Erasmus University, 3000 DR Rotterdam, The Netherlands

VANERMEN H.
Department of Cardiovascular Surgery, O.L. Vreuwziekenhuis, Aalst, Belgium

VAN HAASE R.
Universitair Ziekenhuis Antwerpen, Department of Surgery, Wilrijkstraat 10, 2520 Edegem, Belgium

VAN SWIETEN H.
St. Antonius Hospital, Koekoeslaan 1, 3435 CM Utrecht/Nieuwegein, The Netherlands

VERMEULEN F.
St. Antonius Hospital, Dept. Cardiopulmonary Surgery, Koekoeslaan 1, 3435 CM Utrecht/Nieuwegein, The Netherlands

VIGANO' M.
Divisione di Cardiochirurgica, Policlinico, S. Matteo, 27100 Pavia, Italy

VOLETI C.
Kaiser Foundation Hospital – Dept. of Cardiac Surgery and Division of Cardiology, 1526 – N. Edgemont, Los Angeles, CA 90027, USA

WALPOTH B. H.
Klinik für Thorax-, Herz- und Gefäßchirurgie, Inselspital, 3010 Bern, Switzerland

WALTER P.
Universitair Hospital Antwerpen, Dept. of Cardiac-Surgery, Wilrijkstraat 10, 2520 Edegem, Belgium

WEINHOLD CH.
Department of Cardiac Surgery, University Hospital of Munich, Klinikum Großhadern, Marchioninistraße 15, 8000 Munich 70, FRG

WELLENS F.
Department of Cardiovascular Surgery O.L. Vreuwziekenhuis
Aalst, Belgium

WEST I. E.
Cardiothoracic Unit, St. Thomas Hospital SE1 7EH London,
UK

WIJNEN H. P.
Mèdico-Chirurgicale de Genolier, 1261 Genolier, Switzerland

WILLIAMS B. T.
Cardiothoracic Unit, St. Thomas Hospital SE1 7EH, London,
UK

WINLOVE C. P.
Imperial College of Science and Technology, Prince Consort
Road, London SW7, UK

WOLLENEK G.
II. Chirurgische Universitätsklinik Wien, Spitalgasse 23,
1090 Vienna, Austria

WOLNER E.
II. Chirurgische Universitätsklinik Wien, Spitalgasse 23,
1090 Vienna, Austria

WYNANT H. P.
Department of Cardiovascular Surgery O.L. Vreuwziekenhuis,
Aalst, Belgium

Development of Cardiac Surgery in Europe: Future Demands

M. E. M. MACEDO

It was with a feeling of great honour that I accepted the invitation of Prof. Unger to make the opening remarks to this meeting. And it was a pleasure for the European Society for Cardiovascular Surgery to sponsor this Workshop held in such wonderful surroundings in the presence of so many delegates of the highest level.

Although it is well recognized that many advances which brought cardiac surgery to its present situation and prestige were made in the United States, it must be remembered what has been achieved in the Old World along the same lines. In some cases the idea originated in Europe and was developed elsewhere. In other cases, however, developments of various techniques have been perfected on this side of the Atlantic ocean.

It is not my intention to discuss individual merits or become involved in a discussion of the history of our surgery by going through a series of chronological events. That would be repetitive, long, and fatiguing and these opening remarks should be as short as a *hors-d'œuvre*.

I thought it better to confine my observations to the era of open-heart surgery referring to some of the classical chapters of cardiovascular clinical pathology. I shall mention congenital heart malformations, valvular lesions, aortic aneurysms, myocardial preservation, dysrhythmias, coronary artery disease, and replacement of the diseased heart.

Congenital Heart Disease

The European contributions in this field are dominated by transposition of the great arteries and tricuspid atresia. Some of what will be said about valve surgery can, obviously, be applied to congenital disease involving the heart valves but that, I hope, will be easily understood.

It was in 1958 that Åke Senning [24] brought to the surgical field his clever operation. But, for some reason, it took a long time to become accepted as probably the best way to compensate arterial malformation by redirecting the intraatrial venous circulation. Practically all groups over the world gave preference to Mustard's intraatrial baffle, which appeared just a few years later. But the Leiden group, whose head was Gerald Brom [21], revived the Senning operation less than 10 years ago. Their influence, expertise, and some minor technical details were responsible for the choice of Senning's concept of the operation, which subsequently invaded the world on both sides of the Atlantic.

The Leiden group during these years became a center of activity and cooperation with many other Departments of Pediatric Cardiac Surgery in Europe and elsewhere, from America to Asia. It contributed to establishing and implementing the so-called switch operation in Europe, after the colossal comotion produced in the cardiac surgical world when, at the Second Henry Ford International Symposium in 1975 in Detroit, Adib Jatene reported, with his almost unbelievable simplicity, the first successful clinical case of a surgical dream of many others. In Europe, arterial correction of transposition of great arteries (TGA) has gone through several technical modifications. Among these we wish to mention the work of Magdi Yacoub [1, 2, 7, 28, 29] and his cooperation with the group of A. Bernhard from Kiel, West Germany. Their interest in the anatomic variations of the coronary arteries has continued to be an important source of information. Some other technical alternatives cannot be omitted and I am now thinking of the so-called French connection or maneuver of Yves Lecompte [18].

Tricuspid atresia comes next to mind. It had been dealt with by Glenn's anastomosis or systemic pulmonary connections. Then, 14 years ago, Bordeaux came to the fore, leaving the vineyards in obscurity. The first Anglo-Saxon publication by Francis Fontan and Eugène Baudet [13] from Bordeaux was preceded by a lesser known paper in the French medical literature. And the "Fontan Operation" has been used in many hundreds of patients and was afterwards applied to other congenital malformations like the univentricular heart. An important detail has been stressed by Fontan and subsequently by other surgeons: the valved conduit should be an aortic homograft.

Some modifications of the same principle have been advocated. In Europe we should remember that Viking Björk has insisted on the anastomosis of the right atrial appendage to the outflow of the right ventricle.

Heart Valve Disease

In both acquired and congenital disease there is a great deal of influence of Europe on surgical practice throughout the world. I wish to confine my remarks to the most important innovations brought about by our colleagues in Europe.

The experimental work of Duran and Gunning [11], developed in Oxford, England, on homografts and heterografts to replace a diseased aortic valve dates back to the early sixties. It was published in the Lancet in 1962, and Binet [3], from Paris, was the first to implant a heterograft but only after a long period of work in the laboratory and also in connection with Duran and others.

In 1962, Donald Ross [22], of London, followed soon after by Sir Brian Barratt Boyes, New Zealand, started the clinical use of homografts in the subcoronary position. Ross, Barratt Boyes, and Yacoub have continued to use homografts with various methods of preservation for those valve substitutes. Many other centers have abandoned this type of bioprosthesis but, recently, there has been a revival of confidence and many more Departments are now using homografts.

The first homograft conduit to connect the right ventricle to the pulmonary artery was used, again by Ross [23, 15], in 1964, and the same surgeon is responsible for two other newcomers to the surgical armamentarium: (a) the pulmonary valve autograft in the aortic position as a substitute to a diseased valve, followed by pulmonary valve replacement with an aortic homograft; his experience is impressive and unique; (b) replacement of the aortic root with a valved homograft conduit [12].

In the field of valve replacement with a heterograft the work of Alain Carpentier, Paris, is second to none and his scientific relationship with Edwards Laboratories have been most promising. Marion Ionescu, Leeds, England, has produced, with Shiley Laboratories, another remarkable and popular bioprosthesis constructed with bovine pericardium.

With regard to mechanical disk valves there is hardly any need to remind you of the names of Viking Björk and Victor Hall. It seems that Scandinavia is rather successful in this field. The Shiley Company is responsible for making Björk valves, and their association was the beginning of a colossal number of such valve replacements all over the world.

Atrioventricular valves, if possible, should not be resected. And this is a trend very much born in Europe. Let us remember Geoffrey Wooler [26], who, in the late fifties, in Leeds, England, started doing "his" mitral annulovalvuloplasties; and Norberto de Vega, now in Malaga, Spain, who worked with Wooler, gave a name to "his" tricuspid annuloplasty.

Alain Carpentier is the champion of mitral reconstruction, an operation which is now being used more and more frequently around the world, both in acquired disease [7] and congenital malformations [6] like atrioventricular septal defects. Puig Massana (Barcelona), Paneth (London), and Duran (Santander) have joined the field of creative surgeons engaged in saving the native diseased valve using different reconstructive procedures.

Aortic Aneurysms

Dealing with thoracic aortic aneurysms there are two names to be included on our list of European beginners and developers of techniques. The first is Hugh Bentall [2], from the Royal Postgraduate Medical School, London, who, in 1968, described "his" operation that we all know and many of us have practiced, in ascending aortic aneurysms with aortic insufficiency: the aorta and the valve are replaced and the coronary arteries reanastomosed. The other surgeon who has acquired a formidable and inventive experience in aortic aneurysms is Hans Borst, Hannover, West Germany. But we shall not forget the pioneers who, in the early fifties, used a homograft to replace a segment of the abdominal aorta. They were Jacques Oudot (Leriche's Syndrome) [20] and Charles Dubost (Aneurysm) [9].

In this field, and also in comparable situations, the use of fibrin glue has made life different for surgeons wanting to control troublesome bleeding from a graft or artery. It was originated and is produced in Austria, our host country.

Myocardial Preservation

The work of Dennis Melrose in the fifties is a classic. It was, however, abandoned and new efforts were made in the sixties to protect the myocardium from the ischemia produced by clamping off the aorta. The injection of cardioplegic solutions was brought back to practice by the Hamburg group (Kirsch, Rodewald et al.) and by Bretschneider. The St. Thomas' Hospital team, London (Braimbridge, Hearse et al.), has had, in the middle seventies, a very important influence on propagating this method of myocardial protection associated with well- established constant local pericardial cooling.

Dysrhythmias

The original surgical treatment, to the best of my knowledge, did not start in Europe. But Guiraudon, France, now working in Canada, Hugh Bentall, London, England, Wolfgang Bircks, Düsseldorf, and Hans Borst, Hannover, West Germany, have gained very important experience in this fairly new surgical field.

Coronary Artery Disease

This is the subject which brought us together to Salzburg. Besides the interest that this lovely city is producing in all here present, the fact is that this field of cardiac surgery is going to have an "elitist" treatment here. And, so, I should give it a fairly modest dose in this talk.

Coronary artery surgery was developed to its present state of perfection in the United States in the late sixties. Nevertheless let me remind you of four European achievements. In 1946, my fellow countryman, João Cid dos Santos [8], was the first to "attack" directly and anatomically the patency of an artery. And endarterectomy was born. In 1949, Jean Kunlin [17], from Paris, used a segment of saphenous vein to bypass an obstruction of a peripheral artery. In 1960, Dubost [10], from Paris, relieved for the first time the stenosis of a right coronary artery ostium involved in syphilitic aortitis. In 1961, Åke Senning [25], still in Stockholm, published his case of coronary endarterectomy with patch graft enlargement, under profound hypothermia. The most important aspect of this operation was that angiography located the disease and confirmed the reestablishment of the circulation in the two arteries subjected to this technique (left anterior descending and circumflex). Soon after Favaloro described his operation, a number of European surgeons followed his path. Charles Hahn, Switzerland, Ross, Yacoub, and many others in the United Kingdom, Germany, and France quickly acquired a very important experience. Nowadays, coronary artery surgery occupies 30% – 50%, or more, of the work load in many Departments of Cardiac Surgery.

Cardiac Transplantation

To close this brief account of European developments we cannot forget heart transplantation. The International Society for Heart Transplantation is a fairly new society (1980), meeting once a year, and is basically American although its President is now Terence English, Cambridge, England.

The history of heart transplantation has passed through cycles which are not worth commenting upon at length but has seen its last major advance a few years ago with the appearance of cyclosporin A. One European, Christian Cabrol, from Paris, has never stopped his program of cardiac transplantation, which was initiated in the very early days. Terence English started the project at Papworth, near Cambridge, in England and was followed by Magdi Yacoub at the Harefield Hospital, near London, who now has the second largest experience in the world, obtained in the past 5 years. It includes the highest number of heart-lung transplants. Many others have joined the group of transplant surgeons. Although this is a rather superficial talk I would not like to close without quoting some very important warnings issued by the British Cardiac Society 2 years ago. I do think they should be followed in general by all interested groups or hospitals.

The most important recommendations can be summarized as follows:

1. Cardiac transplantation should be regarded as a service need and must, in no way, intrude on or restrict the expanding facilities for other types of open heart surgery.
2. Intemperate publicity should be avoided.
3. It is strongly recommended that every step should be made to discourage involvement of the media by all concerned.

There are some groups in Europe who have started their own program to develop the artificial heart. Charles Hahn will open in December his new Institut de Recherches Cardiovasculaires in Sion, Switzerland, after a long period of experimental work in more modest premises. Others are also well advanced. However, they have not yet launched their ultimate achievements in clinical application.

Future Demands

Although this is, or at least should be, a free world there is an important idea to bring forward when we discuss *Future Demands.* And that idea is, by no means, different from what does happen in many fields of surgery. It is, however, more visible or more easily felt in very expensive surgery.

Perfectionism is following its path through the efforts of individuals, groups, hospitals, universities, and *countries.* But the benefits therefrom derived to the population should be eventually and gradually extended to all in need and not only to those who have easy access to a well-organized and wealthy enough Health Service, or, somehow, to private institutions which, by definition, can easily afford the best treatment to their paying guests. And after fulfilling the principle that "charity begins at home," we should extend our views to other countries and, of course, to other continents. It might seem ludicrous and on the verge of being ridiculous or pompous to mention heart disease in places where there floats the specter of hunger and unnatural death. But we are not dealing with those problems and our motivation should be within our professional boundaries, increasing our expertise, teaching young people, and extending our services.

Cooperation should be the *message* lit in front of the minds of European cardiac surgeons. The European Society for Cardiovascular Surgery, sponsoring this meeting, should be one of the important links of our surgery in the Old World and contribute to extend its influence and experience to other places even beyond our frontiers in the scope of the general cooperation that seems to be, or at least should be, dominating our minds.

References

1. Arensman FW, Sievers HH, Lang P, Radley-Smith R, Bernhard A, Heintzen P, Yacoub MH (1985) Assessment of Coronary and Aortic Anastomoses after Anatomic Correction of Transposition of the Great Arteries. J Thorac Cardiovasc Surg 90:597–604
2. Bentall H, De Bono A (1968) A Technique for Complete Replacement of the Ascending Aorta. Thorax 23:338
3. Binet JP, Duran CG, Carpentier A, Langlois J (1965) Heterologous Aortic Valve Transposition. Lancet, December 18, 1275
4. Braimbridge MV, Chaven J, Bitensky L, Hearse DJ, Jynge P, Cankovic-Darracott S (1977) Cold Cardioplegia or Continuous Coronary Perfusion? Report on Preliminary Clinical Experience as Assessed Cytochemically. J Thorac Cardiovasc Surg 74:900–906
5. Bretschneider HJ, Hübner G, Knoll D, Lohr B, Nordbeck H, Spieckermann PG (1975) Myocardial Resistance and Tolerance to Ischemia: Physiological and Biochemical Basis. J Cardiovasc Surg 16:241–260
6. Carpentier A, Branchini B, Cour JC, Asfou E, Villani M, Deloche A, Relland J, D'Allaines CI, Blondeau Ph, Piwnica A, Parenzan L, Brom G (1976) Congenital Malformations of the Mitral Valve in Children. J Thorac Cardiovasc Surg 72:854
7. Carpentier A, Chauvaud S, Fabiani JN, Deloche A, Relland J, Lessana A, D'Allaines CI, Blondeau Ph, Piwnica A, Dubost Ch (1980) Reconstructive Surgery of Mitral Valve Incompetence, Ten-Year Appraisal. J Thorac Cardiovasc Surg 79:338–348
8. Dos Santos JC (1977) Note sur la Désobstruction des Anciennes Thromboses Artérielles. Mém Acad Chir 73:409–411
9. Dubost Ch, Allary M, Oeconomos (1951) Anévrysme de l'Aorte Abdominale Traité par Resection et Greffe. Arch Maladies Cœur et des Vaisseaux 44:848
10. Dubost Ch, Blondeau Ph, Pwnica A, Weiss M, Lenfant CL, Passelecq J, Guery J (1960) Syphilitic Coronary Obstruction: Correction under Artificial Heart-Lung and Profound Hypothermia at 10° C. Surg 48:540–547
11. Duran CG, Gunning AJ (1962) A Method for Placing a Total Homologous Aortic Valve in the Subcoronary Position. Lancet, September 8, 488
12. Firmin RK, Edwards MG, Ross DN (1984) Homograft Aortic Root Replacement. Summary of paper presented at the meeting of the Society of Thoracic & Cardiovascular Surgeons of Great Britain and Ireland, Dublin
13. Fontan F, Baudet E (1971) Surgical Repair of Tricuspid Atresia. Thorax 26:240
14. Guilmet D, Bachet J, Goudot B, Laurian C, Gigou F, Bical O, Barbagelatta M (1979) Use of Biological Glue in Acute Aortic Dissection. J Thorac Cardiovasc Surg 77:519
15. Kay PH, Robles A, Ross DN (1985) Fifteen Years Follow Up of 300 Fresh Aortic Homografts in the Right Ventricular Outflow Tract. Summary of paper presented at the meeting

of the Society of Thoracic & Cardiovascular Surgeons of Great Britain and Ireland, London

16. Kirsch U, Rodewald G, Kalmar P (1972) Induced Ischemic Arrest, Clinical Experience with Cardioplegia in Open-Heart Surgery. J Thorac Cardiovasc Surg 63:121–130
17. Kunlin J (1949) Le Traitement de l'Artérite Oblitérante par la Greffe Veineuse. Arch Maladies Cœur et des Vaisseaux 42:371–372
18. Lecompte Y, Zannini L, Hazan E, Jarreau MM, Bex JP, Tu TV, Neveux JY (1981) Anatomic Correction of Transposition of the Great Arteries. J Thorac Cardiovasc Surg 82:629–631
19. Melrose DG, Dreyer B, Bentall HH, Baker JBE (1955) Preliminary Communication, Elective Cardiac Arrest. Lancet, July 2, 21–22
20. Oudot J (1951) Greffe de la Bifurcation Aortique depuis les Artères Rénales jusqu'aux Artères iliaques Externes pour Thrombose Artéritique. Mem Acad Chir (Paris) 77:642
21. Quaegebeur JM, Rohmer J, Brom AG, Tinkelenberg J (1977) Revival of the Senning Operation in the Treatment of Transposition of the Great Arteries. Thorax 32:517–524
22. Ross DN (1962) Homograft Replacement of the Aortic Valve. Lancet, September 8, 487
23. Ross DN, Somerville J (1966) Correction of Pulmonary Atresia with a Homograft Aortic Valve. Lancet, December 31, 1446
24. Senning A (1959) Surgical Correction of Transposition of the Great Vessels. Surg 45:966–980
25. Senning A (1961) Strip Grafting in Coronary Arteries. Report of a Case. J Thorac Surg 41:542–549
26. Wooler GH, Nixon PGF, Grimshaw VA, Watson DA (1962) Experiences with the Repair of the Mitral Valve in Mitral Incompetence. Thorax 17:49
27. Yacoub MH, Radley-Smith R, Maclaurin R (1977) Two-Stage Operation for Anatomical Correction of Transposition of the Great Arteries with Intact Interventricular Septum. Lancet, June 8, 1275
28. Yacoub MH, Radley-Smith R (1978) Anatomy of the Coronary Arteries in Transposition of the Great Arteries, and Methods for their Transfer in Anatomical Correction. Thorax 33:418–424
29. Yacoub MH, Bernhard A, Lange P, Radley-Smith R, Keck E, Stephan E, Heintzen P (1980) Clinical and Hemodynamic Results of the Two-Stage Anatomic Correction of Simple Transposition of the Great Arteries. Circulation 62:1190

Thrombolytic Therapy for Acute Coronary Obstruction: Potential Benefits from Early Reperfusion in Acute Coronary Artery Obstruction

P. G. HUGENHOLTZ

In the past 2 decades, coronary care units (CCUs) have made it possible to recognize and *treat in time* previously fatal arrhythmias during the acute stage of myocardial infarction. This has at least reduced the in-hospital mortality from ±30% to less than 15%. At the same time it has become evident that pump failure, ranging from ventricular dysfunction to acute cardiogenic shock, is now the leading cause of death. Efforts at temporary support of the heart mechanically or through pharmacological means have been largely unsuccessful so that attention is now directed toward *prevention* of ventricular failure and limitation of the myocardial infarct size or even outright prevention of infarction itself. Although experimental data with a variety of pharmacologic agents seemed promising, recent large-scale clinical trials with the early administration of betablockers [1, 2] and calcium antagonists [3–6] have shown no major reduction in mortality and this has helped to refocus attention on earlier reperfusion efforts with streptokinase, a powerful *thrombolytic* agent. The relevance of attempts to improve left ventricular function by reducing the amount of tissue lost to infarction is evident from Fig. 1 a, b, which depicts the general relationship between postinfarction left ventricular ejection fraction, a general expression of left ventricular function, and 1-year mortality. It also shows the benefits which may be expected if ventricular function can be maintained or improved.

The causal role of thrombosis in acute myocardial infarction has for a long time been a matter for debate. Although since Herrick's days it had been assumed that thrombosis was always the *cause* of an infarction, careful postmortem studies in the sixties cast doubt on this theory in that many patients showed infarction without complete obstruction. Some postulated therefore that thrombosis was the sequel of infarction. Such theories, based on postmortem examinations, were corrected through the detailed anatomic studies of Fulton et al. [7] and corroborated by DeWood et al. [8], who showed with coronary arteriography in the first few hours after myocardial infarction that thrombosis was present in nearly all cases. They found in 517 patients studied within 4 h after onset of symptoms a complete *obstruction* in 86%. These data were confirmed in the recent large trial carried out by the Netherlands Interuniversity Cardiological Institute [9], which indicated complete obstruction in 84% of 264 patients who were randomized to early angiography and intracoronary thrombolysis. Similar data were found by others [10–15].

These observations therefore bring three fundamental concepts into focus: First, angiography can be carried out in acute myocardial infarction without major risks; second, thrombosis is present in the majority of cases when studied

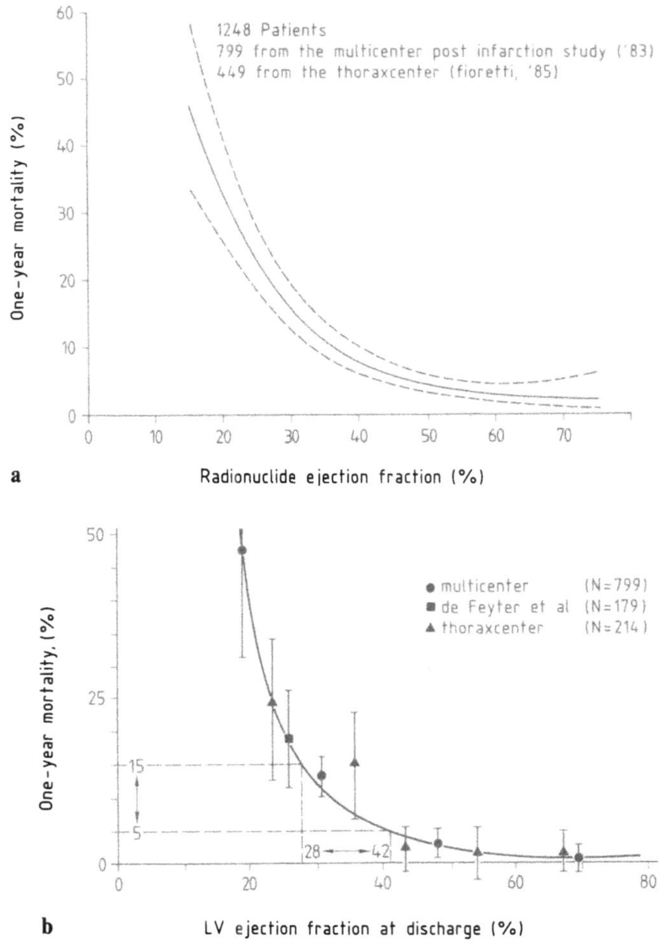

Fig. 1. a Composite of data reported from two studies relating ejection fraction at discharge after acute myocardial infarction with subsequent 1-year survival. **b** It is clear that an improvement in ejection fraction from 28% to 40% could reduce 1-year mortality from 15% to 5%

within the first few hours after symptoms; and, third, the prevalence of complete obstruction declines as the time after the onset of symptoms lengthens. Indeed obstruction was found in only 60% of cases when the interval exceeded 6 h, corresponding to the observations of the pathologists who had found on average complete obstruction in only half of the cases which were usually studied at 12–24 h after onset of symptoms and/or death. It is likely therefore that only in those patients who present themselves in an early stage of acute myocardial infarction for therapy can infarct size be limited by an approach aimed at de-obstruction. Furthermore, from the experiments carried out by the group of Sobel [15], it is evident that early reperfusion will not only limit the ultimate infarct size but will also be able to achieve return toward normal cardiac function and metabolism. Thus all available evidence points toward the need for early de-obstruction.

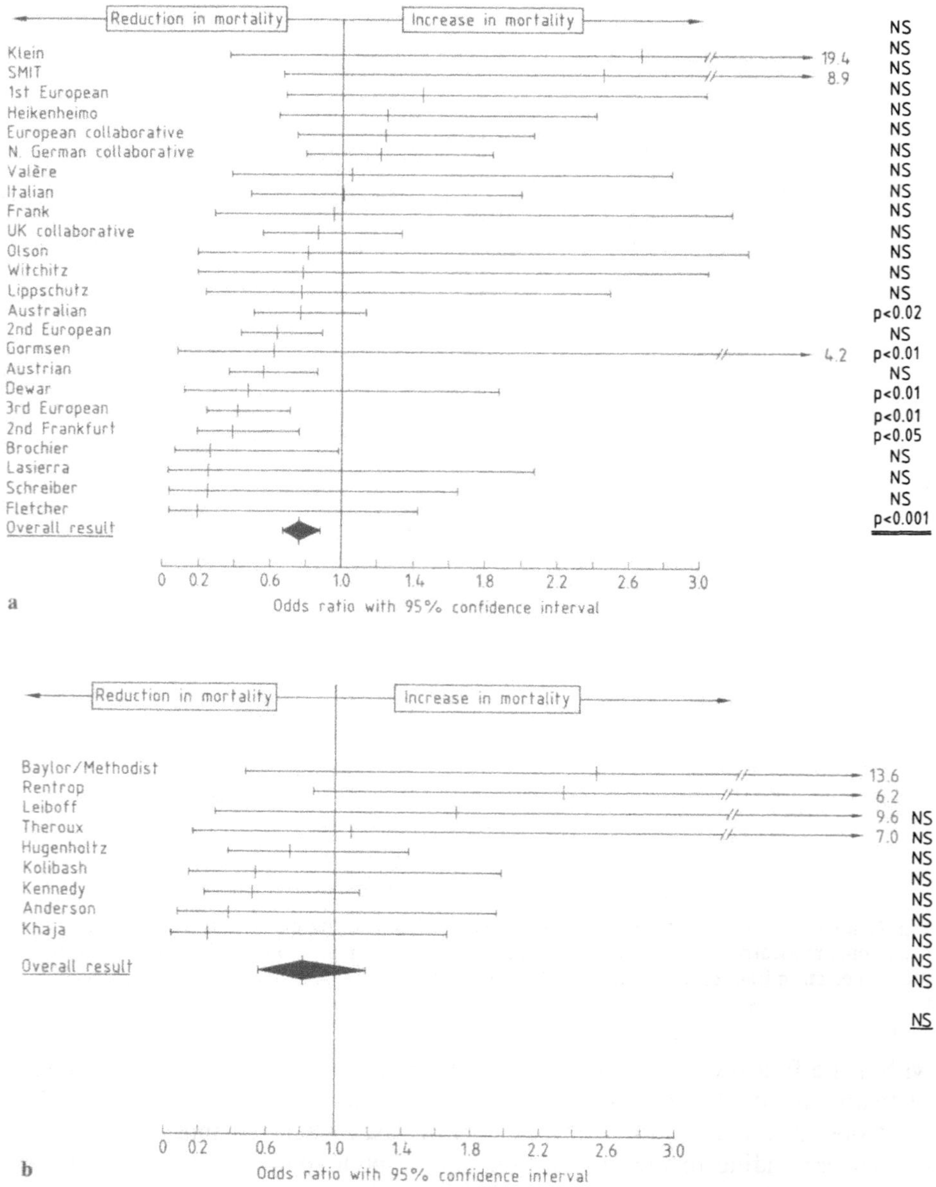

Fig. 2. a The effects of i.v. streptokinase on mortality in 24 trials since 1959. **b** The effects of intracoronary streptokinase on mortality in 9 trials. Reproduced from [22]. (Note that the data for Hugenholtz et al. are incomplete as only half the treated group is included [9])

The feasibility of rapid dissolution of intracoronary thrombi by systemic or selective infusion of thrombolytic substances has been convincingly demonstrated in experimental series and in clinical pilot studies as long as 25 years ago [16–21]. This has led to widespread trials of *intravenous* administration of streptokinase (SK), which was given in varying doses and at varying time intervals, mostly with disappointing or nonsignificant results. This can now bė explained by too small series, poor patient selection, (too) late administration of SK, poor evaluation techniques, and old-fashioned statistical design. In particular, no attempts were made to prove patency of the infarct-related artery by angiography or to the measure infarct size. The earlier experience should therefore be eliminated from current considerations, although Yusuf et al. [22] conclude from a pooled analysis of some 6000 patients in 24 randomized trials with i.v. streptokinase (Fig. 2a) that a reduction in the odds of death by 22% ± 5% can be deduced.

This entire field has now been radically changed by the data from the GISSI (Gruppo Italiano di Streptokinase Sistemica in Infarction) trial [41], an all Italian study, which has shown (Table 2) a highly significant reduction in mortality in those patients who were treated within the first 3 h after onset of symptoms. With the large numbers involved in this trial the reduction in early mortality is statistically highly *convincing.*

The systematic effort at restoration of anterograde flow after *intracoronary* administration was, however, not introduced into clinical practice until 1979 by Rentrop and other workers in Germany [21, 23, 24]. Since then, we have witnessed a dramatic increase in the number of patients with acute ischemic cardiac disorders who have been treated by intracoronary streptokinase infusion [22, 25–27] and the results have given new color to the cheeks of those who advocated the intravenous route, prior to GISSI [41]. A more widespread dissemination of the new technique combining the advantages of early i.v. administration with i.c. lysis and the follow-up treatment of residual coronary artery obstruction [with percutaneous transluminal coronary angioplasty (PTCA) or bypass surgery] now appears to be justified in centers capable of performing these. Its benefits and risks have recently been adequately investigated, as will be shown hereafter. Furthermore it is entirely consistent with experimental evidence [28, 39, 40].

In an Editorial in 1982, in which the literature up to that year was reviewed, various notes of caution were voiced by myself and Rentrop [29] against too much early enthusiasm. We pointed to the main factors which could influence the ultimate outcome positively or negatively. These included: the need to know the time interval between the onset of symptoms and de-obstruction; the extent of restoration of myocardial function in the region perfused by that artery; the functional availability of collateral flow; the best route and optimal amount of the thrombolytic agents; the best agent; their side effects; and the degree to which the usual sequelae of myocardial infarction, such as subsequent angina, reinfarction, and death, could be reduced when compared with a control group, randomly assigned to conventional treatment. These arguments have recently been repeated by Yusuf et al. [22], although their conclusions as to the need for giant trials with thousands of patients to solve these questions are debatable. As long as the true pathophysiological basis for treatment has not been sufficiently clarified and, in fact, varies as the ischemia evolves, among others as function of the available collateral supply, it would seem unwise to lump patient groups with widely varying characteristics together in an effort to reach some form of statistical significance. Rather, therapy should be directed at intervention(s) for a specific derangement. Returning to the editorial question [29]: what *have* we learned from the smaller series and incidental observations in the years since 1980?

Most importantly, *recanalization,* whether by guidewire alone [30, 31] or by clot lysis with streptokinase [9, 15, 26, 32, 33], urokinase, or recombinant tissue plasminogen activator (rtPA) [12, 15, 35–37] (Table 1), has now been shown to limit infarct size provided it is carried out within the first few hours after occlusion onset. An illustration of that experimental observation is shown in Table 1. On the other hand, Reimer et al. [38] and others have confirmed in many animal models that after 6 h of complete ischemia the amount of salvageable myocardium is insignificant. Bergmann et al. [39] have confirmed these findings in closed-chest dogs, employing positron emission tomography to assess [11] C-palmitate uptake by reperfused myocardium. It increased by 76%, as opposed to 15%, when reperfusion was carried out within 2 h rather than 2–4 h after occlusion. These and other studies were, however, performed with animals and since it is now also generally accepted that the functional characteristics of their coronary circulations differ significantly from those of man, it has become clear that no animal model can completely mimick the human situation [28, 39, 40]. Nevertheless, all these data support the concept that reperfusion must be established soon after occlusion, since no major beneficial effects can be expected beyond 3–4 h after onset of ischemia. While data from the pooled analysis by Yusuf [22] suggest that some statistical benefit cannot be excluded when treatment is started late, the numbers are not convincing and recent data from the GISSI trial indicate actual damage by late therapy [41] (Table 2). Rentrop et al. [42], Schwarz et al. [43], and Schröder et al. [44] have also found that while the extent of salvage is less when therapy is started beyond the 4th h after onset of symptoms, late recanalization may still result in some improvement, particularly in those patients in whom collaterals are demonstrable by acute angiography. It is likely that in these patients the evolution of myocardial necrosis, “stuttering necrosis,” is slowed when collateral flow is enhanced early on. Our own data have shown the best improvement in cardiac function, smallest infarct size, and lowest mortality in the subset of 117 patients in whom intracoronary lysis was preceded by i.v. streptokinase. In these lysis was begun at a median of 3 h after onset of symptoms. Angiography before the start of subsequent intracoronary streptokinase showed a patent coronary artery in less then half of these cases, however. This finding supports the notion therefore that lytic therapy works not only through de-obstruction of the main infarct-related vessel but also via improved rheology and reduced viscosity benefiting the collateral bed. In keeping with this is the fact that enzyme washout was highest in those patients who were treated earliest but also occurred in those in whom the infarct-related vessel remained closed. The GISSI data [41], which show a significant mortality reduction after i.v. administration within 3 h of symptoms

Table 1. Clinical course in hospital

	302 patients randomized to		231 patients randomized to		533 patients in total		*P*
	Controls	Intracoronary thrombolysis	Controls	Intravenous + intracoronary thrombolysis	Controls	Thrombolysis	
Number of patients	150	152	114	117	264	269	
Severe heart failure, CCU	8	4	4	6	12	10	
Cardiogenic shock	12	4	12	9	24	13	
Heart failure during reconvalescence	23	17	30	20	53	37	0.05
Ventricular fibrillation	31	20	30	18	61	38	0.01
Pericarditis	23	6	23	13	46	19	0.0004
Bleeding	2	24	5	29	7	53	0.0001
Angina	38	34	17	23	55	57	
Recurrent infarction	3	5	6	7	9	12	
Mortality (14 days)	12	9	14	5	26	14	0.05

Combined data from CCUs, catheterization laboratory, and cardiology ward; *P* values of 0.05 (two-sided) are reported (Fisher exact test); reproduced with permission from the Netherlands Interuniversity Cardiology Institute Trial

Table 2. Data from 11483 patients in the GISSI trial [41]

Hospital mortality when therapy was begun:		i.v. SK 5756	Controls 5727	Difference (*P*)
Within	≦1 h	8.1%	15.3%	<0.002
	≦3 h	8.5%	11.9%	<0.001
	3–6 h	11.3%	12.9%	NS
	12 h	10.6%	12.9%	<0.02
First myocardial infarction		9.7%	12.0	<0.01
Re-infarction		180	92	<0.001
Pericarditis		325	565	<0.001
Left ventricular failure		583	671	NS

together with the drastic reduction in mortality for the i.v. + i.c. streptokinase group from the Netherlands trial, for the first time, confirm the thesis recently proposed by Verstraete [45] that i.v. administration is "the only way." There is, however, one essential difference in that i.v. thrombolysis alone will not "fit the bill" when signs of ischemia persist or return as will be the case in many, if not half, the cases because of the underlying atheromatous lesion.

To clarify these issues, a large-scale investigation into the relevance of intracoronary administration of streptokinase was begun in 1980 at the Thorax Center in Rotterdam and expanded to three other centers so that by 15 March 1985, 533 patients were included in a randomized study [9]. This excludes our earlier pilot trial of 82 patients, whose results in fact mimick the randomized trial. Half of the patients, 264 of the Netherlands Interuniversity Institute Trial, were allocated to conventional treatment in the CCUs and 269 to an attempt at reperfusion. Of these 269, 152 patients were assigned to streptokinase by the intracoronary route only, with 117 receiving 500000 units streptokinase i.v. an average of 100 min prior to administration. This second group was so treated when experience showed us that a significant delay persisted with the preparation of the catheterization laboratory and the introduction of catheters. In more than 80% therapy was begun within 3 h after onset of symptoms. It was shown that mortality at 14 days was 5% in the group assigned to thrombolysis (14 out of 269) versus 9% in the group assigned to thrombolysis (25 out of 264), while at a median of 8 months, mortality was 9% versus 16%, a highly significant reduction in mortality ($P < 0.01$) (Table 1). As stated earlier the mortality in the i.v. + i.c. group was even lower than in the overall group. The *best results* were achieved when spontaneous lysis cases were added to those with lysis and PTCA : 1 death out of 98 cases in 1 year, an observation strongly underpinning the hypothesis that complete revascularization is essential by whatever route. Furthermore, cardiogenic shock, ventricular fibrillation, and pericarditis were half as frequent in the group assigned to thrombolysis (Table 1).

In addition enzyme release (alpha-HBDH) was 30% lower in the treated group, indicating a smaller size of the ultimate infarct. This was also reflected in a marked improvement in left ventricular ejection fraction, which was significantly higher by 7% in the treated group, compared with the control (53% vs. 46%). In the latter group, furthermore, end-diastolic and end-systolic volumes were normal. In addition, throughout the study experience was gained with PTCA, which was carried out in those patients who after initial reperfusion showed significant residual coronary artery obstruction or reocclusion while still in the catheterization laboratory. In this subgroup of patients further reduction of 1-year mortality was achieved. It is of interest to look at other data collected in the same time span at the Thorax Center in patients with unstable angina, a condition which may be considered to be a precursor of acute myocardial infarction. In 136 patients, who had been refractory to intense, often triple, pharmacological treatment, aggressively treated with PTCA, 1-year mortality is now a low 1% with low recurrence of angina or infarction. This indicates the desirability to "clean up" the obstruction when symptoms of ischemia persist regardless of whether prior treatment was vasodilating or thrombolytic. It is the underlying atheromatous obstruction which must be reduced. In this regard we underline the comments by Verstraete [45] that "critical narrowing continues to be a threat to the patient, even after early reestablishment of anterograde flow." The results in the 533 Dutch patients demonstrate that a strategy aimed at early recanalization of the infarct-related artery by both intravenous and intracoronary administration of streptokinase can improve the clinical course and survival in the 1st year after myocardial infarction.

References

1. The MIAMI Trial Research Group (1985) Metoprolol in acute myocardial infarction (MIAMI). Eur Heart J 6:199–226
2. Sleight P (1985) The ISIS trial. Personal communication, Pavia
3. The Danish Study Group on Verapamil in Myocardial Infarction (1984) Verapamil in acute myocardial infarction. Eur Heart J 5:516–528
4. Muller JE, Morrison J, Stone PH, Rude RRE, Rosner B, Roberts R, Pearle DL, Turi ZG, Schneider JF, Serfas DH, Tate C, Schneider E, Sobel BE, Hennekens CH, Braunwald E (1984) Nifedipine therapy for patients with threatened and acute myocardial infarction: a randomized double blind, placebo controlled comparison. Circulation 69:740–747
5. Muller JE and the NAMIS Study Group (1985) Nifedipine therapy for unstable angina and myocardial infarction: randomized double blind evaluations. In: Hugenholtz PG, Goldman BS (eds) Unstable angina. Schattauer, Stuttgart, pp 199–210
6. Sirnes PA, Overskeid K, Pedersen TR, Bathen J, Drivenes A, Froland GS, Kjekshus JK, Landmark K, Rokseth R, Sirnes KE, Sundoy A, Torjussen BR, Westland KM, Wik BA (1984) Evolution of infarct size during the early use of nifedipine in patients with acute myocardial infarction: the Norwegian Nifedipine Multicenter Trial. Circulation 70:638–644
7. Fulton W, Lutz W, Donald KW (1972) Natural history of unstable angina. Lancet 1:860–870
8. DeWood MA, Spores J, Notske R, Mouser LT, Burroughs R, Golden MS, Lang HT (1980) Prevalence of total coronary occlusion during the early hours of transmural myocardial infarction. N Engl J Med 303:897–902
9. Simoons ML, van den Brand M, de Zwaan C, Verheugt FWA, Remme W, Serruys PW, Bär F, Res J, Krauss XH, Vermeer F (1985) Improved survival after early thrombolysis in acute myocardial infarction. Lancet 14:578–582
10. Rentrop P, De Vivie ER, Karsch KR, Kreuzer H (1979) Acute myocardial infarction: intracoronary application of nitroglycerin and streptokinase in combination with transluminal recanalization. Clin Cardiol 5:354–356
11. Serruys PW, van den Brand M, Hooghoudt TEH, Simoons ML, Fioretti P, Ruiter J, Fels PW, Hugenholtz PG (1982) Coronary recanalization in acute myocardial infarction: immediate results and potential risks. Eur Heart J 3:404–415
12. TIMI Study Group (1985) The thrombolysis in myocardial infarction (TIMI) trial: phase I findings. N Engl J Med 312:932–946
13. Schwarz F, Hofmann M, Schuler G, von Olshausen K, Zimmermann R, Kubler W (1984) Thrombolysis in acute myocardial infarction: effect of intravenous followed by intracoronary streptokinase application on estimates of infarct size. Am J Cardiol 53:1505–1510
14. Kennedy JW, Ritchie JL, Davis KB, Stadius ML, Maynard C, Fritz JK (1985) The Western Washington randomized trial of intracoronary streptokinase in acute myocardial infarction. N Engl J Med 312:1073–1078
15. Sobel BE, Geltman EM, Tiefenbrunn AJ, Jaffe AS, Spadaro JJ Jr, Ter Pogossian MM, Collen D, Ludbrook PA (1984) Improvement of regional myocardial metabolism after coronary thrombolysis induced with tissue type plasminogen activator or streptokinase. Circulation 69:983–990
16. Fletcher AP, Alkjaersig N, Smyrniotis FE, Sherry S (1958) The treatment of patients suffering from early myocardial infarction with massive and prolonged streptokinase therapy. Trans Assoc Am Physicians 71:287–293
17. Boucek RJ, Murphy WP Jr (1960) Segmental perfusion of the coronary arteries with fibrinolysis in man following acute myocardial infarction. Am J Cardiol 6:525–533
18. Bolton HE, Tapia FA, Cabral H, Riera R, Mazel MS (1961) Removal of acute coronary thrombus with fibrinolysis, an in vivo experiment. JAMA 175:307–310
19. Breddin K, Ehrly AM, Feckler L et al. (1973) Die Kurzzeitfibrinolyse beim akuten Myokardinfarkt. Dtsch Med Wochenschr 98:861–873
20. Chazov EL, Mareeva LS, Mazaev AV, Sartgoin KE, Sadovshaya M, Ruda Y (1976) Intracoronary administration of fibrinolysin in acute myocardial infarction. Therapevticheskii Arkhiv 48:8

21. Rentrop P, Blanke H, Karsch KR, Weigand V, Kostering H, Oster H, Leitz K (1979) Acute myocardial infarction: intracoronary application of nitroglycerin and streptokinase. Clin Cardiol 2:354
22. Yusuf S, Collins R, Peto R, Furberg C, Stampfer MJ, Goldhaber SZ, Hennekens CH (1985) Intravenous and intracoronary fibrinolytic therapy in acute myocardial infarction: overview of results on mortality, reinfarction and side effects from 33 randomized controlled trials. Eur Heart J 6:556–585
23. Mathey DG, Rodewald G, Rentrop P et al. (1981) Intracoronary streptokinase thrombolytic recanalization and subsequent surgical bypass of remaining atherosclerotic stenosis in acute myocardial infarction: complementary combined approach effecting reduced infarct size, preventing reinfarction, and improving left ventricular function. Am Heart J 102:1194–1201
24. Merx W, Dorr R, Rentrop P et al. (1981) Evaluation of the effectiveness of intracoronary streptokinase infusion in acute myocardial infarction: Postprocedure management and hospital course in 204 patients. Am Heart J 102:1181–1187
25. Ganz W, Nimomiuya K, Hashida J et al. (1981) Intracoronary thrombolysis in acute myocardial infarction: experimental background and clinical experience. Am Heart J 102:1145–1149
26. Kennedy JW, Fritz B, Ritchie J (1982) Streptokinase in acute myocardial infarction: Western Washington randomized trial and progress report. Am Heart J 104:899–902
27. Khaja F, Walton JA, Brymer JF et al. (1983) Intracoronary fibrinolytic therapy in acute myocardial infarction: report of a prospective randomized trial. N Engl J Med 308:1305–1311
28. Schaper W (1983) Natural defense mechanisms to ischemia. Eur Heart J [Suppl D] 4:73–78
29. Hugenholtz PG, Rentrop P (1982) Thrombolytic therapy for acute myocardial infarction: quo vadis? Eur Heart J 3:395–403
30. Rentrop P, De Vivie ER, Karsch KR, Kreuzer H (1978) Acute coronary occlusion with impending infarction as an angiographic complication relieved by a guide wire recanalization. Clin Cardiol 1:101–107
31. Meyer J, Erbel R, Schmitz HJ, Pop T, Meinert T, Schreiner G, Henkel B, Henrichs KJ, Rupprecht HJ, Effert S (1984) Transluminale Angioplastik – Instabile Angina, frischer Infarkt. 50. Jahrestag Deutsche Gesellschaft Herz- und Kreislaufforschung, Mannheim 1984, Z Kardiol 73/II:167–176
32. Markis JE, Malagold M, Parker A, Silverman KJ, Barry WH, Als AV, Paulin S, Grossman W, Braunwald E (1981) Myocardial salvage after intracoronary thrombolysis with streptokinase in acute myocardial infarction. N Engl J Med 305:777
33. Sheehan FH, Mathey DG, Schofer J, Krebber H-J, Dodge HT (1983) Effect of interventions in salvaging left ventricular function in acute myocardial infarction: a study of intracoronary streptokinase. Am J Cardiol 52:431
34. Kambara M, Kawai C, Kammatsuse K, Sato H, Nobuyoshi K, Chino M, Miwa H, Uchida Y, Kodanna K, Mitsudo K, Hayashi T, Kajiwara N, Sekiguchi M, Yasue H (1985) Coronary thrombolysis in urokinase infusion in acute myocardial infarction. A multicenter study in Japan. Cather Cardiovasc Diagn 11:349–360
35. Verstraete M, Bory M, Collen D, Erbel R, Lennane RJ et al. (1985) Randomized trial of intravenous recombinant tissue-type plasminogen activator versus streptokinase in acute myocardial infarction. Lancet 842–847
36. Van der Werf F, Ludbrook PA, Bergmann SR, Tiefenbrunn AJ, Fox KAA, de Geest H, Verstraete M, Collen D, Sobel BE (1984) Coronary thrombolysis with tissue type plasminogen activator in evolving myocardial infarction. N Engl J Med 310:609, 614
37. Van der Werf F, Bergmann SR, Fox KAA, de Geest H, Hoyng CF, Sobel BE, Collen D (1984) Coronary thrombolysis with intravenously administered human tissue type plasminogen activator produced by recombinant DNA technology. Circulation 69:605, 610
38. Reimer KA, Lowe JRE, Rasmussen MM, Jennings RB (1977) The wavefront phenomenon of ischemic cell death. I. Myocardial infarct size versus duration of coronary artery occlusion in dogs. Circulation 56:786–794

39. Bergmann SR, Lerch RA, Fox FAA, Ludbrook PA, Welch MJ, Ter Pogossian MM, Sobel BE (1982) Temporal dependence of beneficial effects of coronary thrombolysis characterized by positron tomography. Am J Med 72:1
40. Hearse DJ, Yellon DM (1981) The borderzone of evolving myocardial infarction: controversy or confusion. Am J Cardiol 47:1321–1334
41. GISSI (Gruppo Italiano di Streptokinase Sistemica in Infarction) (1985) Personal Communication, Milano
42. Rentrop P, Blanke H, Karsch KR, Kaiser H, Kostering H, Oster H, Leitz K (1981) Selective intracoronary thrombolysis in acute myocardial infarction and unstable angina pectoris. Circulation 63:307
43. Schwarz F, Schuler G, Katus H, Hofmann M, Mantley J, Tillmans H, Mehmel HC, Kübler W (1982) Intracoronary thrombolysis in acute myocardial infarction: duration of ischemia as a major determinant of late results after recanalization. Am J Cardiol 50:933
44. Schröder R, Vohringer M, Linderer T, Biamino G, Bruggemann T, Leitner ER (1985) Follow-up after coronary arterial reperfusion with intravenous streptokinase in relation to residual myocardial infarct artery narrowings. Am J Cardiol 55:313–317
45. Verstraete M (1985) Intravenous administration of a thrombolytic agent is the only realistic therapeutic approach in evolving myocardial infarction. Eur Heart J 6:586–593

I. Long-Term Effects of Coronary Artery Bypass Surgery

Long-term Survival After Coronary Bypass: A Study of 1373 Patients

T. ÅBERG, J. RAMSTRÖM, S.-O. NYSTRÖM, A. HALLÉN, G. HELMIUS,
I. CULLHED, L. NORDGREN, and S. BRUNNKVIST

Apart from symptom relief – a readily observable and accepted effect of coronary bypass operations – improvement in long-term survival is an important goal. This effect has been shown in prospective randomized trials to be important in those subgroups of coronary heart disease with a poor survival on medical treatment. Analysis of long-term survival in surgically treated groups without a concomitant medically treated control group may be justifiable, as they have value in providing confirmatory evidence for the general applicability of surgical treatment at a society level. The purpose of this presentation is to analyze our own experience with aortocoronary bypass operations over a period of 15 years.

Material and Methods

From 1970 to 1984, 1373 patients were operated upon for chronic severe and stable angina pectoris with aortocoronary bypass. In the earlier part of the period, only few patients were operated upon each year, increasing markedly over the years. During the same period, 216 patients were operated on for unstable angina. They are not included in the present analysis. Follow-up was made in July 1985, allowing a minimum observation time of 6 months. Average observation time was 50 months, median 44.5 months.

Information about whether the patients were alive or dead and if so the cause of death was obtained from the official Swedish population registry. The information was entered into our prospective data bank. Follow-up is total but for a few foreigners who have been excluded from the study. Survival curves were constructed using the actuarial method for the total material and for pertinent subgroups. Some comparisons were made with published medically treated material.

Left ventricular function was estimated in most patients with either densitometric or planimetric methods. The patients were divided into three groups, those with normal or near normal left ventricle (LV) function, those with moderately depressed LV function, and those with severely depressed LV function. Twenty-six percent had normal LV function, 53% moderately depressed LV function, and 21% severely depressed LV function; 39% had had no clinical myocardial infarctions, 42% had had one, and 19% two or more than two.

Patients were also divided into one-, two, and three-vessel disease and left main stenosis. The criterion was >50% stenosis; 14% of the patients had one-vessel disease, 26% had two-vessel disease, 44% had three-vessel disease, and 16% had left main stenosis. The material was also divided into periods of operation. An early operation group was operated in 1971–1979, one middle group in 1980–1982, and a recent group in 1983–1984. Twenty-nine percent of the patients were operated on during the early period, 36 during the middle, and 35 during the recent period.

The Operation. Operative procedures were standard. Cardioplegic arrest was introduced in 1979. Only few mammary arteries were used during the time of study. An average of 3.1 anastomoses were constructed on an average of 2.2 grafts/patient with an increase during later years. Median cross-clamp time was 64 min, median time on bypass 118 min. The patients were operated upon by eight surgeons.

Results

One-month mortality for the entire material was 3.9%, starting at a rather high level of 8.4% during the first 9 years, declining to the current level of 1.5%. Cause of death is given in Table 1. One hundred and sixteen patients (8.5%) have died during the follow-up period. Most of the decreased patients (74%) died because of heart disease, primarily coronary artery disease. (Vital statistics give 30% as the proportion of deaths due to coronary heart disease in people below 70 years of age in Sweden.) Thus this group of patients still have a proportionately very high rate of death due to the underlying disease in spite of treatment.

Survival Curves. In the following survival curves, total mortality is given, including noncardiac deaths. The proportion of noncardiac deaths was found to be around 25% in all groups larger than 200 patients, but, for clarity, this factor is not discussed further.

The survival curve for the entire material gives an estimated survival of 86% at 5 years and 65% at 10 years. Dividing the material into degree of vessel involvement reveals a higher survival for one- and two-vessel disease and a lower survival for three-vessel disease and left main stenosis (Fig. 1). Survival curves run parallel to each other with similar yearly mortalities.

Table 1. One-month mortality

Reason	Number
Failure of weaning from bypass	20
Arrhythmia + myocardial failure	9
Myocardial failure	16
Postoperative hemorrhage	4
Neurologic complication	3
Sepsis	1
Late tamponade	1

Table 2. Late mortality

Reason	Number
Certain sudden death	20
Certain myocardial infarction	48
Cardiac death, mode uncertain	18
Cerebral hemorrhage or embolus	7
Accidents or suicide	6
Malignancy	13
Miscellaneous	4

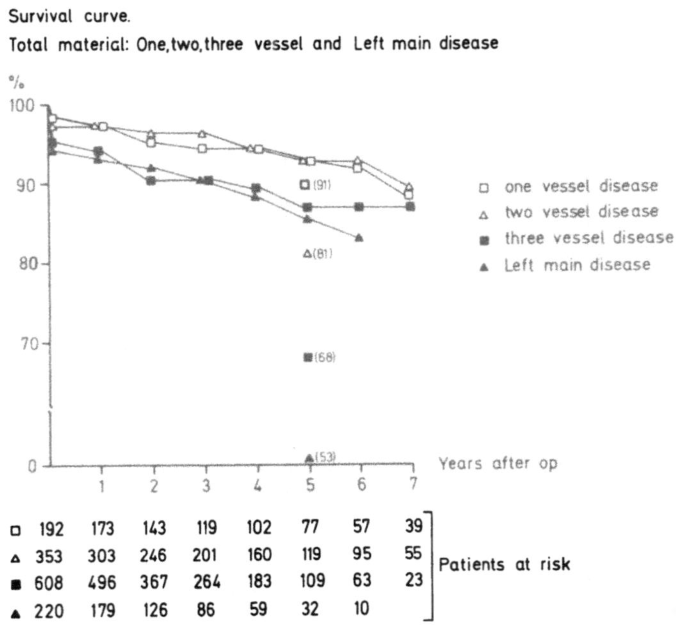

Fig. 1. Survival according to degree of vessel involvement. *Symbols with numbers in brackets* show the mean survival in several medically treated materials [1]. Difference between medical and surgical treatment is greater in left main stenosis and three-vessel disease than in two- and especially one-vessel disease

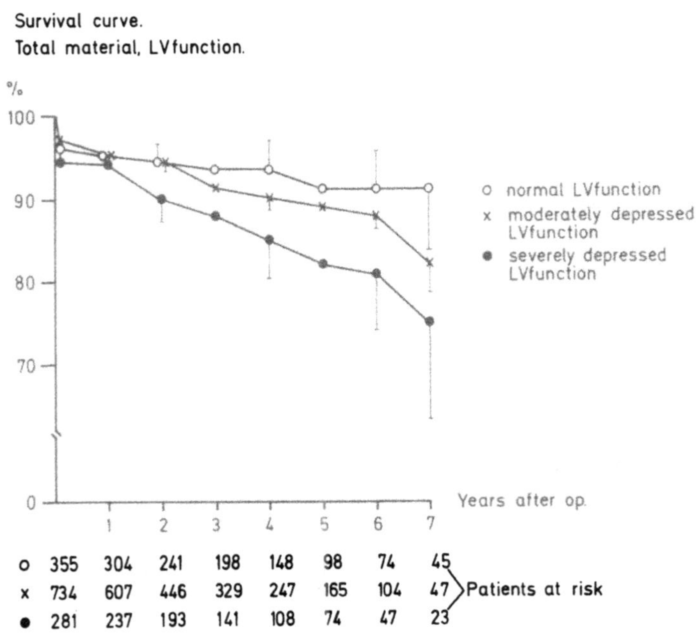

Fig. 2. Entire material divided into degree of left ventricular dysfunction

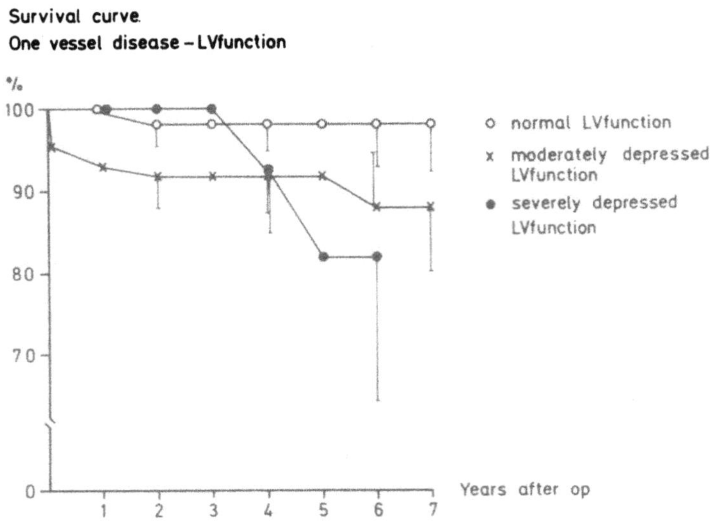

o	73	68	56	45	43	35	29	20	Patients at risk
x	93	81	66	55	47	36	23	17	
•	26	24	21	15	12	6	6		

a

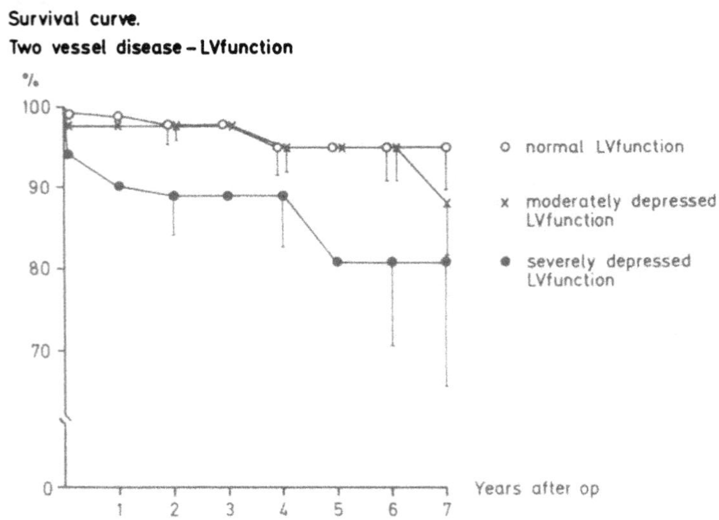

o	99	89	71	62	46	32	29	19	Patients at risk
x	188	158	127	105	84	64	53	31	
•	66	56	49	35	31	24	14	5	

b

Fig. 3a–d. Entire material divided into one-, two-, and three-vessel disease and left main stenosis as well as degree of left ventricular dysfunction

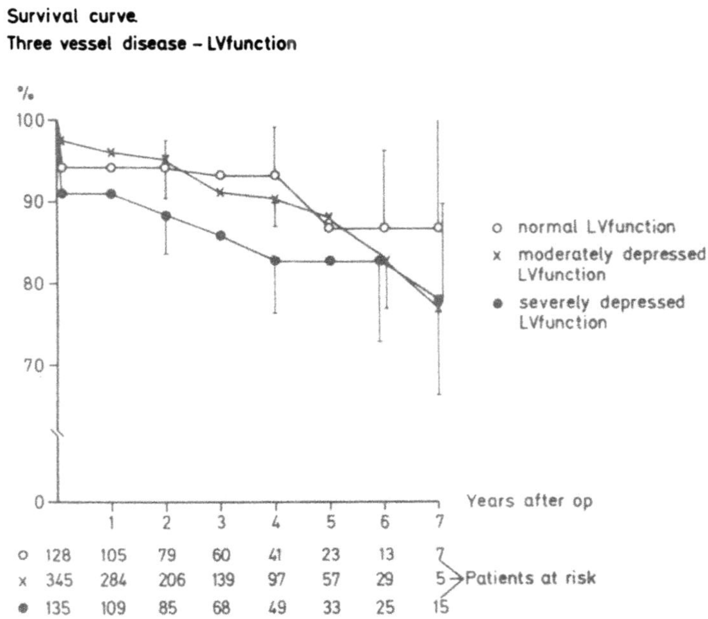
Survival curve
Three vessel disease – LVfunction
%
100
90
80
70
0
1 2 3 4 5 6 7
Years after op
o normal LVfunction
x moderately depressed LVfunction
• severely depressed LVfunction
o 128 105 79 60 41 23 13 7
x 345 284 206 139 97 57 29 5
• 135 109 85 68 49 33 25 15
Patients at risk

c

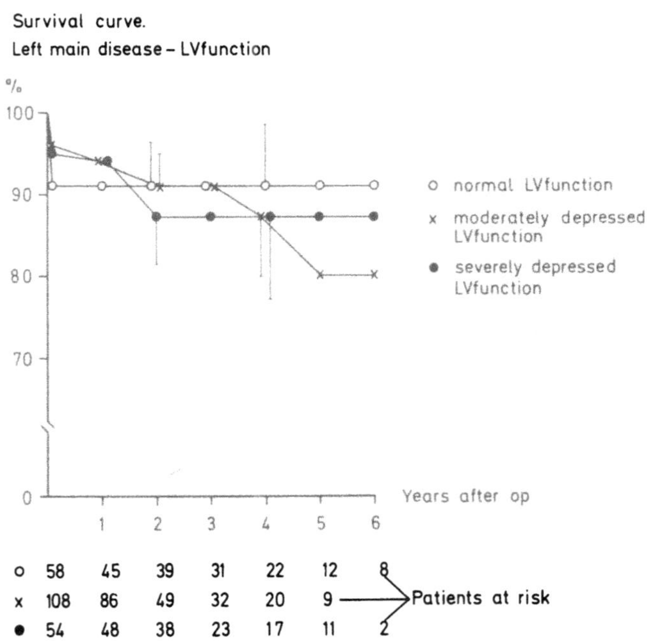
Survival curve.
Left main disease – LVfunction
%
100
90
80
70
0
1 2 3 4 5 6
Years after op
o normal LVfunction
x moderately depressed LVfunction
• severely depressed LVfunction
o 58 45 39 31 22 12 8
x 108 86 49 32 20 9
• 54 48 38 23 17 11 2
Patients at risk

d

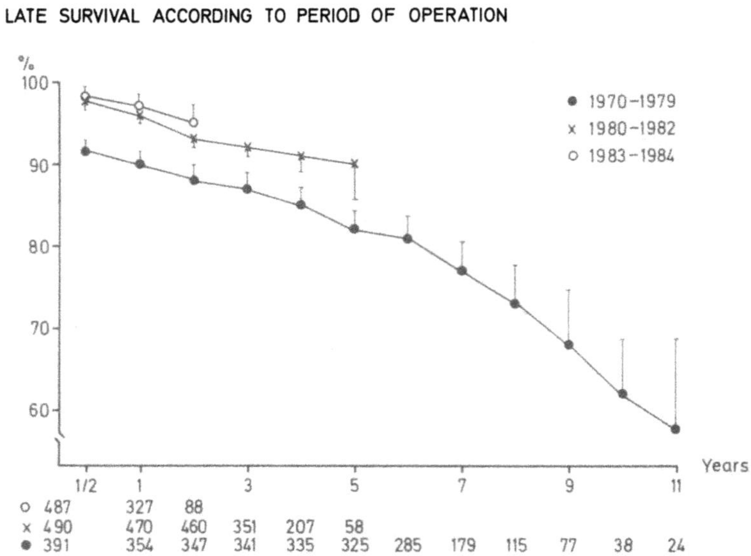

Fig. 4. Entire material divided into period of operation

Dividing the material into patients with normal, moderately depressed, and severely depressed left ventricular function revealed a higher survival during the first 7 years for patients with normal left ventricular function than for the patients with moderately and severely depressed left ventricular function (Fig. 2). Yearly mortality is low in patients with normal LV function (0.6%/year) and higher for patients with moderately depressed (1.3%/year) and severely depressed (2.6%/year) LV function. Further subdivision of the material into degree of vessel involvement *and* left ventricular function substantiated the above findings but for minor variations in the smaller subgroups (Fig. 3).

Dividing the material into period of operation revealed a significantly higher operative mortality in the early group (Fig. 4) and a markedly improved 2- and 5-year survival in the middle and recent operation groups (Table 2). During the first 5–7 years, survival curves tend to be a straight line, indicating a constant yearly mortality rate. After 6–7 years, yearly mortality seems to increase. In the patient group operated on during the earliest period, yearly mortality was 1.5% during the first 6 years and 4% during years 7–11 (Fig. 4). In the early operation group, 34 patients have been reoperated upon (9%).

Discussion

Comparison with Other Material. Our early operation group was operated on during the recruitment period of all three major randomized coronary artery surgery studies. Although the clinical picture was more severe in our patients as the indication for operation was severe angina pectoris, comparisons with this material may be made. Survival in our early operation group is similar to that of the surgical Veterans Administration group, with a 7-year sur-

Table 3. Survival at 2, 5, and 7 years postoperatively in the early, middle, and recent operation groups, divided into one-, two-, and three-vessel disease and left main stenosis (figures are percentages)

	Survival at								
	2 years			5 years			7 years		
	E	M	R	E	M	R	E	M	R
1	94	95	95	89	91	–	89	–	–
2	92	96	98	87	96	–	85	–	–
3	83	92	93	75	87	–	69	–	–
LM	80	88	95	78	88	–	71	–	–
Total	88	93	95	82	90	–	78	–	–

vival rate for all patients of 77% in the Veterans Administration material and 77% in our early operation group. Our markedly superior results in the middle and late operation groups (Table 2) suggest that there is a time factor and a learning curve giving improved surgical results with better familiarity with the operation and with development of improved methods and routines. This suggests that the Veterans Administration surgical results may be judged as inapplicable in coronary artery surgery of today.

On the other hand, the European Coronary Surgery Study group, which treated patients with medium-level angina pectoris (in contrast to our patients with severe angina), had a 5-year surgical survival of 92% compared to 82% in our early, and 90% in our middle, group.

The CASS randomized study, treating patients with only slight symptoms and excluding left main stenosis, had a 7-year survival of 88% compared with 78% in our material.

The main difference between our early and middle recent groups is the 1-month mortality, which was high during earlier years. However, there is a slightly higher medium-term mortality (1–5 years) in the early group compared with later groups, suggesting that the conditions for late survival may have improved in the later material. The cause of this uncertain finding remains speculative. Improved myocardial protection and insertion of more grafts per patient may be possible explanations. In our early operated group, late mortality increased after 5–6 years, reaching an annual mortality of 4% between 6 and 11 years postoperatively. Annual mortality in untreated angina pectoris patients was found to be around 4%. Thus the life-prolonging effect of the operation seems to diminish and possibly cease after several years. The Veterans Administration study drew similar conclusions.

In our material, late survival was markedly influenced by left ventricular function. This finding has been made by several earlier investigations. The lesson of this finding has been to advocate the operation in patients with good LV function before the myocardium suffers from the disease. This notion, however, does not take the limited period during which the operation is effective into consideration. Furthermore, all three major studies have come to similar conclusions: Coronary artery surgery gives a prolonged life in certain subgroups characterized by a poor prognosis on medical therapy. One of the main determinants of prognosis on medical therapy is left ventricular function. As prognosis in patients with normal LV function is good also on medical treatment, and as the life-prolonging effect of surgery becomes smaller within a 10-year period, surgery should be only cautiously advocated in patients with good LV function. The primary treatment in this group may well turn out to be coronary dilatation. Surgical treatment therefore should be shifted more to patients with poor LV function, as the difference between medical and surgical treatment becomes large and important.

Another aim of surgical development must be to increase the time span during which the operation is truly effective. Total revascularization, improved myocardial protection, increased use of internal mammary arteries, better preservation of the vein during the operation, new suture materials, postoperative antithrombocyte treatment, development of artificial grafts, and secondary prevention of the coronary artery disease may all turn out to be the means to reach this goal.

Results of Coronary Revascularization in Patients with Very Poor Versus Normal Left Ventricular Function

B. MOCHTAR, K. LAIRD-MEETER, R. W. BROWER, M. M. P. HAALEBOS, E. BOS, and P. G. HUGENHOLTZ

Introduction

Primary myocardial revascularization is a well-established mode of treatment for patients with angina pectoris caused by significant coronary artery disease. The role of coronary bypass surgery in patients with severe left ventricular dysfunction and disabling angina pectoris remains controversial. In this report we analyze the clinical course of 62 consecutive patients with severe left ventricular dysfunction and disabling angina pectoris who underwent isolated coronary artery bypass grafting (group I). Excluded from this study were patients in whom myocardial revascularization was combined with other procedures. These results were compared with survival of 600 patients with normal left ventricular function who underwent myocardial revascularization at the same time (group II).

Methods

The ejection fraction (EF) was calculated by biplane angiocardiography according to the method of Dodge [3]. Left ventricular dysfunction was defined as an EF of 0.30 or less and normal ventricular function as an EF of 0.55 or more. Group I included 62 patients with a mean age of 55.7 years 93% of which were male (58 patients). All patients had disabling angina pectoris (NYHA III–IV) and 35% (22 patients) also had accompanying symptoms of congestive heart failure. Three-vessel disease was present in 82% of the patients and a main stem lesion in 5%. The mean EF was 0.25. Group II included 600 patients with a mean age of 52.8 years 88% of which were males. Three-vessel disease was present in 42% of the patients [5, 6].

Results

Surgical mortality (28 days) in group I was 4.8% (3 patients), with 13 late deaths (21%). Of the 13 late deaths, 84% (11 patients) were cardiac in origin. The mean follow-up period was 37 months (4–116 months). At follow-up, of 46 remaining long-term survivors, 67% (31/46) were completely asymptomatic (NYHA I) and 26% (12/46) reported improvement in angina (NYHA II), 7%

(3/46) still had disabling angina (NYHA III), and 36% (17/46) were still limited by exertional dyspnea.

Surgical mortality in group II was 1.2% (7 patients) with 23 late deaths. Of the late deaths, 75% were cardiac in origin. The mean follow-up period was 3.5 years (1 – 10 years). At follow-up of the long-term survivors (570 patients), 47% still experienced angina and 37% were limited by dyspnea.

Comparing both groups of patients there were significant differences in surgical mortality (group I, 4.8%, group II, 1.2%) ($P = 0.03$) and long-term survival [group I 5-year survival, 70 (SD, 9%); group II 5-year survival, 95 (SD, 2%) ($P = 0.02$)]. However, no significant difference was found with regard to relief of angina after operation (NS).

Discussion

We therefore conclude that the preoperative EF is an important predictor of survival after aortocoronary bypass grafting, as has been recently reported by Cosgrove, Pigott, Alderman, Myers, and Hochberg [1, 2, 4, 7, 8]. In our series the actuarial survival probability for patients with a poor EF at 5 years was 70 (SD = 9%), significantly lower than those who had a normal EF [95 (SD = 2%)]. We believe that patients in whom severe angina pectoris is the predominant symptom, despite intensive pharmacological therapy, should be operated upon, regardless of poor ventricular function despite the higher operative risk. Predominant ischemic symptoms imply the presence of potential viable myocardium. For the same reason, patients presenting solely with congestive heart failure secondary to irreversible myocardial fibrosis should not be operated upon. Aortocoronary bypass surgery can be performed in patients with severe left ventricular dysfunction with reasonable relief of angina and with an acceptable surgical mortality; however, a low EF is correlated with poorer long-term survival.

References

1. Alderman EL et al. (1983) Results of coronary artery surgery in patients with poor left ventricular function (CASS). Circulation 68:785 – 795
2. Cosgrove DM et al. (1985) Determinants of 10-year survival after primary myocardial revascularization. Ann Surg 202:480 – 490
3. Dodge HT et al. (1960) The use of biplane angiocardiography for the measurement of left ventricular volume in man. Am Heart J 60:762 – 776
4. Hochberg MS et al. (1983) Coronary artery bypass grafting in patients with ejection fractions below forty percent. J Thorac Cardiovasc 86:519 – 527
5. Laird-Meeter K et al. (1983) Angina pectoris, 1 to 10 years after aorto-coronary bypass surgery. Eur Heart J 4:678 – 686
6. Laird-Meeter K et al. (1984) Survival in 1041 patients with consecutive aorto-coronary bypass operations. Eur Heart J 5:35 – 42
7. Myers WO et al. (1985) Surgical survival in the coronary artery surgery study (CASS) registry. Ann Thorac Surg 3:245 – 260
8. Pigott JD et al. (1982) Late results of medical and surgical therapy for patients with coronary artery disease and depressed ejection fraction. Circulation 66/II:220

Progression of Coronary Artery Disease After Bypass Grafting

P. GUITERAS, M. MASOTTI, J. ALTIMIRAS, T. BASSONS, J. M. AUGÉ, C. CREXELLS, and A. ORIOL

Introduction

Aortocoronary bypass grafting influences the natural history of coronary artery disease (CAD). Accelerated atherosclerosis in the proximal segments of grafted arteries has been extensively reported, particularly within the first postoperative year [3–5, 7–10].

Nevertheless, proximal coronary occlusion, due to acute thrombosis [11], is the consequence of the sluggish proximal coronary flow through the baseline stenosis and competitive graft flow. To consider proximal coronary occlusion as a form of CAD progression after surgery may overshadow other forms of progression of atherosclerosis which may be important clues for late graft patency.

This study was focused on analyzing progression of CAD without occlusion after surgical revascularization.

Material and Methods

Since February 1984, a prospective study on aortocoronary graft patency has been underway at our institute. All patients explicitly agree to undergo consecutive cardiac catheterization control before leaving the hospital and 6 months later. This is a preliminary report to study progression of CAD in the first 100 patients (95 men and 5 women, mean age 55.7 ± 7.7 years), 64 of whom were recatheterized 6 months later (Table 1). They received 156 simple and 17 sequential saphenous vein bypasses and 44 left internal mammary (LIMA) conduits. Of these grafts, 108 simple, 11 sequential, and 23 LIMA conduits were restudied 6 months later.

Selective coronary angiograms and graft opacifications were performed and multiple views, including sagittal angulations, were filmed. The same projections were used for the baseline and follow-up angiograms. Two orthogonal views in which the coronary lesions and the grafts could be more clearly seen, particularly at their proximal and distal anastomoses, were projected onto a large white screen and traced on transparent paper. Additionally, a portion of the catheter near its tip end was traced and used to correct the X-ray magnification. The drawings were digitized with a hand-held sonic cursor using the software implemented on a Cardio 200 (Kontron CP/M) microcomputer [13]. Average luminal diameters of the proximal and distal anastomoses, mid-third of the grafts, and the nearest proximal healthy artery; and the narrowest di-

Table 1. Graft, patency, coronary occlusion and progression of CAD

	Average time interval between catheterizations (months)	
	1.5±1.3	6±1.04
No. of patients	100	64
Graft patency rate	189/217 (87%)	123/142 (87%)
Occlusion of grafted artery		
Proximal to graft	52/217 (24%)	32/142 (23%)
Distal to graft	6/217 (3%)	4/142 (3%)
Occlusion of ungrafted artery	0/72	1/50 (2%)
Progression of CAD in grafted artery		
Proximal to graft	4/217 (2%)	7/142 (5%)
Distal to graft	13/217 (6%)	9/142 (6%)
Progression of CAD in ungrafted artery	1/72 (1.4%)	0/50

ameter of each stenosis and arterial bed immediately caudal to the distal graft anastomosis were calculated (Fig. 1). Obstructions of the coronary arteries and the grafts were estimated as the linear percentage of the narrowest luminal diameter of the stenosis to the diameter of the nearest proximal healthy segment. To evaluate the influence of the grafts on CAD progression, each grafted artery was divided into two regions, proximal and distal to the graft.

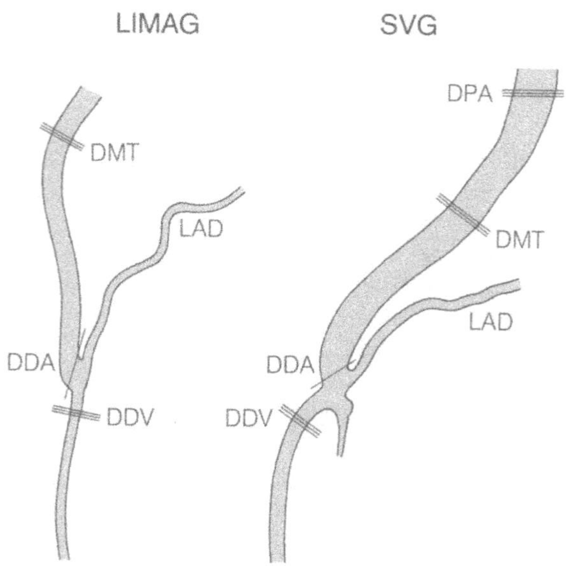

Fig. 1. Drawing from a cineangiogram of a saphenous vein graft (*SVG*) and a left internal mammary artery graft (*LIMAG*) to a left anterior descending artery (*LAD*) in lateral positions. The *thin lines* show where measurements were routinely obtained. *DMT*, diameter of mid-third; *DDA*, diameter of distal anastomosis, *DDV*, diameter of distal vessel; *DPA*, diameter of proximal anastomosis

Table 2. Variables entered in univariate analysis

Clinical ($n = 31$)	Angiographic ($n = 49$)	Surgical ($n = 8$)
Age	Coronary lesions ≧ 50%	Number of grafts
Sex	(1V, 2V, 3V, LMT)	received
Smoking status	Coronary lesions ≧ 70%	Perioperative MI
Serum:	(1V, 2V, 3V, LMT)	∅ distal bed
Cholesterol	Gensini score [a]	Morphology of distal
Triglycerides	Extent score [a]	bed
Glucose	Left ventricular ejection	Type of graft:
Systemic hypertension	fraction [a]	Simple, sequential,
Family history of CAD	Baseline angiogram:	LIMA
Relative obesity	Dominancy	Quality of distal bed
Prior:	Grafted/ungrafted artery	Artery grafted side to
Myocardial infarction	Site, severity, and mor-	side
Congestive heart failure	phology lesion	Endarterectomy
Unstable angina	∅ proximal artery	
Angina class [b]:	∅ and morphology of	
Before CABG	distal bed	
At discharge	First and second control	
At last control	angiograms:	
Duration of angina	Progression of CAD:	
Medical treatment:	In grafted artery	
Before CABG	In ungrafted artery	
After CABG	Site of progression	
Basal ECG	of CAD	
Time from:	Severity:	
CABG to first and last	Of grafted lesion	
control	Of new lesion	
Baseline to first control	∅ distal bed	
	∅ graft (proximal, mid,	
	distal)	
	Graft patency	
	Graft stenosis: site and	
	severity	

CABG, coronary artery bypass graft; ECG, electrocardiogram; ∅, diameter; MI, myocardial infarction; LIMA, left internal mammary artery; V, vessel; LMT, left main trunk

[a] Measured before surgery and at the 1st- and 6th-month controls

[b] Canadian Cardiovascular Society

The severity of CAD was assessed with Gensini's score [12]. The extent of CAD was defined as the number of coronary obstructions of 10% or more severe.

Significant progression of CAD was defined as: (1) a 20% or greater increase in stenosis of a segment narrower than 50%, (2) a 30% or more increase in stenosis of a segment narrowed more than 20% but less than 50%, or (3) a new stenosis of 50% or more in a previously normal coronary segment. Occlusion, that is, the appearance of a new complete obstruction in a segment previously patent, was considered separately, and not counted as progression.

Table 2 lists the clinical, angiographical, and surgical data used in the univariate analysis to determine their influence on progression of CAD. The angiographic variables were measured as stated above. The surgeon measured the distal coronary beds with a probe and subjectively reported their quality.

Data were related to CAD occlusion and CAD progression or their absence, using Chi-square statistics if categorical, and the unpaired t-test or one-way analysis of variance if continuous. Significant differences were finally entered to develop a multivariate logistic regression model for the absence/or progression of CAD. The goodness-of-fit of the final model was assessed by Hosmer's and Brown's tests [16]. A P value of 0.05 was accepted for each test.

Results

Graft patency, coronary occlusion, and progression of CAD are summarized in Table 1.

Figures 2 and 3 show that coronary occlusion was almost exclusively proximal to the graft at both the first and 6-month controls. The same figures show that while coronary occlusion was almost exclusively proximal, CAD progression was often immediately caudal to the distal graft anastomosis. Finally, Fig. 4 shows more frequent progression of CAD in grafted than nonbypassed arteries.

Factors Influencing Progression of Atherosclerosis

Progression of atherosclerosis in patients can be seen in Table 3.

At the 6-month control, none of the seven patients receiving a single graft experienced progression of CAD and only two had proximal coronary occlusion.

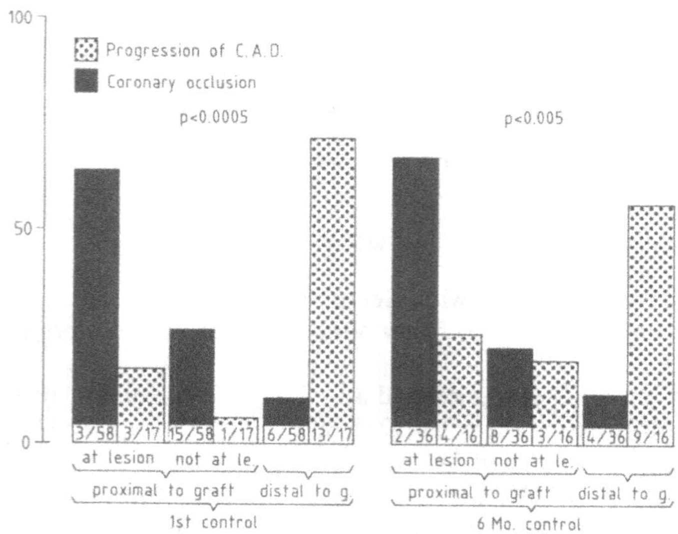

Fig. 2. Coronary occlusion was significantly more frequent than progression of coronary artery disease in both controls. While coronary occlusion was proximal from the distal end of the graft anastomosis, progression of CAD tended to be distal to the graft

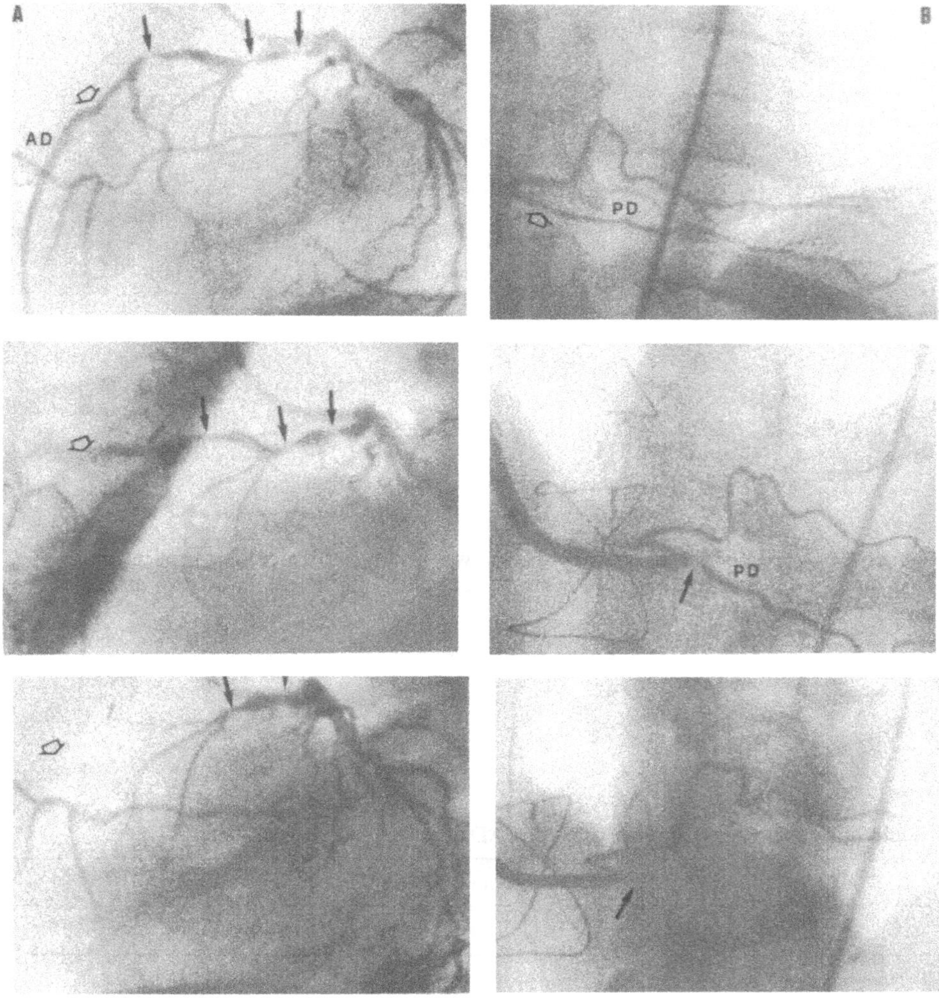

Fig. 3. A *From top to bottom:* LAD in lateral position. Male with two proximal and a mid-LAD stenosis (*arrows*) before CABG; he received a LIMA conduit. At the first postoperative control (*middle*) competitive flow beyond the mid-third stenosis is seen (*open arrow*). At the 6-month control (*bottom*) the LAD has occluded proximal to the graft at the level of the second proximal lesion. **B** *From top to bottom:* right coronary artery in the right anterior oblique position. Male with a distal occlusion of his RCA with a good distal bed (1.6 mm diameter). He received a simple saphenous vein graft to the posterior descending artery (*PD*). At the first control an 86% stenosis has developed just distal to the graft (*arrow*). At the 6-month control, the posterior descending artery has occluded and only the posterolateral branches are seen retrogradely

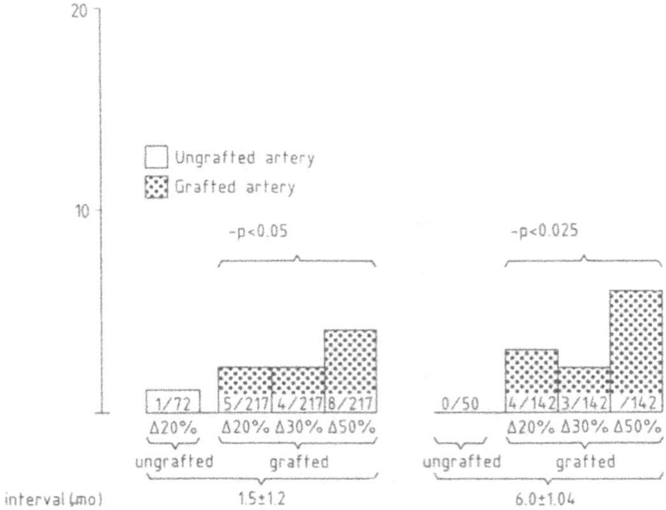

Fig. 4. Progression of coronary artery disease was significantly more frequent in the grafted than the ungrafted arteries at both controls, regardless of the criteria used to measure progression of CAD

Table 3. Factors related to progression of CAD after surgery (patients)

Univariate analysis			
	No progression	Progression	*P*
First control ($n = 60$):			
Sex: female/male	0/46	4/14	0.0021
Age (years)	59.4±7.6	53.7±7.8	0.02
Six-month control ($n = 42$):			
≧ two grafts per patient	21/28 (75%)	14/14 (100%)	<0.05
Incomplete revascularization	12/28 (43%)	1/14 (7%)	<0.05
Graft occlusion or stenosis	5/28 (18%)	6/14 (43%)	0.07

Logistic regression analysis		
	β-coefficient	*P*
Six-months control ($n = 42$):		
Age (years)	0.216	0.0119
Incomplete revascularization	2.853	0.0001
Grafts per patient: 4	−3.828	0.0001
3	−1.933	0.0001
2	−4.41	0.0001
Constant	−7.065	

Table 4. Factors related to progression of CAD after surgery (arteries)

Univariate analysis

	No progression	Progression	*P*
First control ($n = 159$):			
Diseased distal bed (angio)[a]	64/141 (45%)	13/18 (72%)	<0.05
Diseased distal bed (surgery)	68/128 (54%)	15/17 (88%)	0.005
Endarterectomy	21/141 (15%)	5/18 (28%)	0.0005
Severity of grafted lesion (%)[a]	79.9±19.5	89.8±14.9	0.041
∅ distal bed (mm)[b]	1.8± 0.5	1.0± 0.5	0.00001
Six-months control ($n = 106$):			
Simple saphenous graft	65/90 (72%)	15/16 (94%)	0.07
New stenosis in the graft	2/90 (2%)	3/16 (19.4)	<0.005
∅ distal bed (mm)[b]	1.7±0.6	1.0± 0.6	0.03

Logistic regression analysis

	β-coefficient	*P*
First control ($n = 135$):		
∅ distal bed (mm)[b]	2.205	0.00001
Diseased distal bed (surgery)	−0.731	0.045
Constant	−0.886	
Six-months control ($n = 88$):		
∅ distal bed (mm)[b]	1.22	0.021
Type of graft: simple saphenous	−2.144	0.056
LIMA	5.649	0.056
Constant	5.717	

∅, diameter; LIMA, Left internal mammary artery

[a] At baseline coronary angiogram

[b] At first angiographic control

However, progression of atherosclerosis was seen in 14 patients who received two or more grafts. On the contrary, revascularization had been more frequently incomplete in patients free of progression. Graft occlusion or stenosis favored progression of the disease. An acceptable logistic model inversely related age and incompleteness of revascularization to CAD progression and directly to the number of grafts received per patient.

Progression of atherosclerosis in arteries can be seen in Table 4. The logistic model retained only diseased and narrow distal beds as independent factors favoring progression of CAD.

At the 6-month control, the logistic regression showed that a narrow distal bed and simple saphenous grafting favored CAD progression.

Discussion

Accelerated atherosclerosis in the grafted arteries immediately after surgery has been extensively reported in the literature [3–5, 7–10, 15]. For lesions of similar severity, the annual incidence of progression of atherosclerosis in medically treated patients has been reported between 24% and 35% [2, 3, 6, 14] but 50%–62% in grafted arteries [3–5, 7–10, 15]. The actual difference may be greater, since most reported series in medically treated patients have been retrospective, and therefore sequential catheterization has been biased by symptoms. Nevertheless, progression of atherosclerosis in grafted arteries appears to level off between 5 and 10 years after surgery [5], and only in grafted arteries with closed grafts does progression of atherosclerosis remain higher than in ungrafted arteries (93% vs. 47%, respectively).

Most authors have considered coronary occlusion as a form of progression of atherosclerosis [3–5, 7–10, 15]. Coronary occlusion is usually an acute phenomenon always due to luminal thrombosis [1, 11], while coronary artery disease (CAD) is usually a progressive multistage phenomenon [5]. Since proximal flow in the grafted coronary artery is compromised by the preoperative stenosis and the bypass flow [9], proximal coronary occlusion occurs early, and often regardless of the severity of the baseline lesion. We thus decided to analyze coronary occlusion apart from CAD progression.

In this study, occlusion of grafted arteries was more frequent than progression of CAD at both the first (27% vs. 8%) and second controls (26% vs. 11%). Our incidence of CAD progression in grafted arteries is less than that reported by others [3–5, 7–10], even if occlusion is considered as a form of atherosclerotic progression. This may be due to the fixed, relatively short interval between the angiographic controls, or to the fact that the second study was not prompted by symptoms, or to a less-evolutive atherosclerosis.

Occlusion in the grafted artery tended to be an early event, almost exclusively at the level of the preoperative lesion proximal to the distal graft anastomosis, as extensively reported by others [3–5, 7–10], while progression of CAD was more frequent in the last control and distal to the graft anastomosis. Similar incidence of distal progression of CAD at the 6-year angiographic control was reported by Bourassa et al. [4], who emphasized that proximal coronary occlusion is the most frequent event within the 1st year although it remains stable thereafter.

Progression of CAD after surgery was influenced neither by the accepted coronary risk factors nor by the extent and severity of baseline CAD. Since the time interval between sequential catheterization was fixed we could not detect the obvious influence of time on CAD progression.

The deleterious effect of the completeness of revascularization and the number of grafts received on CAD progression were to be expected. Young age has also been reported to favor CAD progression in medically treated patients [17]. Since the time interval between sequential angiograms was short, the effect of progression of CAD and coronary and graft occlusion on symptoms, although apparent, did not reach statistical significance. Progression of CAD was influenced by the choice of a too narrow or diseased distal bed, sometimes requiring endarterectomy.

Since in medically treated patients CAD develops proximally, at the junctions of the segments moved by the cardiac contraction and their branches entering into the myocardium, it seems logical that the site for developing future atheromatous lesions will now be moved distally to the graft implant. The graft itself will play the role of an epicardial vessel with the remaining artery acting like a myocardial branch.

References

1. Barger AC, Beeuwkes III R, Lainey LJ, Silverman KH (1984) Hypothesis: vasa vasorum and neovascularization of human coronary artery arteries. N Engl J Med 310:175
2. Bemis CE, Gorlin R, Kemp HG, Herman MV (1973) Progression of coronary artery disease. Circulation 47:455
3. Ben ZVI, Hildner FJ, Javier RP, Fester A, Samet P (1974) Progression of coronary artery disease. Cinearteriographic and clinical observations in medically and surgically treated patients. Am J Cardiol 34:295
4. Bourassa MG, Campeau L, Lesperance J, Grondin CM (1982) Changes in grafts and coronary arteries after saphenous vein aortocoronary bypass surgery: results at repeat angiography. Circulation 65 (II):90
5. Bourassa MG, Enjalbert M, Campeau L, Lesperance J (1984) Progression of atherosclerosis in coronary arteries and bypass graft: ten years later. Am J Cardiol 53:102C
6. Bruschke AVG, Proudfit WL, Sones EM Jr (1973) Progress study of 590 consecutive nonsurgical cases of coronary disease followed 5 to 9 years. II. Ventriculographic and other correlations. Circulation 47:1154
7. Campeau L, Crochet D, Lesperance J, Bourssa MG, Grondin CM (1975) Postoperative changes in aortocoronary saphenous vein grafts revisited. Circulation 52:369
8. Cashin WL, Sanmarco ME, Nessim SA, Blankenhorn DH (1984) Accelerated progression in atherosclerosis in coronary vessels with minimal lesions that are bypassed. N Engl J Med 311:824
9. Cipriano PR, Sacks AH, Reitz BA (1980) The effect of stenosis of bypass grafts on coronary flow. Circulation 62:61
10. Cosgrone DM, Loop FD, Sheldon WC (1982) Results of myocardial revascularization. A 12 year experience. Circulation 65 (II):37
11. Falk E (1983) Plaque rupture with severe preexisting stenosis precipitating coronary thrombosis. Characteristics of coronary atherosclerotic plaques underlying fatal occlusive thrombi. Br Heart J 50:127
12. Gensini GC, Kelly AE (1972) Incidence and progression of coronary artery disease. Arch Intern Med 129:814
13. Harrison DG, White CW, Hiratzka LF, Doty DB, Barnes DH, Easthan CL, Marcus ML (1984) The value of lesion cross-sectional area determined by quantitative coronary angiography in assessing the physiologic significance of proximal left anterior descending coronary arterial stenosis. Circulation 69:IV
14. Kramer JR, Matsuda Y, Mulligan JC, Aronow M, Proudfit WL (1981) Progression of coronary atherosclerosis. Circulation 63:519
15. Lawrie GM, Lie JT, Morris GC, Beazley HL (1976) Vein graft patency and intimal proliferation after aortocoronary bypass. Am J Cardiol 38:856
16. McCullagh P, Nelder A (1983) Generalized linear models. University Press, Cambridge
17. Moïse A, Theroux P, Taeymans Y, Descoings B, Lesperance J, Waters DD, Pelletier G, Bourassa MG (1983) Unstable angina and progression of coronary atherosclerosis. N Engl J Med 309:685

Left Ventricular Systolic Function and Diastolic Filling Before and After Coronary Artery Bypass Surgery

P. BRUGGER, K. LUDWIG, F. LOHFEYER, F. UNGER, and G. KLEIN

Bypass surgery dramatically alters the symptomatic status of many patients and prolongs life in some. It has been well documented in some studies that after revascularization exercise tolerance improves even when antianginal medications are reduced [13, 18, 21]. There is also general agreement that aortocoronary bypass surgery improves angina pectoris in a high percentage of patients [10].

There have been other studies showing that global and regional systolic left ventricular function during exercise improve with successful bypass grafting of significantly stenosed, major epicardial-coronary arteries [2, 6, 7, 9, 17, 21]. Because the diastolic function is more sensitive than the systolic function, we examined in 23 patients with coronary artery disease the diastolic function noninvasively by the parameters peak filling rate and time to peak filling rate before and after coronary artery bypass surgery. Beyond that we determined the ejection fraction (EF) at rest and during exercise.

The purpose of our investigation was to determine the left ventricular systolic and diastolic function in patients who had diminished left ventricular function as well as exercise-induced ischemia before surgery, subsequently had an uncomplicated bypass operation, and were symptomatically improved after surgery.

Patients and Methods

The study comprised 23 patients (22 men and 1 woman, age range 33–66 years, average age 52 years, with confirmed coronary artery disease). Seventeen had already suffered a myocardial infarction; of these 6 in an inferior and 11 in an anterior wall. Twenty-two patients with no cardiovascular disease served as a control group.

The analysis of left ventricular function was carried out with a nuclear stethoscope (BIOS) a mobile gamma-ray measuring probe. The measurements were performed in the prone position after prior intravenous administration of 10–15 mCi 99m-technetium.

In this nuclear medical technique, the ventricular volumes were detected analogously to radionuclide ventriculography. All patients underwent bicycle exercise testing before and after revascularization.

For detection of the left ventricular systolic function the ejection fraction and of the diastolic function the parameters peak filling rate (PFR) and time to

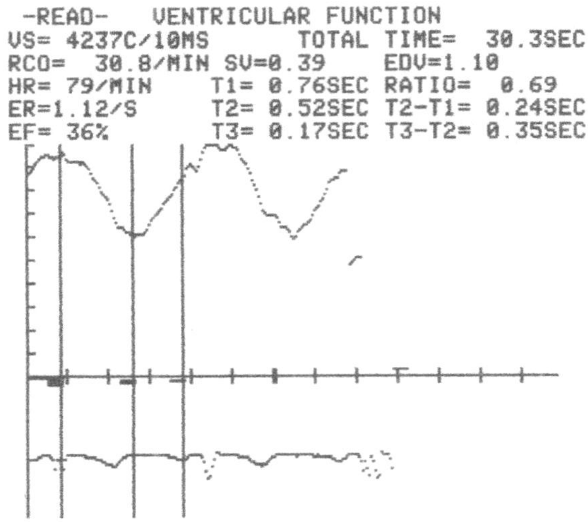

Fig. 1. Computer printout of ventricular function with two time curves. Manifestation of various functional parameters including EF and TPFR

peak filling rate (TPFR) were determined (Fig. 1). The PFR and the TPFR are measurements of the left ventricular relaxation time and of the rapid filling phase. The PFR is defined as the maximum steep rise in the rapid filling phase and the TPFR as the time to PFR.

The results were analyzed statistically by means of the paired Student *t*-test. Correlations between nuclear stethoscope and contrast ventriculography were made by linear regression analysis.

Results

As a whole, 23 patients with coronary artery disease (CAD) were investigated before and after revascularization. The PFR and TPFR were determined as parameters of diastolic function and the EF as a parameter of systolic function. After coronary artery bypass surgery there was a nonsignificant increase of the EF at rest from 49% ± 11% to 51% ± 7% and a significant rise of the EF during exercise from 38% ± 14% to 62% ± 11% ($P < 0.0001$) (Fig. 2).

Of special interest was the diastolic function, which showed a significant increase of the PFR from 2.37 ± 0.63 EDV/s to 2.88 ± 0.68 EDV/s (End Diastolic Volume) ($P < 0.025$) (Fig. 3) The TPFR also showed a significant improvement of the left ventricular diastolic function, decreasing significantly from 196 ± 33 ms to 138 ± 39 ms ($P < 0.005$) (Fig. 4).

In the control group of 22 patients there was a significant rise in EF at rest to exercise from 70% ± 9% to 81% ± 8% ($P < 0.001$) and a normal diastolic function at rest with a PFR of 3.65 ± 1.0 EDV/s and a TPFR of 135 ± 44.0 ms.

In a comparison between left ventricular ejection fraction measured by the nuclear stethoscope and contrast ventriculography, in another study [3] in 34 patients with CAD we found a good correlation, with a correlation coefficient of $r = 0.89$ (Fig. 5).

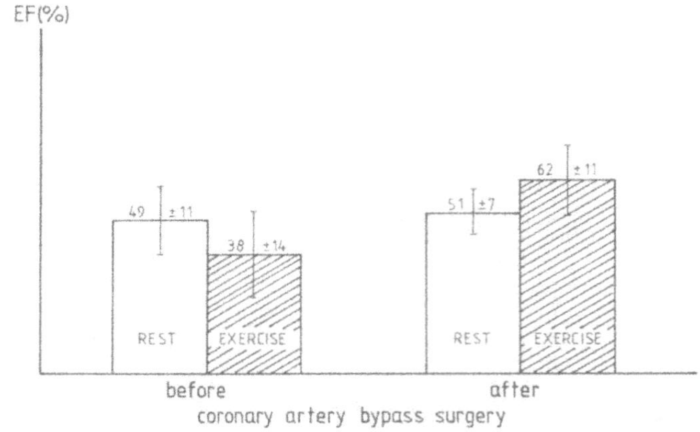

Fig. 2. Effect of revascularization on ventricular systolic function at rest and during exercise

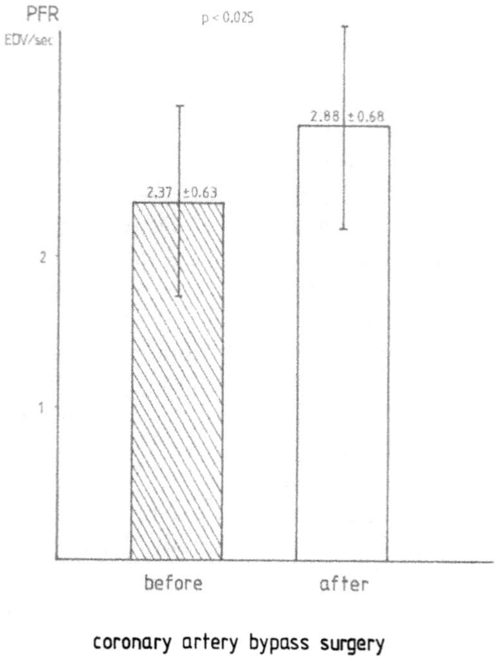

Fig. 3. Diastolic filling behavior (peak filling rate) in 23 patients before and after coronary artery bypass surgery

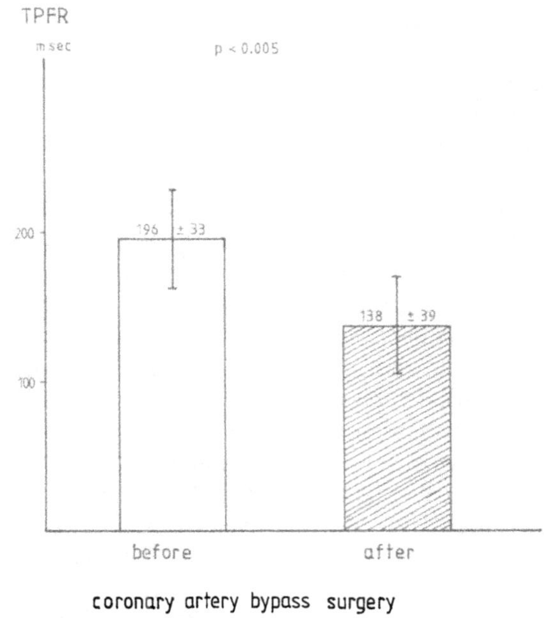

Fig. 4. Diastolic filling behavior (time to peak filling rate) in 23 patients before and after coronary artery bypass surgery

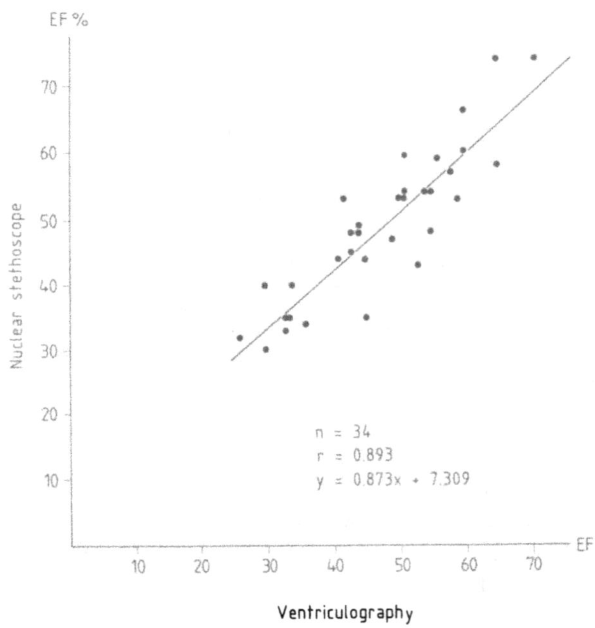

Fig. 5. Correlation between left ventricular ejection fraction measured by the nuclear stethoscope and contrast ventriculography in patients with coronary artery disease

Discussion

Coaxial (nonimaging) and imaging radionuclide techniques have been used extensively to study postoperative changes in left ventricular function in patients undergoing cardiac surgery [1, 11, 12, 14, 19, 20, 22, 23], most frequently in terms of left ventricular ejection fraction. Such investigations have generally shown a reduction in ejection fraction immediately after coronary bypass grafting, with return to preoperative baseline levels by 24 h to 7 days [11, 14, 20, 22]. A more complete longitudinal study demonstrated no serial change in resting ejection fraction but a significant postoperative increase in ejection fraction response to exercise [1]. Similar results were presented by Kent et al. [17], who had found that coronary artery bypass surgery does not predictably improve myocardial function at rest but does improve the function of myocardial segments with exercise-induced myocardial ischemia. On the basis of the results presented in this study, similar improvement of myocardial ischemia has been found. In the patients who had clinically successful results after bypass surgery, the mean EF during exercise increased significantly from 38% ± 14% to 62% ± 11% after surgery whereas the ejection fraction at rest stayed nearly unchanged. Moreover, the diastolic function at rest improved significantly as seen by the filling parameters PFR changing from 2.37 ± 0.63 EDV/s to 2.88 ± 0.68 EDV/s, and TPFR changing from 196 ± 33 ms to 138 ± 39 ms.

These data show that abnormal left ventricular systolic function during exercise and diastolic function can be greatly improved by reavscularization.

It is known that the mechanism of the augmentation of the EF is the significant increase in end-diastolic volume and preload not a reduction in systolic volume as occurs in normal individuals [8, 19].

The enhancement in relaxation is probably due to the correction of multiple biochemical and mechanical abnormalities that occur during preoperative ischemia [5]. These altered filling dynamics after revascularization allow an increased amount of blood to enter the left ventricle despite an even greater reduction in filling time. Left ventricular filling is a dynamic process involving the interaction of active and passive properties of the atria and ventricles [24].

The left ventricular myocardium consists of muscle and interstitial connective tissue. Whereas the percentage of the latter is low in normal left ventricle, there is a fibrotic transformation of the heart muscle in patients with CAD [15]. This leads to a restricted systolic and diastolic function. This function disorder can be demonstrated by the abnormal filling parameters PFR and TPFR. In this connection an earlier study appears worth mentioning where we found an abnormal PFR and/or prolonged TPFR in 85.9% of our patients with coronary artery disease [4]. The decreased PFR and the increased TPFR in our coronary patients may reflect the abnormally stiff ventricle frequently seen in coronary artery disease. Even in the absence of clinical infarction intraoperative transmural biopsies have shown the frequent occurrence of increased interstitional fibrosis and myocardial hypertrophy in these patients [16]. Possibly the significant improvement of the diastolic function at rest may be explained by the disappearance of silent ischemia after revascularization.

This study demonstrates that coronary artery bypass surgery improves left ventricular systolic function during exercise and diastolic function at rest significantly.

References

1. Austin EH, Oldham HN, Sabiston DC, Jones RH (1983) Early assessment of rest and exercise left ventricular function following coronary artery surgery. Ann Thorac Surg 35:159
2. Barry WH, Pfeifer JF, Lipton MJ, Tilkan AG, Hultgren HN (1976) Effects of coronary artery bypass grafting on resting and exercise hemodynamics in patients with stable angina pectoris: a prospective, randomized study. Am J Cardiol 37:823
3. Brugger P (1985) Linksventrikuläre diastolische Funktion und ventrikuläre Arrhythmien bei koronarer Herzkrankheit. Z Kardiologie 74:512–518
4. Brugger P, Lässer W, Kullich W, Stoiberer I, Klein G (1985) Nuclear medical determination of left ventricular diastolic function in coronary heart disease. Clin Cardiol 8:353–355
5. Brutsaert DL, Rademakers FE, Sys SU (1984) Triple control of relaxation: implications in cardiac disease. Circulation 69:190
6. Bussmann WD, Mayer V, Kober G, Kaltenbach M (1979) Ventricular function at rest, during leg raising and physical exercise before and after aortocoronary bypass surgery. Am J Cardiol 43:488
7. Campeau L, Elias G, Esplugas E, Lesperance J, Bourassa MG, Grondin CM (1974) Left ventricular performance during exercise before and one year after aortocoronary bypass surgery for angina pectoris. Circulation 50 [suppl II]:II-103
8. Carroll JD, Hess OM, Hirzel HO, Turina M, Krayenbuehl HP (1985) Left ventricular systolic and diastolic function in coronary artery disease: effects of revascularization on exercise-induced ischemia. Circulation 72 [1]:119–129
9. Chesebro JH, Ritman EL, Frye RL, Smith HC, Vlietstra RE, Pluth JR (1982) Left ventricular performance before and after aortocoronary artery bypass surgery. Circulation 65 [suppl II]:II-98
10. Council on Scientific Affairs (1979) Indications for aortocoronary bypass graft surgery. JAMA 343:2709
11. Czer L, Hamer A, Murphy F, Bussell J, Chaux A, Bateman T, Matloff J, Gray RJ (1983) Transient hemodynamic dysfunction after myocardial revascularization. J Thorac Cardiovasc Surg 86:226
12. Ellis RJ, Mangano DT, van Dyke DC (1979) Relationship of wedge pressure to end-diastolic volume in patients undergoing myocardial revascularization. J Thorac Cardiovasc Surg 78:605
13. Frick MH, Harjola PT, Valle M (1983) Persistent improvement after coronary bypass surgery: ergometric and angiographic correlations at 5 years. Circulation 67:491
14. Gray R, Maddahi J, Bermann D, Raymond M, Waxman A, Ganz W, Matloff J, Swan JC (1979) Scientigraphic and hemodynamic demonstration of transient left ventricular dysfunction immediately after uncomplicated coronary artery bypass grafting. J Thorac Cardiovasc Surg 77:504
15. Hess O (1982) Diastolische Funktion des linken Ventrikels. In: Thieme Copythek. Thieme Stuttgart; 98–99
16. Hess OM, Schneider J, Carroll JD, Eqloff L, Turina M, Krayenbuehl HP (1983) Myocardial structure of LV segments with and without exercise-induced wall motion abnormalities in patients with coronary artery disease. J Am Coll Cardiol 1:734
17. Kent KM, Borer JS, Green MV, Bacharach SL, McIntosh CL, Conkle DM, Epstein SE (1978) Effects of coronary-artery bypass on global and regional left ventricular function during exercise. N Engl J Med 298:1434
18. McIntosh HD, Garcia JA (1978) The first decade of aortocoronary bypass grafting, 1967–1977. A review. Circulation 57:405

19. Miller DC, Daughters GT, Derby GC, Mitchell RS, Ingels NB, Stinson EB, Alderman EL (1985) Effects of early postoperative volume loading on left ventricular systolic function (including left ventricular ejection fraction determined by myocardial marker) after myocardial revascularization. Circulation 72 [suppl II]: II-207
20. Phillips HR, Carter JE, Okada RD, Levine FH, Boucher CA, Osbakken M, Lappas D, Buckley M, Pohost GM (1983) Serial changes in left ventricular ejection fraction in the early hours after aortocoronary bypass grafting. Chest 83:28
21. Rahimtoola SH (1982) Postoperative exercise response in the evaluation of the physiologic status after coronary bypass surgery. Circulation 65 [suppl II]: II-106
22. Reduto LA, Lawrie GM, Reid JW, Whissenand HH, Noon GP, Kanon D, DeBakey ME, Miller RP (1983) Sequential postoperative assessment of left ventricular performance with gated cardiac blood pool imaging following aortocoronary bypass surgery. Am Heart J 101:59
23. Weisel RD, Burns RJ, Baird RJ, Hilton JD, Ivanov J, Mickle DA, Teoh KH, Christakis GT, Evans PJ, Scully HE, Goldman BS, McLaughlin PR (1983) A comparison of volume loading and atrial pacing following aortocoronary bypass. Ann Thorac Surg 36:322
24. Yellin EL, Sonnenblick EH, Frater RWM (1980) Dynamic determinants of left ventricular filling: an overview. In: Baan J, Arntzenius AC, Yellin EL (eds) Cardiac dynamics. Nijhoff, The Hague, pp 145–158

Radionuclide Study of Left Ventricular Wall Motion Before and After Coronary Bypass Surgery

E. Astorri, M. Busi, G. A. Contini, G. Gavaruzzi, and P. P. Ferretti

The purpose of this study was to assess global and regional left ventricular function in patients undergoing coronary artery surgery. Using gated radionuclide ventriculography, we evaluated the left ventricular performance before and 6 months after myocardial revascularization.

Patients and Methods

Fity-eight patients, 51 males, 7 females, ranging from 36 to 69 years old, gave their informed consent to the study when in schedule for myocardial revascularization. Forty-four patients had unstable angina, while 14 had stable effort angina and 34 patients had evidence of previous myocardial infarction (MI), 23 inferior and 11 anterior or anterolateral.

Six patients had significant single-vessel disease (left anterior descending, LAD), while 18 had two-vessel disease (including LAD) and 34 had coronary three-vessel disease.

Myocardial revascularization was performed by one (6 patients), two (17 patients), three (13 patients), four (14 patients), five (6 patients), and six (2 patients) coronary artery bypass grafts. All the surgical procedures were performed in general hypothermia (27° ± 2° C); myocardial preservation was obtained by local cooling and ischemic cardioplegic arrest with hyperpotassic, slightly alcalotic and hyperosmotic solution.

Gated radionuclide left ventriculography was performed in all patients 2–3 days before and 6 months after myocardial revascularization. Blood pool visualization was achieved by in vivo labeling autologous red blood cells with 20–25 mCi ^{99m}Tc; the patients were examined in 35°–45° left anterior oblique projection and 15° caudal tilting, using a large-field gamma camera (LFOV Searle), linked to a compatible computer (PDP 11/34 Digital Equipment Corp.).

Parameters computed by this technique included: global ventricular ejection fraction (EF); regional ejection fractions, namely anteroseptal (AS-EF), apical (AP-EF), and inferoposterior (IP-EF); peak ejection rate (PER); and peak filling rate (PFR) [3].

Data were analyzed by *t*-test using paired data and by linear regression analysis as appropriate.

Results

Six months after surgery all but five patients were in fairly good clinical condition, they could perform normal physical activities, and many of them returned to work. Five patients had angina pectoris on strong exertion, but of a lesser degree than before operation. Two of these patients suffered a perioperative myocardial infarction.

Before surgery, global EF was seen in all but 13 patients (≧50%). There was a close correlation between data obtained by contrast and radionuclide angiography ($r = 0.87$; $P < 0.001$).

Table 1. Global and regional left ventricular performance before (A) and after (B) myocardial revascularization (see text)

	A	B	*t*-test
Fifty-eight patients			
EF (%)	55.8 ±13.5	57.2 ±14.4	NS
AS-EF (%)	58.4 ±15.0	44.4 ±14.5	$P<0.05$
AP-EF (%)	67.5 ±20.7	70.8 ±19.5	NS
IP-EF (%)	56.1 ±12.5	68.5 ±16.0	$P<0.001$
PER (s^{-1})	3.11± 0.92	3.26± 0.92	NS
PFR (s^{-1})	2.52± 0.89	2.85± 0.96	$P<0.01$
Group I (LAD + diagonals) (7 patients)			
EF (%)	62.0 ±19.6	58.4 ±20.5	NS
AS-EF (%)	54.5 ±21.5	47.4 ±15.6	$P<0.05$
AP-EF (%)	69.0 ±32.6	68.0 ±29.6	NS
IP-ER (%)	64.0 ±14.3	63.0 ±19.2	NS
PER (s^{-1})	3.07± 0.94	3.13± 0.98	NS
PFR (s^{-1})	2.82± 0.89	2.69± 1.07	NS
Group II (LAD + LCA) (14 patients)			
EF (%)	57.3 ±10.1	58.1 ±12.4	NS
AS-EF (%)	50.7 ±10.6	48.3 ±12.8	NS
AP-EF (%)	69.6 ±16.5	72.6 ±13.2	NS
IP-EF (%)	55.0 ±10.0	67.4 ±16.5	$P<0.05$
PER (s^{-1})	3.07± 0.65	3.31± 1.08	NS
PFR (s^{-1})	2.59± 0.98	2.90± 0.86	NS
Group III (LAD + RCA) (16 patients)			
EF (%)	52.4 ±15.6	55.1 ±17.0	NS
AS-EF (%)	46.4 ±17.5	42.0 ±16.6	$P<0.05$
AP-EF (%)	61.4 ±20.4	65.6 ±19.9	NS
IP-EF (%)	57.3 ±16.3	71.1 ±18.4	$P<0.001$
PER (s^{-1})	2.89± 0.88	3.31± 1.17	$P<0.05$
PFR (s^{-1})	2.47± 0.94	2.81± 1.14	$P<0.05$
Group IV (LAD + LCA + RCA) (21 patients)			
EF (%)	54.8 ±11.2	57.9 ±11.9	NS
AS-EF (%)	46.2 ±13.2	42.7 ±13.9	NS
AP-EF (%)	70.1 ±19.3	74.6 ±19.3	NS
IP-EF (%)	53.2 ± 9.4	69.0 ±13.1	$P<0.001$
PER (s^{-1})	3.31± 1.11	3.25± 0.58	NS
PFR (s^{-1})	2.43± 0.84	2.93± 0.88	$P<0.01$

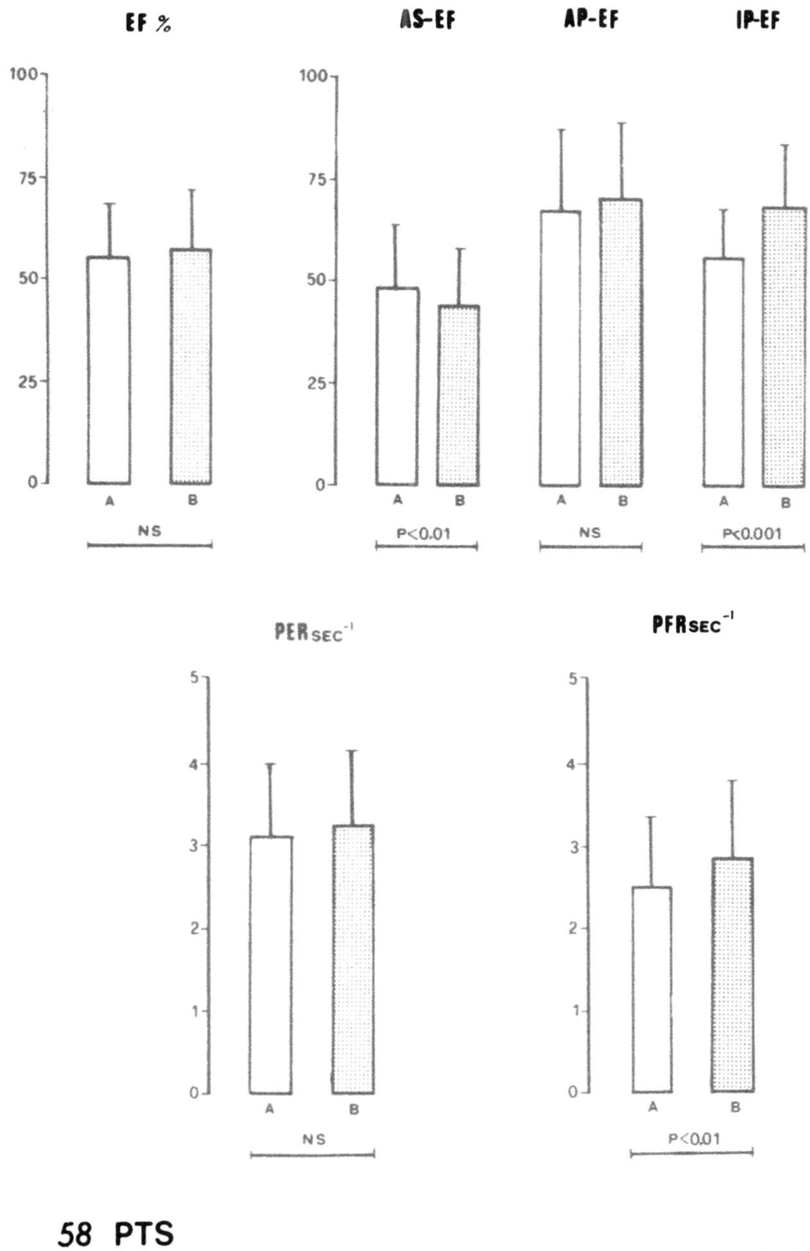

Fig. 1. Global (*EF*) anteroseptal (*AS-EF*), apical (*AP-EF*), inferoposterior (*IP-EF*) ejection fractions, peak ejection rate (*PER*), peak filling rate (*PFR*) before (*A*) and 6 months after (*B*) coronary artery bypass surgery. Mean values ± SDs are shown

After surgery, EF was found slightly and not significantly increased (Fig. 1, Table 1). AS-EF was slightly but significantly impaired, AP-EF was slightly improved, and IP-EF had a remarkable and highly significant improvement of regional kinetics. PER showed a slight increase; PFR had a very significant improvement.

According to the site and the number of implanted grafts, patients were divided into four groups. Group I: seven patients who had grafts on the LAD and diagonals – global and regional EF were impaired; PER and PFR did not change (Fig. 2). Group II: 14 patients who had grafts on the LAD and left circumflex artery (LCA) – EF was unchanged, while IP-EF was significantly raised. Group III: 16 patients who had grafts on the LAD and right coronary artery (RCA) – AS-EF was significantly impaired, while EF and AP-EF increased; IP-EF, PER, PFR showed a significant rise. Group IV: 21 patients who had grafts on the three coronary vessels – EF and IP-EF significantly increased (Table 1).

Relations between prepostoperative changes of different parameters have been studied. There was a significant direct linear correlation between the size and the direction of the variation of AS-EF and IP-EF (Δ AS-EF = 0.36; Δ IP-EF = 8.47; $r = 0.49$; $n = 58$; $P < 0.001$).

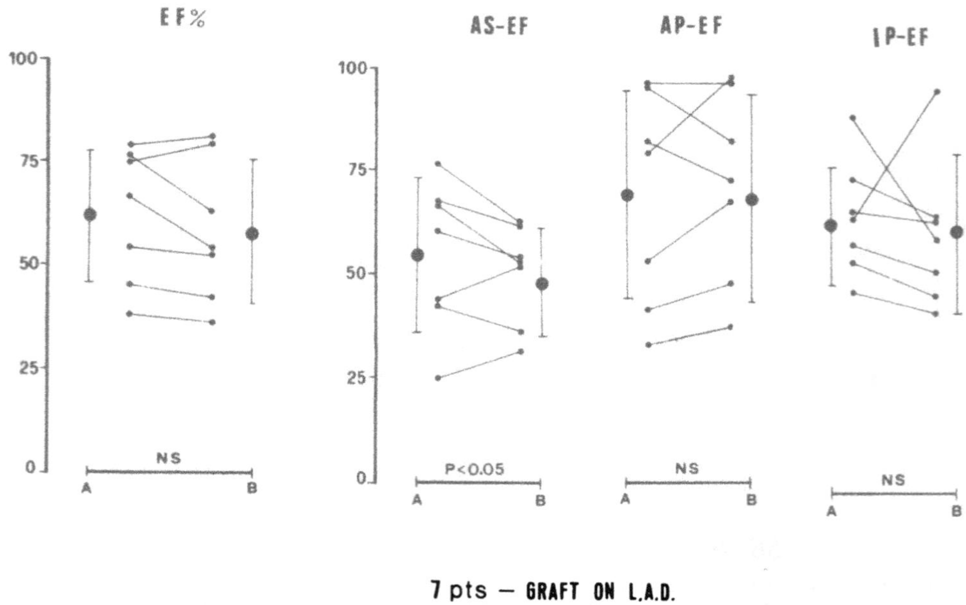

Fig. 2. EF, AS-EF, AP-EF, IP-EF, in each patient who had grafts implanted on the LAD before (*A*) and 6 months after (*B*) coronary artery bypass surgery. Mean values ± SDs are shown (abbreviations are the same as for Fig. 1)

Discussion

The various parameters considered in the analysis of left ventricular function showed a change in global and regional performance 6 months after revascularization. No significant changes of global EF were found in comparison with preoperative values, although actually EF slightly increased. These results are concordant with the results of other studies [2, 7]; as in those studies ventricular function was not extremely damaged before operation.

Regional wall motion had different patterns of change. The slight but significant impairment of AS motion agreed with the angiographic and echographic findings of a paradox septal movement after cardiopulmonary bypass [4]. While AP-EF slightly increased, IP motion showed a clear-cut and highly significant improvement (Fig. 1). The improvement of the IP sector was constant in groups II, III, and IV. Only in group I, concerning patients who had grafts on LAD, we did find a slight impairment of IP motion (Fig. 2). There was an obvious correspondence between the site of the bypass grafts and the behavior of regional IP kinetics. The finding of a direct significant correlation between the size and the direction of changes in AS and IP motion could indicate that the increase of IP motion was not compensatory because of the decrease of AS motion. On the contrary, the trend of IP variation parallels that of AS variation. It could suggest that reperfusion exerts a comparable influence on both the regional kinetics.

Twenty-three patients had a previous inferior MI. Only in 15 of these patients was complete revascularization of the peri-infarction area feasible. The greatest rises in IP wall motion were observed in this group [5]; while in the other eight patients, who had incomplete revascularization, a modest and not significant variation of IP motion was observed (Fig. 3). Among the 11 patients with previous anterior MI, an increase of EF, AP-EF, and IP-EF was observed.

In a previous work [1] we found an increase of PER and PFR shortly after operation; this result could be explained by an increase of sympathetic tone after the stress of surgery. It is likely that nervous adrenergic tone was back to baseline 6 months after operation; nevertheless, PFR was still improved, suggesting the achievement of a better ventricular compliance. PFR improved more than EF and PER. Impairment of left diastolic ventricular filling is an early abnormality in coronary patients with still normal systolic function; our data seem to confirm that this is a reversible disturbance related to myocardial ischemia.

Myocardial revascularization, by means of coronary artery bypass graft, achieved a better perfusion of ischemic myocardium, restoring its contractile state. The best improvements were observed in the most damaged areas [6, 7]. In the patients with the worst evolution of the observed parameters, there was a good correlation between clinical picture, radionuclide investigation, and coronary angiography.

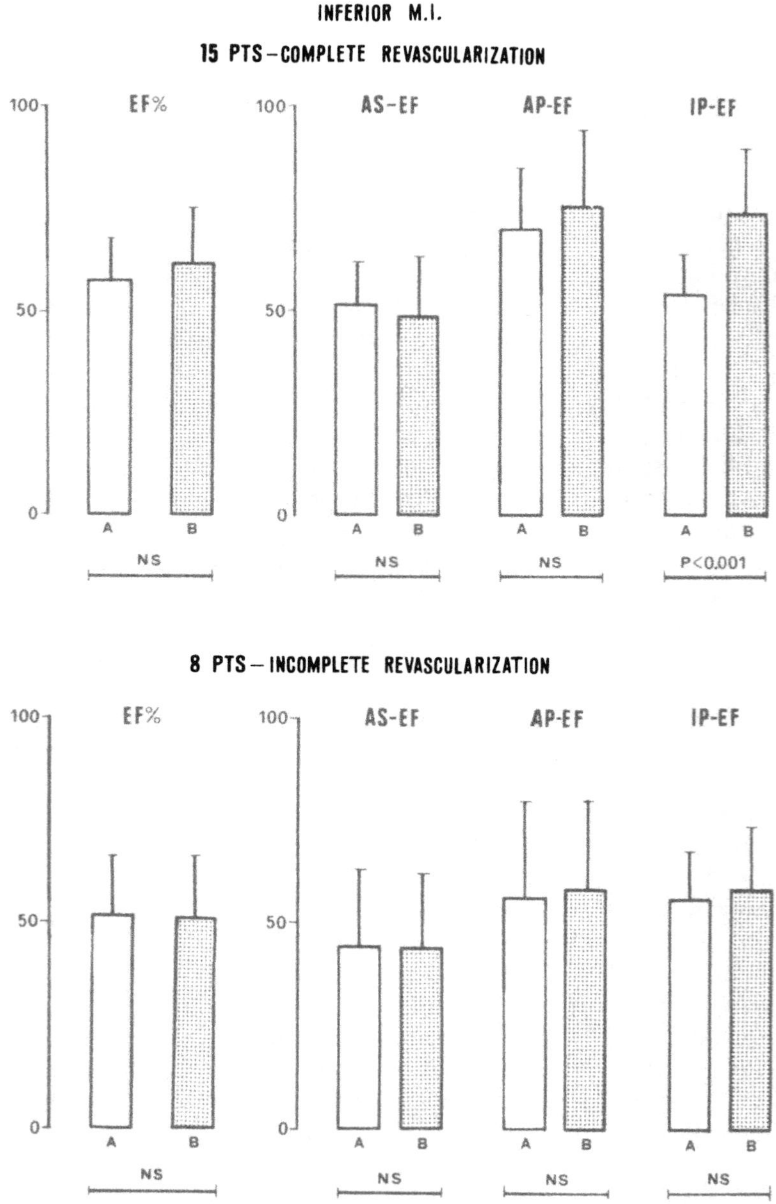

Fig. 3. EF, AS-EF, AP-EF, IP-EF in 23 patients with previous inferior myocardial infarction, before (*A*) and 6 months after (*B*) coronary artery bypass surgery. Mean values ± SDs are shown (abbreviations are the same as for Fig. 1)

References

1. Astorri E, Busi M, Contini GA, Ugolotti G, Restori E, Ferretti PP (1984) Short-term radionuclide study of ventricular function after coronary bypass surgery. In: Unger F (ed) Coronary artery surgery. Springer, Berlin Heidelberg, pp 206–210
2. Austin EH, Oldham HM Jr, Sabiston DC Jr, Jones RH (1983) Early assessment of rest and exercise left ventricular function following coronary artery surgery. Ann Thorac Surg 35:159–169
3. Ferretti PP, Restori E, Astorri E, Gavaruzzi G, Calbiani B, Ugolotti G (1983) Radioventricolografia sinistra all'equilibrio. Clin Ter Cardiovasc 6:321–330
4. Freeman MR, Gray RJ, Berman DS, Maddahi J, Raymond MJ, Forrester JS, Matltoff JM (1981) Improvement in global and segmental left ventricular function after coronary bypass surgery. Circulation 64 [suppl 2]:34–39
5. Lindsay J Jr, Nolan NG, Kotlyaron EV, Goldstein SA, Schoolmeester LW, Bacos JM (1982) Radionuclide ventriculography following coronary bypass surgery: correlation with arteriographic findings. Ann Thorac Surg 33:238–243
6. Mintz LJ, Ingels NB, Daughters GT, Stainson EB, Alderman EL (1980) Sequential studies of left ventricular function and wall motion after coronary arterial bypass surgery. Am J Cardiol 45:210–216
7. Rogers WS, Hood WP Jr, Mantle JA, Baxley WA, Kirklin JK, Zorn JL, Nath HP (1984) Return of left ventricular function after reperfusion in patients with myocardial infarction: importance of subtotal stenoses or intact collaterals. Circulation 69:338–349

Coronary Artery Bypass in Patients with Left Main Disease: Long-Term Results

G. Minzioni, T. Ragni, C. Goggi, P. Spreafico, and M. Vigano

Introduction

Left main coronary artery disease (LMCAD) is a particularly severe form of coronary artery disease (CAD); its frequency ranges from 5% of 7% in patients with CAD [4, 6, 7] and virtually all published reports show a grim natural history: the survival rate of medically treated patients with LMCAD ranges from 65% to 57% at 2 years [9, 16], from 49% to 46% at 5 years [3, 13], and from 13% to 31% after 10 years [19]. Coronary artery bypass grafting (CABG) is generally accepted as the treatment of choice in these patients and randomized studies of large series have shown a significantly better prognosis for the operated patients, with 88% or 86% survival at 4 years [5, 7]. The data obtained from our experience with 155 consecutive cases of LMCAD treated by CABG form the basis of this report.

Patients and Methods

From January 1977 to August 1984, 155 patients with significant stenosis of the left main coronary artery (LMCA) were operated upon at the Division of Cardiac Surgery, Policlinico S, Matteo, Pavia Italy. Mean age was 55 years (range 37–76); there were 15 female patients (10%) angina was stable in 22 patients, unstable in the remaining 133 (11 of whom had Prinzmetal's variant form). Coronarographic studies showed that the mean stenosis of the LMCA was 77%, with complete occlusion in five cases. The right coronary artery was involved in 101 patients (65%), with total occlusion in 36. Mean ejection fraction was 48% (range 22%–77%). Ninety patients (62%) had suffered a myocardial infarction prior to surgery. At operation 450 coronary artery bypass crafts (CABG) were performed; the CABG/patient ratio was 2.9. There were 7 single CABGs (4.5%), 38 double CABGs (24.7%), 71 triple CABGs (46.1%), and 38 quadruple or more CABGs (27.4%). In one patient with ostial stenosis a patch enlargement of the LMCA with no CABG was performed. One hundred and fifty-five grafts were performed on the left anterior descending artery in 149 patients; the circumflex artery was grafted 124 times, the right coronary artery 105 times (in 101 patients), and the diagonal branches 66 times. Other cardiac procedures were associated with CABG in 31 patients: 20 left ventricular plications or resections, 21 endoarteriectomies, and 3 valve replacements. Actuarial survival curves were obtained according to the Kaplan-Meyer method [10]; confidence limits of 70% were computed using the Greenwood formula [1] and the differences between groups were tested by the log-rank (Mantel-Henszel) test [17].

Results

There were six hospital (within 30 days) deaths: five patients could not be weaned from the pump, one patient died on day 3 owing to an acute myocardial infarction, and another patient suddenly died on day 20 at home after a normal postoperative course. A previous large myocardial infarction was present in five of the six fatal cases, and in three patients a ventricular resection was associated with the CABG. Disease of the right coronary artery was also present in five of these patients. There were five male patients (hospital mortality for male, 3.5%) and one female (hospital mortality for female, 6.6%).

Hospital complications included six (3.9%) myocardial infarctions (fatal in one case), postoperative hemorrhage in seven patients, and sternal infection in one patient.

Follow-up information on all the 149 survivors was obtained from hospital records, questionnaires, and telephone interviews; mean follow-up time was 36 months (range 1 to 101). There were 11 late deaths, 4 of which were due to malignancy or stroke; a new myocardial infarction developed in six patients. To evaluate the influence of preoperative variables (age, sex, ejection fraction, left ventricular end diastolic pressure, previous myocardial infarction, right coronary artery disease or associated procedure) we tested the cumulative probability of "being alive" and "being alive and angina free" for the subgroups according to the variables described.

The actuarial survival curve for the whole population of operated patients shows 92% (confidence limit 70% = ±2%) survival rate at 4 years and 84% (CL 70% = ±7%) at 6 years postoperatively, accounting for 2.6% linearized mortality rate (see Fig. 1). These results are confirmed by other surgical series reported by Chaitmann et al. [5] (92% at 3 years), Takaro et al. [20] (88% at 42 months), Farinha et al. [7] (86% at 56 months) and Loop et al. [14] and Killen et al. [11] (88 at 5 years).

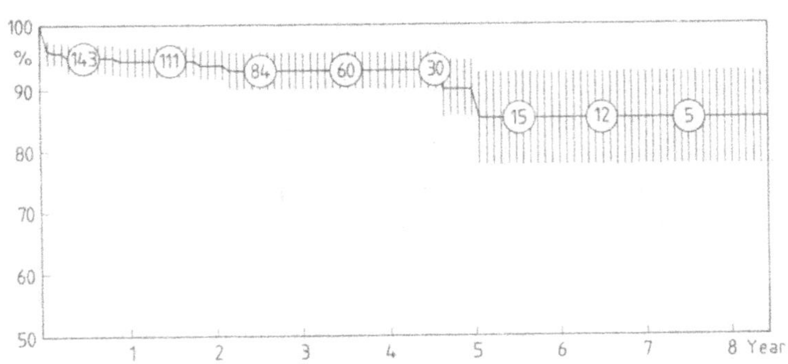

Fig. 1. Actuarial survival of the patients operated on, including operative mortality

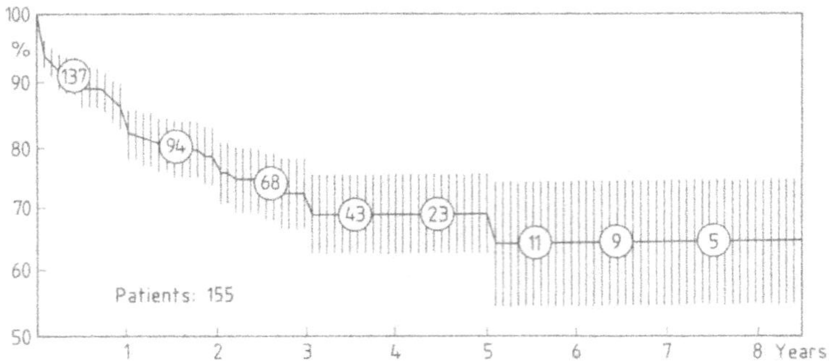

Fig. 2. Cumulative probability of being alive and angina free, including operative mortality

The cumulative probability of being alive and angina free is 68% after 4 years and 63% after 6 years for our patient population (see Fig. 2).

Six years after surgery, higher survival rates were observed in the group of patients without preoperative myocardial infarction (88% vs. 82%), with no right CAD (88% vs. 76%), with an ejection fraction equal to or higher than 45% (87% vs. 78%), with severe (greater than 75%) narrowing of the LMCA (85% vs. 79%), and without combined procedures (85% vs. 83%). These differences are not statistically significant. The same conclusions apply to the cumulative probability of being alive and asymptomatic: the best results are obtained in the patients without myocardial infarction (69% vs. 60%), with no right CAD (66% vs. 55%), with EF $\geqq$ 45% (77% vs. 46%), and with severe (> 75% stenosis of the LMCA (79% vs. 55%; $P = 0.04$).

Discussion

Coronary artery bypass surgery in patients with LMCAD significantly improves survival and lessens symptoms. Some studies [4, 20] have shown that statistically significant improvement in survival is limited to the subgroup of patients with associated right CAD, particularly when left ventricular impairment is present. However, although not at a statistically significant level, survival was improved in all patients, even in the subgroup with a nonstenotic dominant right coronary artery, or with a stenotic dominant right coronary artery and normal left ventricle, or LMCA stenosis of 50% – 59% and normal or mildy abnormal left ventricle. Surprisingly, in our experience (and in contrast with most series) the patients with severe LMCA stenosis fared better than the others; considering the low level of probability of such a hypothesis, the P value (0.04) should not be considered as significant. This result cannot be explained by the coexistence of variables favoring the good outcome of this subset of patients. Considering the severe prognosis of patients with LMCAD when medically treated, we suggest, on the basis of our data and in accord with previous and larger studies, that CABG be performed in all patients with LMCAD, with acceptable risk and good long-term results.

References

1. Anderson RP, Bonchek LI, Grunkemeier GL, Lambert LE, Starr A (1974) The analysis and presentation of surgical results by actuarial methods. J Surg Res 16:224
2. Anderson RP, Rahimtoola SH, Bonchek LI, Starr A (1974) The prognosis of patients with coronary artery disease after coronary bypass operations. Time-related progress of 532 patients with disabling angina pectoris. Circulation 50:274
3. Campeau L, Corbara F, Crochet D, Petitclerc R (1978) Left main coronary artery stenosis. The influence of aorto coronary bypass surgery on survival. Circulation 57:1111
4. Chaitman BR, Rogers WJ, Davis K, Tyras DH, Berger R, Bourassa MG, Fisher L, Hertzberg VS, Judkins MP, Mock MB, Killip T (1980) Operative risks in left main coronary artery disease (CASS). N Engl J Med 303:953
5. Chaitman BR, Fisher LD, Bourassa MG, Davis K, Rogers WJ, Maynard C, Tyras DH, Berger RL, Judkins MP, Ringqvist I, Mock MB, Killip T (1981) Effect of coronary bypass surgery on survival in subsets of patients with left main coronary artery disease. Report of the Collaborative Study in Coronary Artery Surgery (CASS). Am J Cardiol 48:765
6. DeMots H, Rosch J, McAnulty JH, Rahimtoola SH (1977) Left main coronary artery disease. In: Rahimtoola SH (ed) Coronary bypass surgery. Davies, Philadelphia, p 201
7. Farinha JB, Kaplan MA, Harris CN, Dunne EF, Carlish RA, Kay JH, Brooks S (1978) Disease of the left main coronary artery. Surgical treatment and long term follow up in 267 patients. Am J Cardiol 42:124
8. Jeffery DL, Vijayanagar R, Bognolo DA, Eckstein PF, Spoto E Jr, Natarajan P, Willard EH, Connar RG (1983) Surgical treatment of 200 consecutive patients with left main coronary artery disease. Ann Thorac Surg 36:193
9. Jones EL, King III SB, Craver JM, Douglas JS, Kaplan JA, Morgan EA, Brown CM, Bradford JM, Hatcher CR (1980) The spectrum of left main coronary artery disease. Variable affecting patient selection, management and death. J Thorac Cardiovasc Surg 79:109
10. Kaplan EL, Meier P (1958) Non-paremetric estimation from incomplete observations. J Am Stat Assoc 53:457
11. Killen AD, Reed WA, Kindred L, McConahay DR, Arnold M (1980) Surgical therapy for left main coronary artery disease. J Thorac Cardiovasc Surg 80:255
12. Killip T, Ryan TJ (1985) Randomized trials in coronary bypass surgery. Circulation 71:418
13. Lim JS, Proudfit WL, Sones FM (1975) Left main coronary arterial obstruction: long-term follow-up of 141 non-surgical cases. Am J Cardiol 36:131
14. Loop FD, Cosgrove DM, Lytle BS, Thurer RL, Suripfendorfer C, Taylor PC, Proudfit WL (1979) An 11 year evolution of coronary surgery (1967–1978). Ann Surg 190:444
15. Loop FD, Lytle BW, Sheldon WC (1980) Hard and soft data on treatment of left main coronary lesions. Am J Cardiol 45:524
16. Oberman A, Kouchoukos NT, Harrell RR, Holt JH, Russel RO, Rackley CE (1976) Surgical versus medical treatment in disease of the left main coronary artery. Lancet 2:591
17. Peto R, Pike C, Armitage P, Breslow NE, Cox DR, Howard SV, Mantel N, McPherson K, Peto J, Smith PG (1977) Design and analysis of randomized clinical trials requiring prolonged observations of each patient. Br J Cancer 35:1
18. Pierpont GL, Kruse M, Ewald S, Weir EK (1985) Practical problems in assessing risk for coronary artery bypass grafting. J Thorac Cardiovasc Surg 89:673
19. Rahimtoola SH, Grunkemeier G, Tepley J, Lambert L, Thomas DR, Yuen-Fure S, Staa A (1981) Changes in coronary bypass surgery leading to improved survival. JAMA 246:1912
20. Takaro T, Peduzzi P, Detre KM, Hultgren HN, Murphy ML, Van der Bel-Kahn J, Thomsen J, Meadows WR (1982) Survival in subgroups of patients with left main coronary artery disease. Veteran Administration cooperative study of surgery for coronary artery occlusive disease. Circulation 66:14

Loss of Improvement After Myocardial Revascularization: 11-Year Follow-up

I. SHEIBAN, G. P. TREVI, D. CASAROTTO, P. BENUSSI, A. SCURO, R. ACCARDI, A. MOTTA, G. PUGLIESE, A. MARINI, and A. BENINI

Introduction

Coronary artery bypass grafting is effective treatment for angina pectoris in selected patients with coronary artery disease. After this procedure symptoms improve, and exercise tolerance is enhanced [1, 2]. In patients who have received maximal drug therapy and yet remain intolerably symptomatic, bypass surgery is a definite therapeutic advantage at least for some years [3–17]. Results from randomized trials indicate that angina may recur in 3%–5% of patients each year [1].

In this study we report on our experience with a series of patients who underwent myocardial revascularization, to give a further contribution to late results of coronary bypass surgery. Furthermore, we sought to identify preoperative factors which might give an indication of the late outcome of surgery.

Materials and Methods

The study includes 162 patients, 142 males and 20 females, aged between 30 and 69 years (mean age, 51.9 years), operated on between January 1973 and January 1984.

The collection of data ended in June 1985, giving a potential follow-up period of 16–132 months, with an average of 56.4 months. Included in this study were patients who had effort angina before surgery and pure bypass surgery. There were unselected consecutive patients. All patients were periodically checked by the same medical staff at the same center. Seventy-five patients underwent postoperative control coronary arteriography and graft opacification studies at 10–130 months after operation.

The functional class was determined prior to the first angiography by the same three observers according to the New York Heart Association Functional Classification (NYHA class) as applied to angina by the Canadian Cardiovascular Society [18]. Improvement was defined as the complete disappearance of angina or a decrease in severity by at least two functional classes. Deterioration or loss of improvement meant appearance of angina or increase of severity by at least two functional classes.

Selective graft opacification and coronary arteriography were obtained in at least four views in patients who underwent angiographic control. The changes were considered significant in the grafts with a narrowing greater than 50% to total obstruction. Significant changes in unbypassed major coronary arteries and in the distal segments of grafted arteries were the appearance of a new stenosis reducing the luman by ≧ 50% and the progression of a preexisting narrowing of more than 50% to subtotal or total occlusion.

Results

The course of angina after operation is described in Fig. 1. There is a progressive loss of improvement which is more evident in the 7th year after surgery; however, at 11 years after operation, functional improvement is maintained in 76.2% of patients, with 69.2% of patients completely free of angina at 10 years after operation (Fig. 2). Reappearance of angina in this later group (patients with total relief of symptoms after myocardial revascularization) was mostly encountered in patients with severe preoperative functional class. At 8 years after operation, 78.8% and 59.2% of patients who underwent surgery respectively in III and IV NYHA class were completely free of angina (Fig. 3).

Correlation between diffusion of coronary stenosis and late operative results indicates that total relief of angina or functional class improvement is not related to the number of coronary vessels involved (Fig. 4). Reappearance of angina is independent from diffusion of coronary lesions, but mostly occurs in patients

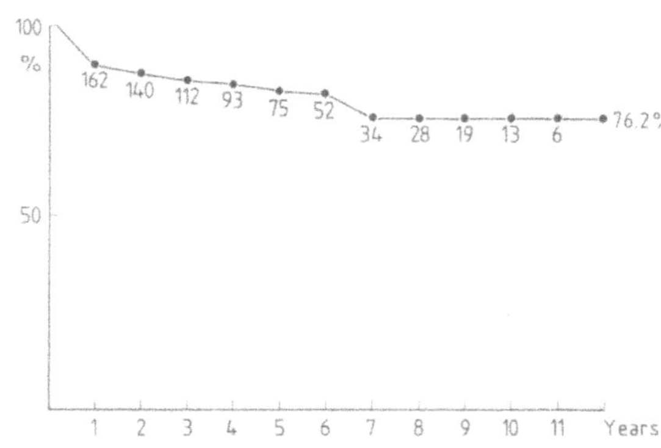

Fig. 1. Improvement of NYHA class after operation

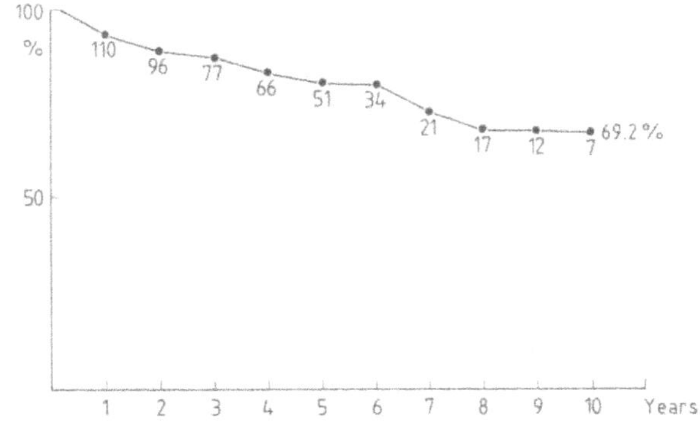

Fig. 2. Absence of angina after operation

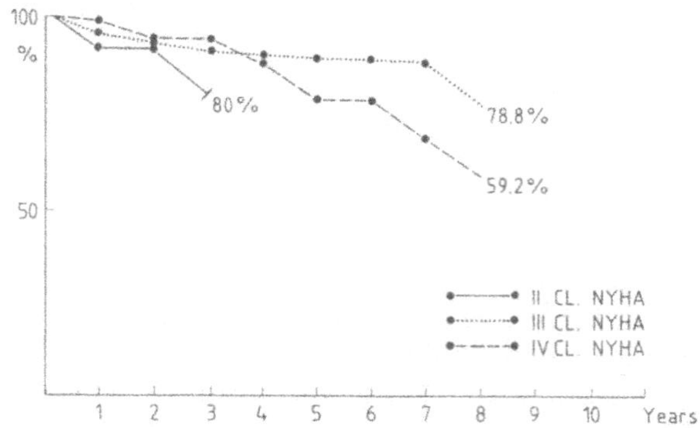

Fig. 3. Correlation between preoperative NYHA class and reappearance of angina after operation

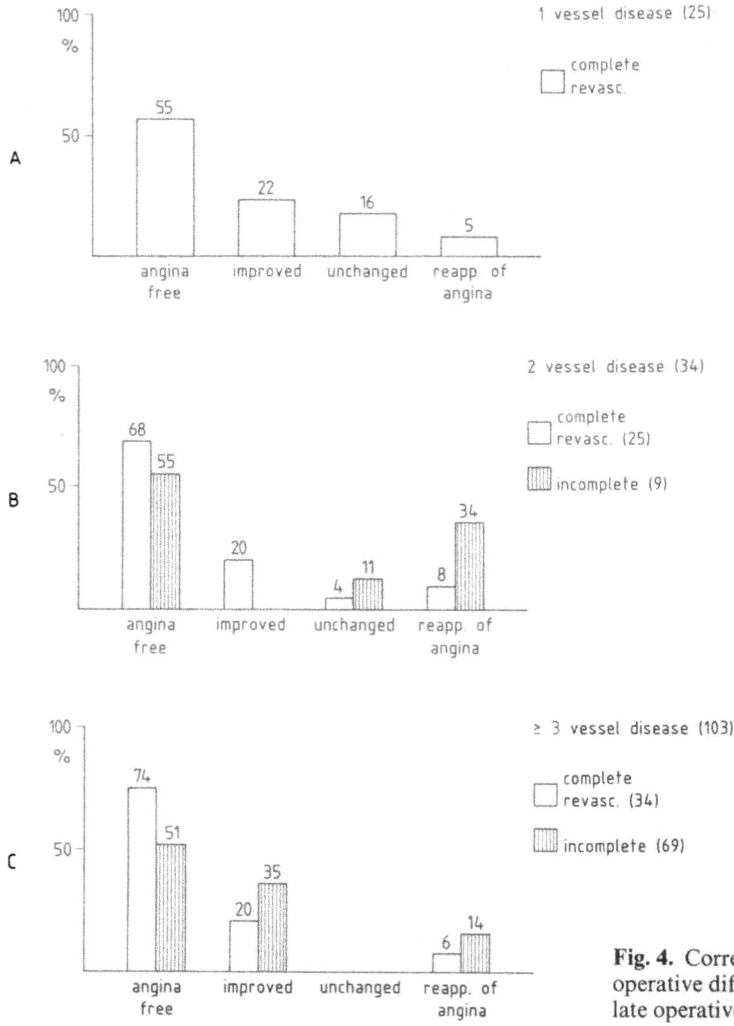

Fig. 4. Correlation between preoperative diffusion of CAD and late operative results

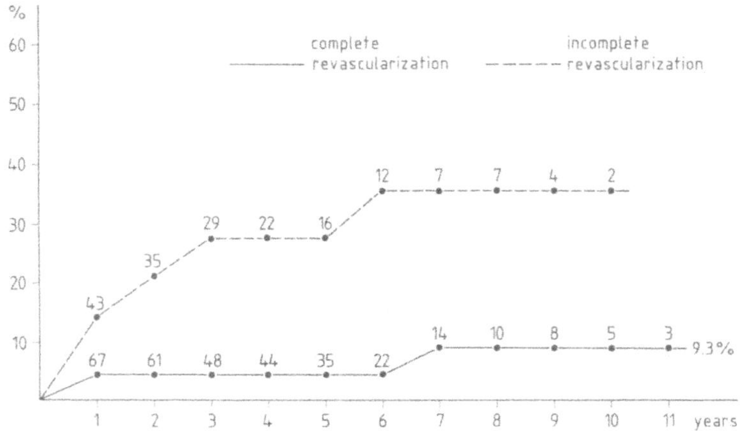

Fig. 5. Reappearance of angina in asymptomatic patients correlated to the type of revascularization performed

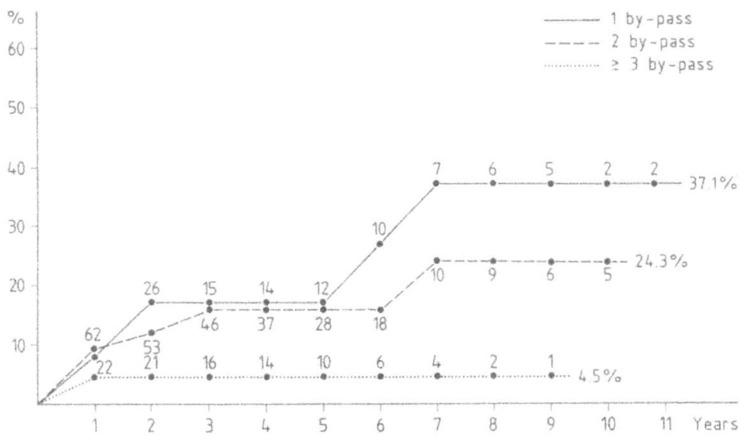

Fig. 6. Reappearance of angina in asymptomatic patients correlated to number of grafts received

who had received "incomplete" revascularization. In fact 11 years after surgery, 35.1% of patients with "incomplete" revascularization (who were totally free of angina) complained on reappearance of angina, while only 9.3% of those with "complete" revascularization had reappearance of angina in the same period of follow-up (Fig. 5). Moreover, reappearance of angina was closely related to the number of grafts received (Fig. 6), confirming indirectly that long-term relief of angina is related well to "completeness" of revascularization.

Of 75 patients who underwent angiographic control (10–130 months after surgery), 46 had all the grafts patent, 15 had all the grafts occluded and 14 had patent and occluded grafts.

The majority of patients with patent grafts mantained the improvement obtained by surgery. However, 18 patients of this group had deterioration of func-

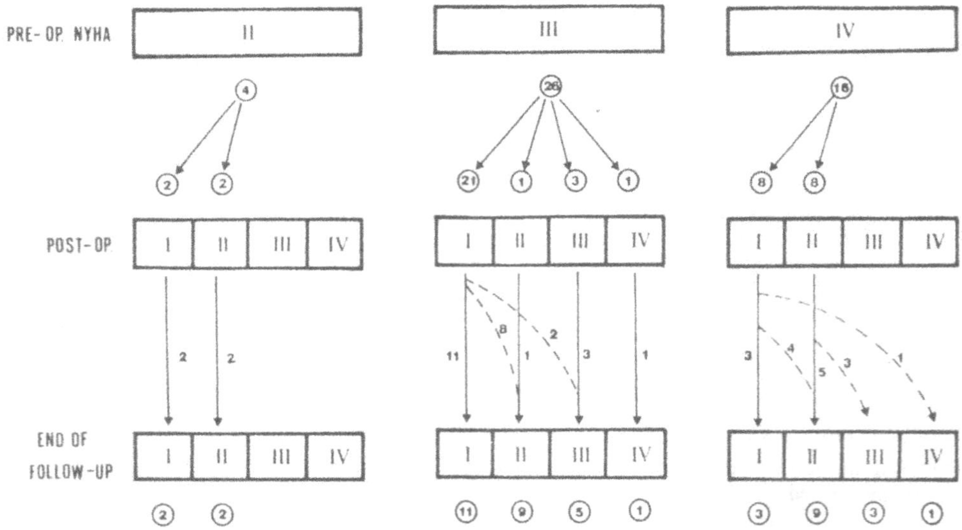

Fig. 7. Modifications of NYHA class in patients with patent grafts

tional class despite patency of all the grafts implanted (Fig. 7). Twelve of these 18 patients displayed progression of coronary artery disease on the native coronary vessels (not grafted). The other six patients displayed persistence of collaterals directed to the grafted vessel or retrograde opacification on the grafts during injection of contrast medium selectively in the grafted vessels, suggesting an insufficient perfusion pressure into the grafts.

Discussion

Several authors reported a decrease of complete and partial improvement of angina from 80%–85% at 1 year after surgery to 60%–70% at 2–3 years postoperatively [1, 17, 19, 20]. It is apparent that the results could vary according to definition of improvement of angina. Campeau et al. [21] reported that in their experience, where improvement is defined as improvement by at least one functional class, the improvement rate at 7 years after surgery was 75.8%.

However, the significance of this slight improvement by only one functional class is questionable because of the difficulties of assessing such a subjective parameter. This slight degree of improvement may be a placebo effect or the result of combined drug therapy prescribed in the majority of these partially improved patients [22]. Thus assessment of long-term results of myocardial revascularization is better defined by evaluating patients with total relief from angina after surgery.

The results obtained from this study indicate that angina will recur or deteriorate at 4.6%/year, in accordance with the National Institutes of Health Consensus Development conference Statement. Angina will mostly recur in patients operated on in advanced functional NYHA class and in those recieving "incomplete" revascularization. Better long-term results are obtained in patients with "complete" revascularization and consequently in those with a large number of grafts.

Graft patency is mostly accompanied by persistence of clinical improvement obtained by surgery [21, 23–26]; however, angiographic controls confirm that angina may also recur in patients with patent grafts and it is mostly due to progression of coronary stenosis on the native (not-grafted) coronary vessels or to graft dysfunction. Of 18 patients with reappearance of angina, despite patency of all the grafts, 12 displayed progression of coronary aterosclerosis on the native coronary vessels, while the other 6 patients of this group displayed persistence of coronary collaterals directed to the grafted vessels and retrograde opacification of the grafts after contrast medium was selectively injected into the grafted vessel. These angiographic findings can be explained by a "dysfunction" of the bypass due to insufficient perfusion pressure into the grafts, which may cause reduction of flow through the graft and consequently may explain reappearance of angina in these patients. Analysis of our data and those of other authors suggests that:

1. Preoperative NYHA class does not influence the short-term outcome of aortocoronary bypass surgery; late recurrence of angina after operation is more observable in patients with advanced preoperative NYHA class.
2. There is a slow but constant loss of improvement obtained by aortocoronary bypass surgery which becomes more evident 7 years after operation.
3. Relief of angina is better maintained in patients who undergo "complete" than those with "incomplete" revascularization.
4. There is no observable correlation between preoperative left ventricular function and diffusion of coronary-artery disease and persistence of improvement after myocardial revascularization.
5. Patency of the grafts is mostly accompanied by clinical improvement. Recurrence of angina in patients with patent grafts is mostly due to progression of coronary atherosclerosis on the native coronary arteries (not bypassed) or to graft "dysfunction" with insufficient perfusion pressure into the graft.

References

1. National Institute of Health (1982) Consensus development conference statement on coronary by-pass surgery. Scientific and clinical aspects. Circulation 65 [suppl II]: 126
2. McNeer JF, Margolis JR, Lee KL, Kisslo JA, Peter RN, Kong Y, Behar VS, Wallace AG, McCants CB, Rosati RA (1978) The role of the exercise test in the evaluation of patients for ischemic heart disease. Circulation 57:64
3. McIntosh HD, Garcia JA (1978) The first decade of aortocoronary bypass grafting. 1967–1977. A review. Circulation 57:405
4. McIntosh HD, Wright KE Jr, Wray NP (1976) Indications for saphenous vein aortocoronary by-pass surgery. Argero Rev I: 183
5. Favaloro RG (1979) Direct myocardial revascularization: a ten year journey. Myths and realities. Am J Cardiol 43:109
6. Coronary Artery Surgery Study (CASS) (1983) Quality of life in patients randomly assigned to treatment groups. Circulation 68 [5]:951–960
7. Rahimtoola SH (1982) Coronary by-pass surgery for chronic angina – 1981. A perspective, Circulation 65 [2]:225–241

8. Murphy ML, Hultgren HN, Detre K, Thomsen J, Takaro T and participants of the Veterans Administration Cooperative Study (1977) Treatment of chronic stable angina. A preliminary report of survival data of the randomized Veterans Administration Cooperative Study. N Engl J Med 297:621
9. Read RC, Murphy ML, Hultgren HN, Takaro T (1978) Survival of men treated for chronic stable angina pectoris. A cooperative randomized study. J Thorac Cardiovasc Surg 75:1
10. Takaro T, Hultgren HN, Lipton MJ, Detre KM and participants in the study group (1976) The Veterans Administration Cooperative randomized study of surgery for coronary arterial occlusive disease. II. Subgroup with significant left main lesions. Circulation 54 [suppl III]:III-107
11. Hultgren HN, Takaro T, Detre K and participants in the VA Cooperative Study (1977) Veterans Administration Cooperative study of surgical treatment of stable angina: preliminary results. In: Rahintoola SH (ed) Coronary bypass surgery. Davies, Philadelphia, p 119
12. Detre K, Hultgren HN, Takaro T (1977) Veterans Administration Cooperative study of surgery for coronary arterial occlusive disease. III. Methods and baseline characteristics, including experience in medical treatment. Am J Cardiol 40:212
13. Peduzzi P, Hultgren HN (1979) Effect of medical vs surgical treatment on symptoms in stable angina pectoris. The Veterans Administration Cooperative study of surgery for coronary arterial occlusive disease. Circulation 60:888
14. Veterans Administration Cooperative Study (1980) Surgery for coronary arterial occlusive disease. Use of nominative clinical parameters to characterize prognosis in patients with angina pectoris, treated medically or surgically. Am J Cardiol 45:456 (abstract)
15. Detre K, Peduzzi P, Murphy M, Hultgren H, Thomson J, Oberman A, Takaro T (1986) Effect of bypass surgery on survival of patients in low- and high-risk subgroups delineated by the use of simple clinical variables. The Veterans Administration Cooperative Study group for surgery for coronary arterial occlusive disease. Circulation. (In press)
16. European Cooperative Surgery Study Group (1979) Coronary artery bypass surgery in stable angina pectoris: survival at two years. Lancet 1:889
17. European Coronary Surgery Study Group (1980) Prospective randomized study of coronary artery bypass surgery in stable angina pectoris. Second interim report. Lancet 2:491
18. Bourassa MG, Lesperance J, Corbara F, Saltiel J, Campeau L (1978) Progression of obstructive coronary artery disease 5 to 7 years after aortocoronary bypass surgery. Circulation 58 [suppl 1] I-III
19. Johnson MD, Kayser KL, Pedraza PM (1984) Angina pectoris and coronary bypass surgery: patterns of prevalence and recurrence in 3105 consecutive patients followed up to 11 years. Am Heart J 108:1190–1197
20. Lawrie GM, Morris GC Jr, Calhoon JF, Safi H, Zamora JL, Beltengady M, Baron A, Silvers A, Chapman DW (1982) Clinical results of coronary by-pass in 500 patients at least 10 years after operation. Circulation 66 [suppl I]: 1982
21. Campeau L, Lesperance J, Hermann J et al. (1979) Loss of the improvement of angina between 1 and 7 years after aortocoronary bypass surgery. Correlations with changes in vein graft and in coronary arteries. Circulation 60 [suppl I]: I-I
22. Campeau L, Heitz A, Crochet D, Lesperance J (1976) Long-term improvement of effort angina following aortocoronary saphenous vein bypass graft surgery: increased myocardial blood flow or pain denial placebo effect. Ann Roy Coll Physicians Surg Can 9:13
23. Grondin CM, Lesperance J, Bourassa MG et al. (1974) Serial angiographic evaluation in 60 consecutive patients with aortocoronary artery vain graft 2 weeks, 1 year and 3 years after operation. J Thorac Cardiovasc Surg 67:I
24. Uthaner DF, Robert EW, Alderman EL, Wexler L (1979) Long-term serial angiographic study after coronary artery by-pass surgery. Circulation 60:250
25. Hamby RI, Aintablian A, Handler M et al. (1979) Aortocoronary saphenous vein bypass grafts. Long-term patency, morphology and blood flow patients with patent grafts early after surgery. Circulation 60:901
26. Robert EW, Guthaner DF, Wexler L, Alderman EL (1978) Six year clinical and angiographic follow-up of patients with previously documented complete revascularization. Circulation 58 [suppl I]: 1-194

Abstract

Progression of Coronary Artery Disease (CAD) After Bypass Grafting (CABG)

P. GUITERAS, M. MASOTTI, J. ALTIMIRAS, T. BASSONS, J. M. AUGÉ, C. CREXELLS, and A. ORIOL

Sequential coronary angiograms were performed on 100 consecutive patients 1.3 months before and 0.3 months after and on 59 patients 6.3 months after CABG. Quantitative assessment was used to define progression of CAD as: (1) Any lesion to total obstruction (25% of the arteries), (2) Δ 20% in lesions > 50% (3% of arteries), (3) Δ 30% in lesions < 50% (2% of arteries), or (4) Δ 50% for normal segments (4% of arteries). Logistic regression found progression related to:

First check after CABG	*P*
Graft flow at first check	0.00001
RCA > LAD > LCX	0.0002
Gensini score before CABG	0.0008
Quality of distal bed	0.0002
Check 6.3 months after CABG	
Number of lesions before CABG	0.0017
Graft flow at first check	0.014
Graft flow at 6-month check	0.015
CAD progression at first check	0.021
Quality of the distal bed	0.039

Thus: (1) Progression of CAD during the first 6 months after surgery is fast and (2) the extent of CAD before surgery, quality of the distal bed, and patency of the graft determine progression of CAD after surgery.

Heart Transplantation for End Stage Coronary Heart Disease: A 4-Year Experience

H. REICHENSPURNER, B. M. KEMKES, G. OSTERHOLZER, and B. REBLE

Introduction

Coronary heart disease (CHD) represents one of the main causes of death in modern civilisation. Conservative and operative therapy have improved during recent years. Coronary artery bypass graft (CABG) surgery and percutaneous transluminal coronary angioplasty (PTCA) help to prevent angina pectoris and lethal myocardial infarction. Nevertheless there has still been no therapy for patients with progressive distal coronary atherosclerosis, which has no indication for CABG or PTCA. Since heart transplantation (HTx) has become an accepted clinical method during the past 15 years, it could be the choice therapy for these patients [1].

Patients

During the past 5 years 62 HTx were performed at the Munich University Hospital. Fortytwo patients suffered from congestive cardiomyopathy, eleven from CHD, three had previous valve replacements, and one suffered from morbus Uhl, a congenital degeneration of the right ventricle [2]. Combined heart-lung transplantation was carried out in three patients with primary pulmonary hypertension (Fig. 1) [3].

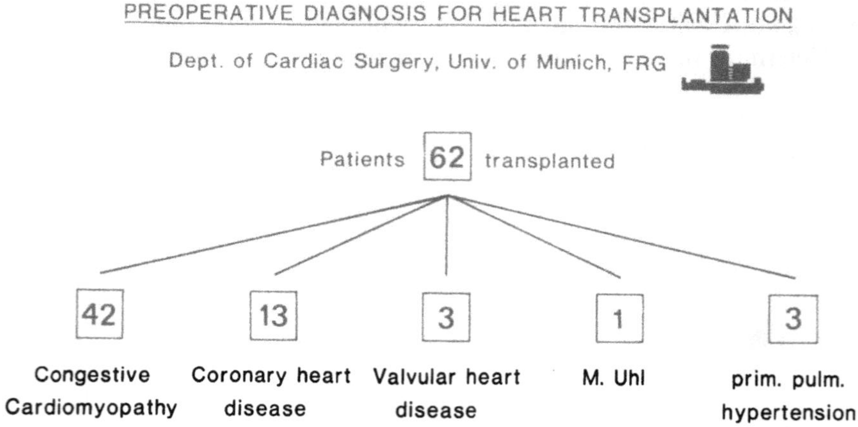

Fig. 1. Primary diagnoses of the transplanted patient at the University of Munich

Table 1. Results of coronary angiography and ventriculography in eleven patients who were given transplants because of coronary heart disease

Patient	Sex	Age (yrs) at operation	Coronary arteries		Ventricular aneurysm	EF (%)	Outcome
			Stenosis	Occlusion			
L. J.	M	32	LAD		+	19	Alive
G. W.	M	44	RCA/CX	LAD		30	Alive
K. H.	M	37	LAD	RCA		20	Died
V. L.	M	41	LAD/CX	RCA		12	Alive
S. H.	M	45	LAD/CX			20	Alive
S. F.	M	35		LAD		35	Alive
K. S.	M	49		LAD		15	Died
B. W.	M	47	LAD/RCA	CX		35	Alive
W. B.	F	35		LAD	+	25	Alive
O. T.	M	44	LAD/RCA	DIAG.		13	Alive
E. W.	M	44	CX	RCA/LAD		18	Alive

The age of the patients suffering from CHD ranged from 33 to 49 years (Table 1). In all cases the coronary angiogram showed severe distal stenoses or occlusions of the main coronary arteries and the history revealed severe myocardial infarction. A left ventricular aneurysm appeared after occlusion of the left anterior descending artery (LAD) in two patients. The LAD occlusion was reopened by thrombolytic drugs in patient No. 1. The ejection fraction in all cases ranged between 11% and 35% (mean, 18.5%) and the cardiac index was 1.75 liters/min/m^2 on average. The ages of the donors ranged between 15 and 37 years. Seven hearts were retrieved by distant organ procurement (mean distance, 480 km; mean ischemic time 162 min). The HTx were performed according to the technique of Lower and Shumway [4].

Immunosuppressive Regimen

All patients were treated with ciclosporin (5–14 mg/kg body wt. loading dose, continued according to a serum trough level of 80–150 ng/ml) and prednisone (2.0 mg/kg body wt. per day tapered down to 0.15 mg/kg body wt. per day within 6 weeks). Patient No. 1 was treated with conventional immunosuppression consisting of azathioprine, prednisone, and antithymocyte globulin until postoperative day 27. Because of the suspicion of gastrointestinal perforation a laparotomy was necessary and the immunosuppressive therapy was changed to ciclosporin.

Rejection Monitoring

The diagnosis of acute rejections (AR) was based on cytoimmunological monitoring (CIM) of the peripheral blood and on a computerized high-frequency ECG (HF-ECG) [5, 6]. The CIM values, whether activated lymphocytes or lymphoblasts, are visible in the mononuclear concentrate of peripheral blood. In the case of an activation of the peripheral lymphocytes, monoclonal antibodies against T-helper and T-suppressor cells are used to differentiate acute rejections from infections [5]. The HF-ECG is very sensitive to frequency spectrum changes and amplitude changes of the QRS complex. The patient is treated with 1 g methylprednisolone/day for 3 days in the case of cell activation in CIM combined with typical changes of the QRS complex in the HF-ECG. After this therapy a control endomyocardial biopsy (EMB) is performed. The patient is treated with additional antithymocyte or antilymphocyte globulin in the case of ongoing AR according to the presence of T or B lymphoblasts in the CIM [6].

Results and Discussion

Nine of the eleven CHD patients given transplants are currently alive, with postoperation times spanning from 5 years to 18 months (Fig. 2). Cause of death was cardiac fibrillation of unknown cause 228 days postoperatively in one case. The second patient was switched from ciclosporin therapy to conventional immunosuppression because of renal insufficiency depending on severe glomeruloscerosis due to ciclosporin. Thereafter he developed severe leukopenia and died from septicemia 2.5 years postoperatively. The resulting 1-year survival rate is 91%, which is high compared with patients who are given transplants for other kinds of cardiac dysfunction [7].

The average rate of rejections was 1.1 AR/patient. The sensitivity of CIM and EMB was 95%. The sensitivity of the HF-ECG was 100%. Using this type of monitoring the number of invasive EMBs were reduced from 12–16 to 2–4 biopsies per patient within the first 3 months postoperatively. This corresponds to a reduction of 75% compared with routinely biopsied patients [8]. The rate of lethal AR was 0% in these cases. This is a major improvement compared with other clinical studies [1]. Infectious complications were caused by herpes simplex virus ($n = 3$), mycobacterium tuberculosis ($n = 1$), pneumatosis cystoides intestinii ($n = 1$), legionellosis ($n = 1$), non-A-non-B hepatitis ($n = 1$), and *Candida* septicaemia ($n = 1$). Chronic graft atherosclerosis remains a limiting factor for long-term surveillance after HTx. A coronary angiogram performed every

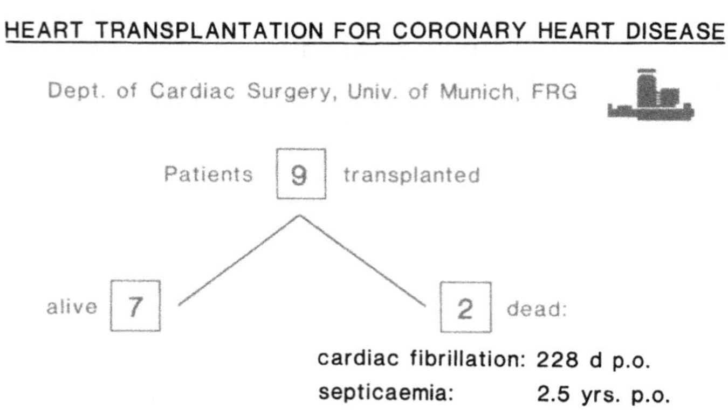

Fig. 2. Surveillance after cardiac transplantation for coronary heart disease

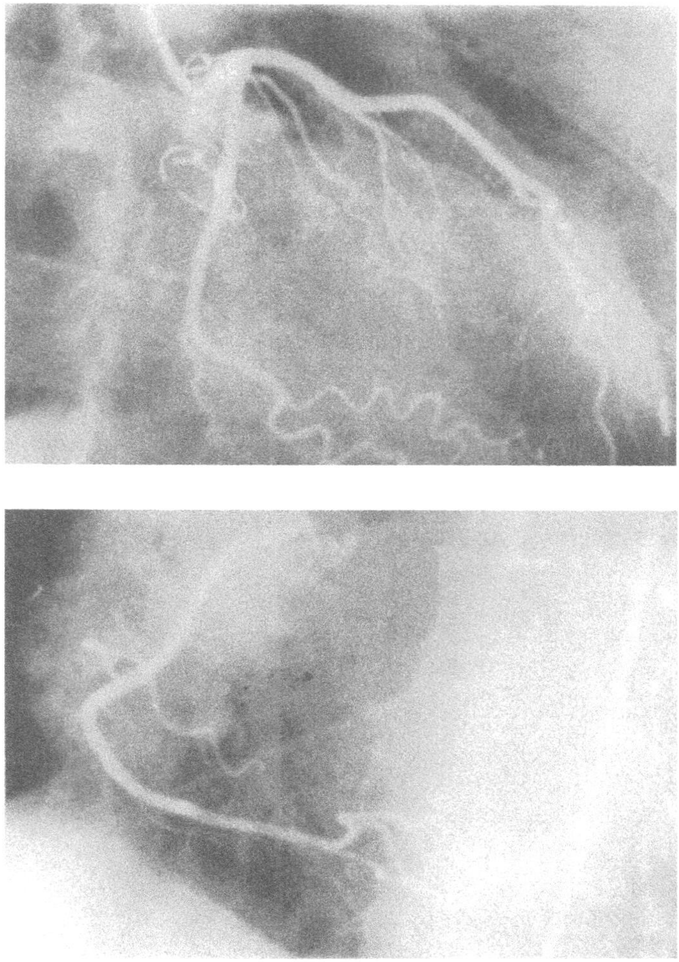

Fig. 3. Coronary angiography 1 year after heart transplantation because of coronary heart disease

year is mandatory because of the lack of symptoms in a denervated transplanted heart (Fig. 3). In this study no graft atherosclerosis was found after transplantation.

Conclusion

Cardiac transplantation represents a therapeutic alternative for patients under 55 years of age with progressive distal atherosclerosis, when neither PTCA nor CABG are feasible. The 1-year survival rate of 91% justifies the use of this clinical method. These clinical results are confirmed by the experience of Stanford University [1].

Up to now 73 HTx were performed at our unit with further more 6 patients, suffering from coronary heart disease.

References

1. Jamieson SW, Oyer PE, Baldwin J et al. (1984) Heart transplantation for end stage ischemic heart disease: the Stanford experience. Heart Transplant 3:224
2. Reichart B, Überfuhr P, Welz A et al. (1983) Heart transplantation at the University of Munich – The first one and a half years. Heart Transplant 2:266
3. Reichart B, Reble B, Kemkes BM et al. (1984) Die beiden ersten Herz-Lungentransplantationen in Deutschland. MMW 126:1316
4. Lower R, Stofer RC, Shumway NE (1960) Studies on orthotopic homotransplantation of the canine heart. Surg Forum 11:18
5. Reichenspurner H, Ertel W, Hammer C et al. (1984) Immunologic monitoring of heart transplant patients under cyclosporine immunosuppression. Transplant Proc 16:1251
6. Reichenspurner H, Kemkes BM, Osterholzer G et al. (1985) Particular control of infection and rejection episodes after 4 years cardiac transplantation. Tex Heart Inst J 13:5
7. Kaye MP, Elcombe SA, O'Fallon WM (1985) The International Heart Transplantation Registry. Heart Transplant 4:290
8. Baumgartner WA, Borkon SM, Achuff SC et al. (1985) Heart and heart-lung transplantation: development, organization and initiation. Heart Transplant 4:197

Intraarterial Digital Subtraction Angiography for Postoperative Determination of Aortocoronary Bypass Graft Patency*

K. H. HAUENSTEIN, G. NÖLDGE, B. URBANYI, G. SPILLNER, and V. SCHLOSSER

Introduction

Efforts have been made in recent years to establish a postoperative control method to determine the patency of aortocoronary bypass grafts by the development of noninvasive procedures. According to the literature, graft occlusion is expected to occur in 8%–20% of grafts [3, 4, 10] during the first days or weeks after operation. In about another 10% low to middle grade stenoses are visualized at the proximal and distal anastomoses without any clinical symptoms. None of these noninvasive procedures such as directional Doppler sonography [15], myocardial scintigraphy [11], and angio-sequence CT [2, 7, 9, 14, 17] are able to visualize the graft through its whole course. The quality of the distal anastomoses, which is decisive for the prognosis of the bypass, cannot be judged. Even with transvenous digital coronary angiography, demonstration of the distal anastomoses is not satisfactorily possible [6].

There is no doubt that the morphological structures after revascularization are demonstrated best by conventional selective coronary angiography. However, this method seems to be too invasive, time-consuming, and costly as a routine postoperative control. Moreover, the complication rate of 2%–3% [10] excludes it as an early routine method. In contrast to this procedure, intraarterial digital subtraction angiography (DSA) with nonselective injection of small quantities of a nonionic contrast medium with low iodine content in the aortic bulb is a new method giving comparably clear results with a significantly lower risk.

Material and Method

For the investigations we used standard DSA equipment (DVI-2 V, Philips) for peripheral vessel studies with a maximal imaging rate of 3/s. The monitor was 23 cm in diameter. Modern F-5-pigtail catheters (Mallinckrodt) with a length of 110 cm were introduced via the femoral artery in the aortic bulb, to inject 30 ml 40% nonionic contrast medium (Solustrast 200®) with a flow rate of 16 ml/s. Four different standardized positions were used for the visualization of the course of the grafts: 90° right (Fig. 1) or left (Fig. 2) and 60° right or left

* Dedicated to Professor Wenz on his 60th birthday.

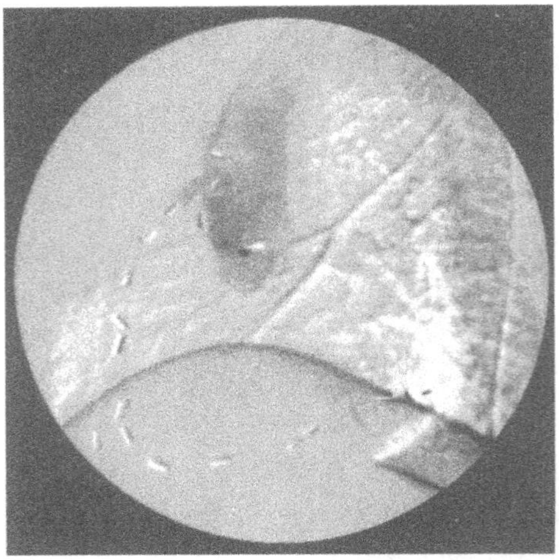

Fig. 1. Ninety-degree right lateral position. Occlusion of a jump graft 1 cm after its origin. The course of the occluded part is marked by numerous clips

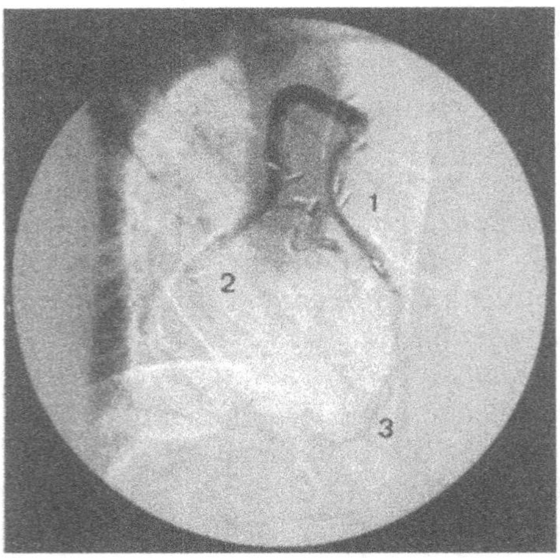

Fig. 2. Ninety-degree left lateral position. Single graft to the LAD (*1*); jump graft to the RCA and CX (*2*); original coronary vessels (*3*)

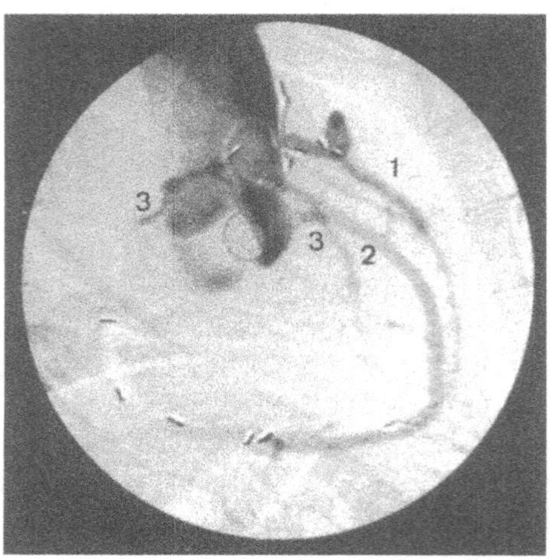

Fig. 3. Sixty-degree left lateral position. Single graft to the LAD (*1*); single graft to the CX (*2*); original coronary vessels (*3*)

(Fig. 3) lateral position. In most of the patients two series were necessary for exact demonstration of the bypasses; only in some special cases was a third run needed. During the past 7 months we examined 148 patients (115 male, 33 female) who had undergone aortocoronary bypass surgery. The examination was performed in the early postoperative period (5th – 21st postoperative day). The age of the patients ranged from 38 to 68 years. Three hundred and nine grafts with 430 distal anastomoses were implanted (206 single grafts, 89 jump grafts with two and 14 with three distal anastomoses). The right coronary artery (RCA) was involved in 94, the left coronary artery system (LCA) in 336 grafts. In nine cases the internal mammary artery (IMA) was used as a bypass to the LAD.

Results

In all cases determination of the function of the proximal anastomoses and the patency of the grafts through their whole course was possible (Table 1). Total or partial occlusions of single-, jump-, or sequential grafts were found in 10% (Table 2). Eighty percent of distal anastomoses could be visualized well or very well (Fig. 4a, b); 16% of the distal anastomoses were satisfactorily delineated. Only in 4% was the distal anastomosis not visible. Four of the 14 internal mammary artery bypasses to the LAD were occluded. In all cases with well or very well visualized distal anastomoses the connected coronary vessel showed excellent perfusion. In our patient group, no serious complications occurred; one patient showed disorientation for a few days without neurological deficits.

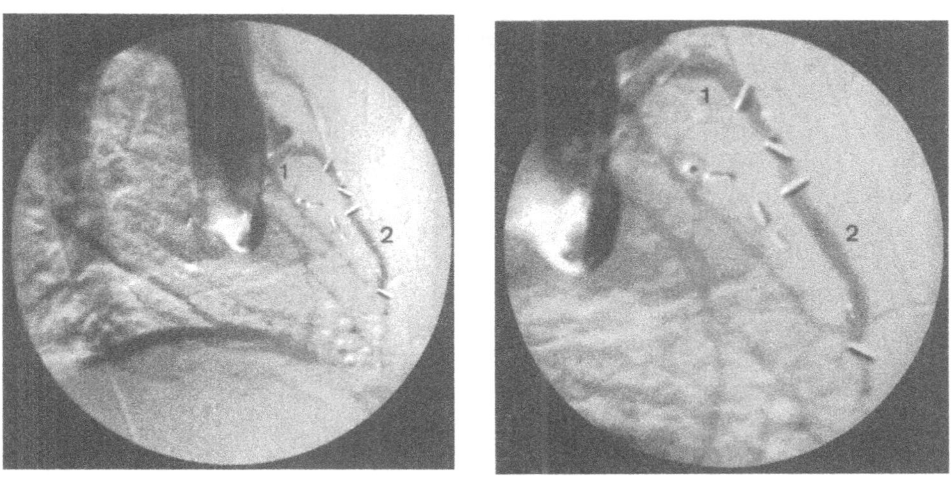

a b

Fig. 4. a Sixty-degree left lateral position. Single graft to the LAD (*1*); single graft to the RCA (*2*). **b** Enlargement of the anastomoses

Table 1. Aortocoronary bypasses (148 patients)

Number of bypasses (total)	309
With 1 distal anastomosis	206
With 2 distal anastomoses	89
With 3 distal anastomoses	14

Table 2. Aortocoronary bypasses (430 distal anastomoses)

Right coronary artery	94
Occluded	10 (10.6%)
Left coronary artery	336
Occluded	33 (10.0%)

Discussion

All previously applied noninvasive methods like computed tomography [2, 7, 9, 14, 17], myocardial scintigraphy [8, 11], or Doppler sonography [15] were not able to give adequate information about the patency of the whole aortocoronary graft and its proximal and distal anastomosis. With transvenous DSA [12, 13] it has also not been possible to judge adequately the patency and course of the graft and particularly the situation at the distal anastomosis. The introduction of the imaging of coronary grafts postoperatively without superselective catheterization of coronary ostia with the intraarterial digital subtraction technique allows a simultaneous not superimposed visualization of all grafts and anastomoses with a low risk. This was possible with a 90° or 60° right or left lateral position of the patient. The same technique was used for the demonstration of the patency of mammary artery bypass grafts.

This is a valid method for the radiologist which gives sufficient information about the patency of the grafts and the function of the anastomoses [5, 16, 18]; it is a very important and helpful postoperative method regarding the prognostic judgment of the bypasses.

In 96% the patency of the distal anastomoses could be proved; in 80% adequate judgment of the distal anastomoses and the connected coronary artery vessel was possible.

The spatial resolution, however, is still better in conventional coronary angiography than in the DSA technique concerning the visualization of the smaller and smallest coronary vessels [1]. But for the evaluation and postoperative control of venous grafts, which generally have a larger diameter, intraarterial DSA is very satisfactory, with a low rate of complications. The method described represents a procedure of low risk with high sensitivity and sensibility for visualization of aortocoronary and internal mammary artery bypass grafts, especially in the early postoperative period.

References

1. Birnbaum D, Banzer D (1984) Imaging of coronary grafts without catheterisation of coronary ostia. In: F Unger (ed) Coronary artery surgery. Springer, Berlin Heidelberg New York Tokyo, pp 240–245
2. Daniel GW, Döhring W, Stender HS, Lichtlen PR (1983) Value and limitations of computed tomography in assessing aortocoronary bypass graft patency. Circulation 67 [5]:983–987
3. Grondin CM, Lesperance J, Bourassa MG, Pasternac A, Campeau L, Grondin P (1974) Serial angiographic evaluation in 60 consecutive patients with aortocoronary artery vein grafts 2 weeks, 1 year and 3 years after operation. J Thoracic Cardiovasc Surg 67:1
4. Guthaner DF, Robert FW, Aldermann EL, Wexler L (1979) Long-term serial angiographic studies after coronary bypass surgery. Circulation 60 [2]:250–258
5. Hauenstein KH, Schlosser V, Roeren T, Kauffmann GW, Urbanyi B (1985) Intraarterielle DSA zur Kontrolle aortocoronarer Gefäßbrücken – eine Alternative zur Coronarangiographie. Radiologe 25:247–250
6. Heuser I, Krestin GP, Hannekum H, Wimmer G (1985) Darstellung aortokoronarer Venenbrücken mit der digitalen Subtraktionsangiographie. Dtsch Med Wochenschr 110:243–247
7. Heuser L, Lackner K, Hauser H (1982) Validität der Computertomographie bei der Darstellung offener und verschlossener aortokoronarer Venenbrücken (ACVB). Fortschr Roentgenstr 137:619
8. Kolibash AJ, Call TD, Bush CA, Tetalman MR, Lewis RP (1980) Myocardial perfusion as an indicator of graft patency after coronary artery bypass surgery. Circulation 61:882
9. Kruger RA, Mistretta CA, Houk TL, Kubal W, Riedeer SJ, Ergun DL, Shaw CG, Lancaster JC, Rowe GG (1979) Computerized fluoroscopy techniques for intravenous study of cardiac chamber dynamic CS. Invest Radiol 14:279
10. Lichtlen PH, Engel HJ (1979) Risiken und Komplikationen der Koronarangiographie. Straube, Erlangen
11. Lösse B, von Lierde C, Rafflenbeul D, Krönert H, Bircks W, Feinendegen LE, Loogen F (1981) Wert der Thallium-201-Myocardszintigraphie für die Beurteilung des Funktionszustandes aortokoronarer Bypass-Gefäße. Z Kardiol 70:231–237
12. Luska G, Hendrickx P, Kuhl A, Lichtlen P, Stender HS (1984) Kontrolle von aortokoronaren Venenbypassgrafts (ACVB) mit Hilfe der peripher venösen digitalen Subtraktionsangiographie. Röntgenstrahlen 52:20–23
13. Luska G, Hendrickx P, Kuhl A, Lichtlen P (1985) Periphervenöse digitale Subtraktionsangiographie (DSA) zur Kontrolle von aortokoronaren Venenbypassgrafts (ACVB). Fortschr Röntgenstr 142:35–40
14. Mühlberger V, zur Nedden D, Knapp E, Unger F, Scharfetter H, Braunsteiner H (1981) Computertomographische Darstellung aortokoronarer Venengrafts – Vergleich mit der selektiven Koronarangiographie. Z Kardiol 70:377–379
15. Pisko-Dubienski A, Braid RJ, Wilson DR (1975) Noninvasive assessment of aortocoronary saphenous vein bypass graft patency using directional Doppler. Circulation 52:188–197
16. Schlosser V, Hauenstein KH, Bonzel T, Santana A, Spillner G, Urbanyi B (1985) Die Bedeutung der digitalen Subtraktionsangiographie (DSA) zur Überprüfung koronarchirurgischer Ergebnisse. Herz-Kreislauf 652–655
17. Urbanyi B, Wimmer B, Wink K, Santana A, Spillner G, Schlosser V (1984) Evaluation of aortocoronary graft patency with computed tomography. In: F Unger (ed) Coronary artery surgery. Springer, Berlin Heidelberg New York Tokyo pp 197–200
18. Witte G, Jacobs G, Grabbe E, Rödiger W, Kalmar P, Bücheler E (1984) Arterielle DSA zur Darstellung des aortokoronaren Venenbypass. Fortschr Röntgenstr. 140 [3]:251–253

II. Percutaneous Transluminal Coronary Angioplasty

Emergency Coronary Surgery Following Unsuccessful Angioplasty: Postoperative Results as a Function of Preoperative Status

J. PALENKER, A. SCHIESSLER, B. HEMPEL, A. JOHN, and E. S. BÜCHERL

During 1984/1985 17 patients were operated on in our hospital on an emergency basis for complications resulting from balloon dilatation of the coronaries.

We carried out this study with the aim of finding a correlation between the preoperative condition of the patient and the operative results. The patients were between 39 and 64 years of age, average 58.2 years, which is 4 years above the average age of our total number of patients.

All 17 patients survived operation. The indications for operation were as in Table 1: 12 patients had severe angina pectoris with typical ECG changes and 5 patients had been resuscitated from a state of circulatory collapse due to ventricular fibrillation. Of these five patients four were admitted with stable circulatory status, while one patient was admitted in an unstable stage, with circulatory shock and tachycardia.

Among the group of 12 patients with severe angina pectoris uneasy changes, 3 had acute construction of a coronary thrombus, 1 had a broken guide wire lying in the ostium of the right coronary artery, and another had a dissection of the left coronary in the region of the proximal left anterior descending artery (LAD). Preoperative management consisted of one or more of the following:

(1) pharmacological support, (2) thrombolytic treatment, (3) mechanical support methods, and (4) pacemakers.

All the patients were given a preoperative nitroglycerine infusion and six were also given a catecholamine infusion. All were also heparinized; in addition three patients had streptokinase infused into the coronaries. Two patients also had small catheters placed in their coronaries to keep the lumen open. An in-

Table 1. Preoperative status of the patients and indications for surgery

	No. of patients
Group I	
Severe angina pectoris	12
ECG alterations (ischemic signs)	12
Group II	
Resuscitation	
a) Resuscitation, intubation, pharmacological support Stable circulation	4
b) Resuscitation, intubation, pharmacological support Unstable circulation (cardiogenic shock)	1

traaorta balloon pump was not used. Two patients also had emergency temporary pacemakers put in.

It is interesting to go into details of the operative treatment undertaken (Table 3).

Ten patients had bypasses put only on the diseased vessel, one also had an additional bypass on the diagonal branch. Seven patients had bypasses performed on other vessels as well, and a total of seven patients had thrombendarterectomy of the vessels performed. On the whole nine patients were given single coronary bypass, five a double bypass, and three a triple bypass operation.

Reperfusion times give us a rough idea of the damage and dysfunction of the myocardium (Table 4).

Table 2. Preoperative treatment

	No. of patients
1. *Pharmacological support*	
Adrenergic agents	6
Nitroglycerine	17
2. *Thrombolysis*	
Intracoronary (streptokinase)	3
Systemic (heparin)	17
3. *Mechanical devices*	
Intraluminar perfusion catheters	2
Intraaorta balloon pump	–
4. *Pacemaker*	

Table 3. Operative procedure – methods of revascularization

	No. of patients
1. Grafting only the diseased vessel	10
2. Grafting of other stenotic / occluded vessels	7
3. Thrombectomy (additional TEA)	6

Table 4. Reperfusion time in the extracorporeal circulation

Longest time, 130 min
Shortest time, 14 min
Mean reperfusion time, 34 min
Group I (patient with angina pectoris)
Mean reperfusion time, 26 min
Group II (patient after reanimations)
Mean reperfusion time, 62 min
a) Mean reperfusion time, 40 min (preoperative stable state)
b) Reperfusion time, 130 min (preoperative unstable status)

Reperfusion time ranged from 14 to 130 min. The first group of patients who were admitted only with angina pectoris had shorter reperfusion times compared with the second group, who were admitted after ventricular fibrillation in stable or unstable circulatory status. The one patient who came in a state of cardiogenic shock was reperfused for a period of 130 min. In the first group of patients there was a correlation between the length of the reperfusion time and the postoperative rise of cardiac enzymes in blood as a result of coronary obstructions and myocardial ischemia. When the aortic clamp was removed only one patient went into ventricular fibrillation, the one who was admitted with cardiogenic shock; all the others showed either spontaneous onset of sinus rhythm or nodal rhythm going on into sinus rhythm. Two patients had implantation of temporary epicardial pacemaker electrodes because of sinus bradycardia.

One patient from group I and three from group II required circulatory support with catecholamines. Dopamine was the drug of choice and one patient of group II who came in cardiogenic shock in addition had adrenaline infusion.

The period of postoperative ventilation ranged from 7 to 60 h. The group I patients could nearly all be extubated after a period of 12 h, but those in group II required longer ventilation. Only one of the group II patients could be extubated within the first 24 h. Only the patient who was admitted with cardiogenic shock required catecholamine support for longer than 24 h.

In summary we can state the following: there were no deaths, even in the patients who were operated on within 3 h on an emergency basis following failure of balloon angioplasty. Patients who had cardiac arrest or ventricular fibrillation or who were admitted in an unstable circulatory state required longer reperfusion times and catecholamine support, and also longer ventilation periods. Postoperatively only one patient was in a confused and irritable state for 3–4 days; there was no lasting damage in any other organ than the heart.

From these results it is clear that those patients who are operated on early and who had no cardiac arrest did not differ significantly in their postoperative course from our elective coronary artery patients. Our operative techniques and myocardial protection contributed to the short reperfusion times and short catecholamine support for less than 1 h. In other words these patients compare well with our elective coronary patients. Only in those patients who were admitted with an unstable circulatory state or cardiogenic shock can one expect significant myocardial damage and relatively more postoperative complications.

Emergency Coronary Artery Bypass Grafting in Patients with Acute Myocardial Ischemia After Percutaneous Transluminal Coronary Angioplasty

B. RIGLER, D. BRANDT, H. GOMBOTZ, W. KLEIN, and J. KRAFT-KINZ

Myocardial injury from failed percutaneous transluminal coronary angioplasty (PTCA) is an infrequent but serious complication presenting a spectrum from anginal pain alone to severe transmural myocardial infarction with hypotension, shock, and cardiac arrest. Prevention of myocardial necrosis and preservation of left ventricular function requires immediate restoration of coronary artery blood flow. With patients refractory to medical therapy, urgent emergency myocardial revascularization is the accepted therapy of this complication.

Methods and Patient Data

From April 1980 through October 1985 emergency operations were carried out in 20 patients due to complicated PTCA, representing 8.2% of the entire series of 252 patients with attempted angioplasty. During the first years of the PTCA program surgical support involved complete coronary artery bypass grafting facilities in a standby position. Since 1985 the angioplasties were scheduled between two elective surgical procedures and started when the first patient was to come of the pump. The decision for surgical intervention was based on the angiographic appearance of occlusion or dissection of the instrumented coronary artery and on the clinical symptoms of acute myocardial ischemia refractory to medical therapy. Bypass grafting (aortocoronary bypass graft) was performed in a standard manner – after immediate institution of the extracorporeal circulation (ECC), the distal anastomoses were created at first in the infarcted or instrumented area using cold cardioplegic arrest. Performance of distal anastomoses was followed by cardioplegic graft perfusion, completion of revascularization, and reperfusion on ECC. The intraaortic balloon pump was not used as routine in the preoperative period. Postoperative management included controlled respirator therapy during the first 12–24 h, inotropic support with dopamine and/or dobutamine as well as afterload reduction in hypertensive patients by administration of nitroglycerin. Evidence of perioperative myocardial infarctions was determined by postoperative electrocardiographic changes and elevations in myocardial (CKMB) and total serum creatine kinase (CPK).

Among the 20 patients who underwent emergency operations there were 16 male and 4 female patients aged 40–72 years (mean, 57 years). All patients had normal left ventricular function and severe angina despite medical therapy. Nine (45%) patients had one-vessel disease, 10 (50%) had two-vessel disease,

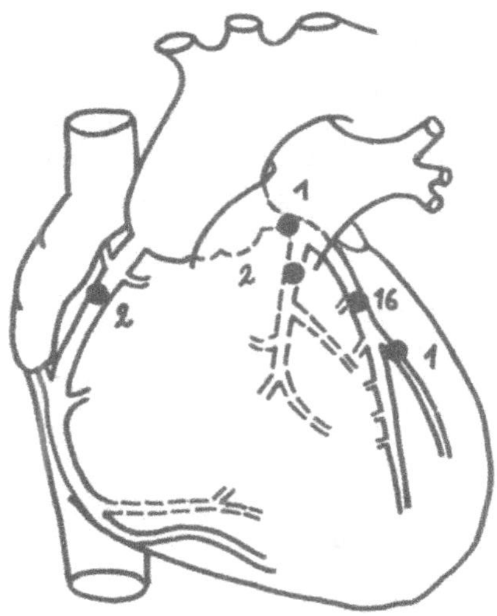

Fig. 1. Site of attempted PTCA

and 1 suffered from isolated left main coronary artery disease (LMCAD). Eight patients presented with a history of myocardial infarction. One patient had undergone a previous bypass graft procedure; another was on a hemodialysis program. Twenty-two PTCA attempts were made in the 20 patients, the majority of the procedures being in the left anterior descending (LAD) branch (Fig. 1). Symptoms of myocardial ischemia occurred in two patients after initially successful PTCA, in 15 patients after failed PTCA, and in 3 instances following attempted angioplasty. A delay between the onset of symptoms of ischemia and PTCA of 30 min to 8 h was seen in 4 patients. The ischemic

Table 1. Onset of symptoms of myocardial ischemia following PTCA

	During	Delayed
PTCA failed (dissection)	2	1
(occlusion)	12	–
PTCA successful	–	2
PTCA attempted (occlusion)	2	1
N patients	16	4

Table 2. Acute myocardial ischemia after PTCA: indication for emergency surgery

Indication	*N*
Chest pain alone	7
Chest pain + ST segment ↑	13
Hypotension (shock)	8 (3)
Cardiac arrest	4

symptoms appeared in the majority (80%) of the angioplasty procedures immediately after PTCA (Table 1). Thirteen (65%) patients developed ST-segment elevations on ECG; in seven (35%) instances anginal pain alone remained refractory to drug therapy, streptokinase treatment, and repeated angioplasty. Eight patients were found hypotensive, three in severe cardiogenic shock and four suffering episodes of cardiac arrest (Table 2).

Results

Nineteen patients could be revascularized up to 12 h after PTCA. The patient who had undergone previous ACBG surgery died prior to the institution of ECC despite prompt insertion of the intraaortic balloon pump. When he arrived at the theater he was in severe cardiogenic shock, developing several episodes of cardiac arrest. He died after unsuccessful resuscitation during thoracotomy. The relationship between obstructive coronary artery lesions (more than 60%) and instrumented and revascularized coronary arteries is shown in Table 3. Fourteen patients had double vein grafts and five had single vein grafts. The graft per patient relationship was 1.7 and 17 of the 19 survivors had complete revascularization.

At operation four patients showed discolored and acinetic areas of myocardium distal to the injured arteries. Mean revascularization time was 161 min, ranging from 110 to 290 min. Mean aortic cross-clamping time and duration of ECC were 26.6 and 73 min respectively. Reperfusion time averaged 20.6 min and varied from 13 to 60 min, with prolonged reperfusion in 3 patients.

Morbidity and mortality of the emergency operations are summarized in Table 4. Mortality was 5% on account of one death prior to ECC institution. No patient required insertion of the intraaortic balloon pump in the postoperative period. All the revascularized patients are alive, with a mean follow-up of 11.8 (1 – 55) months, 89% presenting free of anginal pain and 2 reporting dyspnea on moderate exertion. Thirty-seven percent of the patients developed perioperative new Q-wave infarctions. The incidence of Q-wave infarction was higher in patients with preoperative ST-segment elevation but did not correlate with the revascularization time. Four of the seven ECG infarctions were considered to be small according to the ECG findings. Two of the three patients with large

Table 3. Relationship between diseased, instrumented, and revascularized CAs in 19 patients with acute myocardial ischemia following PTCA

Site of CAD	Diseased CA	Instrumented CA	Revascularized CA
LMCA	1	1	2 (LAD, LCX)
LAD	15	15	15
Diagonal B.	6	1	8
RCA	6	2	4
LCX	4	2	4
	32	21	33

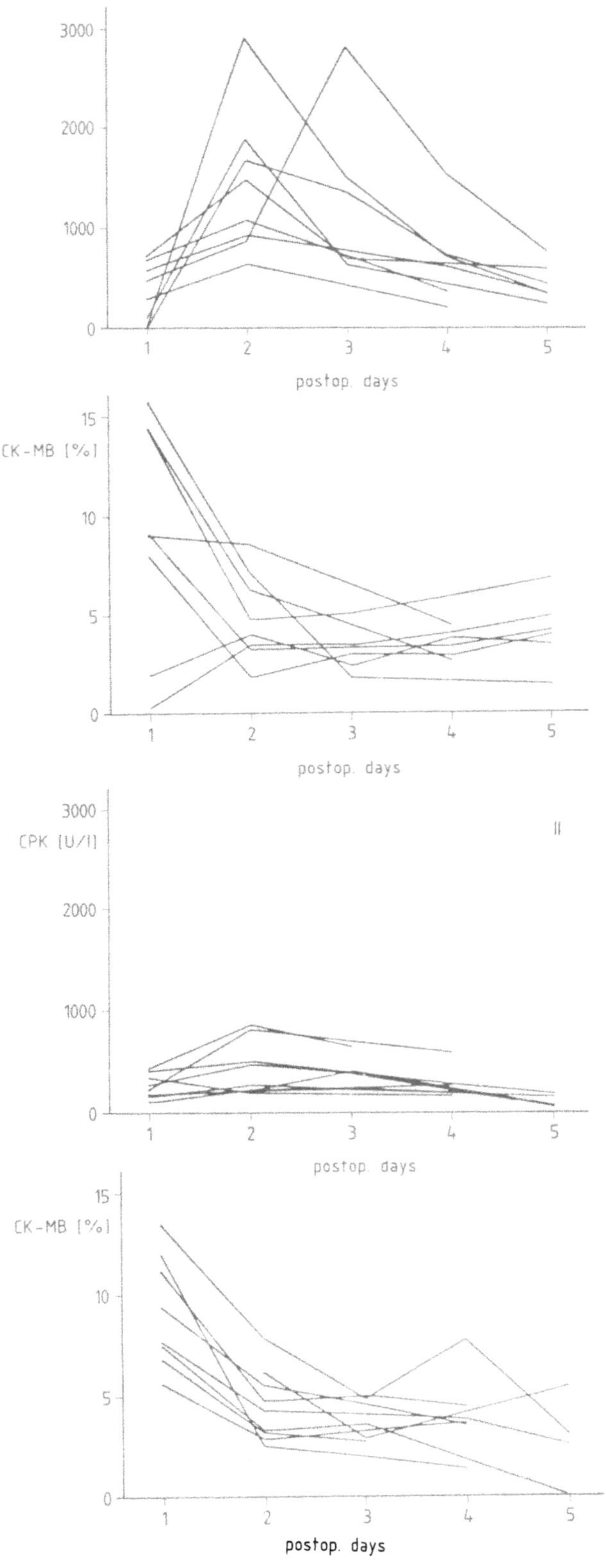

Fig. 2. Pattern of postoperative (CPK, MB) serum enzyme activities in 17 revascularized patients. (*I*, patients with myocardial necrosis; *II*, patients without myocardial necrosis). CK-MB expressed as a percentage of CPK

Table 4. Morbidity and mortality of emergency ACBG patients (AMI/PTCA) April 1980 to October 1985

N patients	20
Death (prior to ECC)	1 (5%)
Alive	19
Perioperative new Q-wave infarctions	7 (37%)
Angina free	17 (89%)
Dyspnea at exertion	2
Late sternal fistulas	1

Mean follow-up 11.8 (1–55) months

Table 5. Postoperative findings

ECG	Pat + ST ↑ *N*=12	Pat – ST ↑ *N*=7
New Q-wave infarction	5	2 (37%)
Site of infarction		
Supraapical	2	2
Anterolateral	2	
Posteroseptal	1	
Size of infarction		
Small	2	2
Large	3	

ECG infarctions had bypass graft occlusion documented angiographically early in the postoperative period. Either of these patients received saphenous vein grafts with a varicose wall because of severe bilateral varicosis (Table 5).

With regard to the postoperative serum enzyme activities of CPK and CK-MB (expressed as a percentage of total CPK), which were available in 17 patients in the postoperative period, we found the peak values mainly around the second postoperative day. Maximum serum enzyme activities of CPK and CK-MB averaged 855.2 (155–2895) U/liter and 51.4 (12–134) U/liter respectively. Minor differences could be seen in patients with preoperative myocardial infarction and anginal pain alone. However, 52% of the 19 patients showed elevated serum enzyme activities indicative of myocardial necrosis (Fig. 2).

Discussion

Initially restricted to patients with single-vessel disease, PTCA is now in use in patients who are in a higher risk category due to previous bypass graft procedures and/or multiple-vessel disease. Despite growing experience with angioplastic techniques, myocardial injury continues to occur, requiring emergency operations in 2.8%–21% of the series reported more recently [1, 3]. The indication for emergency operation depends on the clinical symptoms of acute myocardial ischemia in conjunction with the angiographic evidence of a centrally occluded or dissected coronary artery. Careful monitoring is necessary in the case of clinically silent dissection. In patients with delayed onset of myocardial ischemia angiographic restudy is recommended to assess the amount of myocardium in jeopardy – a viewpoint which is debatable if further delay seems unavoidable by the catheterization restudy itself.

In contrast to elective bypass grafting emergency interventions following complicated PTCA are associated with higher mortality (5%) and morbidity [4, 5]. Preoperative usage of heparin, aspirin, or streptokinase usually affects coagulation parameters, leading to a reexploration rate more than that of elective ACBG. With perioperative myocardial infarctions, varying proportions are reported in the literature, ranging from 6% to 70% [1, 3, 6, 7]. Thirty-seven percent of our patients sustained new Q-wave infarctions and three of them were considered to be small according to the ECG findings. Although difficult to interpret, analysis of postoperative serum enzyme activities indicated at least discrete myocardial necrosis in 52% of the patients. The incidence of enzyme or ECG infarctions did not correlate with the time elapsed between PTCA, onset of ischemic symptoms, and restoration of blood flow.

On the other hand, with emergency bypass grafting we have been able to avoid myocardial necrosis, even in patients with long-lasting revascularization time up to 260 min.

With myocardium in jeopardy because of complicated PTCA any delay should be avoided due to the unpredictable natural course – about 20% of our patients suffered episodes of cardiac arrest prior to ECC institution, with one death. Patients at risk should be scheduled carefully and the beneficial effects of the intraaortic balloon pump should be kept in mind [2, 5]. Despite the remarkable incidence of perioperative myocardial infarctions all surviving patients showed significant improvement in hemodynamics, suggesting salvage of ischemic myocardium, and none of the patients required postoperative intraaortic balloon pump support.

References

1. Abi-Mansur P, Curling PE, Grüntzig AR (1985) Impact of balloon angioplasty (PTCA) on cardiac anesthesia practice. Presented at 7th Annual Meeting of the Society of Cardiovascular Anesthesiologists, Phoenix, Arizona (Abstract book) page 20
2. Block PC (1985) Emergency surgery after percutaneous transluminal coronary angioplasty: he who calls the tune has to pay the piper. Ann Thorac Surg 40:1
3. Brahos GJ, Baker NH, Gene-Ewy H, Moore PJ, Thomas JW, Sanfelippo PM, Mc Vicker RV, Johnson-Fankhauser D (1985) Aortocoronary bypass following unsuccessful PTCA: experience in 100 consecutive patients. Ann Thorac Surg 40:7
4. Jones EL, Craver JM, Grüntzig AR, King SB III, Douglas JS, Bone DK, Guyton RG, Hatcher CR (1982) Percutaneous transluminal coronary angioplasty: role of the surgeon. Ann Thorac Surg 34:493
5. Murphy DA, Craver JM, Jones EL, Curling PE, Guyton RA, King SB II, Grüntzig AR, Hatcher CR (1984) Surgical management of acute myocardial ischemia following percutaneous transluminal coronary angioplasty. J Thorac Cardiovasc Surg 87:332
6. Rigler B, Stenzl W, Tscheliessnigg KH, Gombotz H, Brandt D, Metzler H, Hiotakis K, Klein W (1985) Ergebnisse der dringlichen aortocoronaren Bypasschirurgie bei Patienten mit akuter Myokardischämie nach perkutaner transluminaler Koronarangioplastik. WMW 19/ 20:494
7. Satter P, Scherer D (1984) Ergebnisse notfallmäßig durchgeführter aorto-coronarer Bypass-Operationen nach transluminalem Angioplastieversuch. Presented Second Cardiovascular Symposium Zürs (personal communication)

Percutaneous Transluminal Coronary Angioplasty in Progressive Myocardial Ischemia: Medium-term Results

N. Spampinato, C. Gagliardi, P. Stassano, V. de Amicis, M. Chello, G. Jannelli, F. di Lello, P. Pepino, A. Musumeci, and G. Ricciardi

Introduction

Percutaneous transluminal coronary angioplasty (PTCA) has undergone a major evolution since 1977, when Gruentzig and coworkers [3] made their first balloon dilatation. The success rate with PTCA has improved, ranging from 60% to about 90%, as the experience of operators (learning curve) and availability of materials have increased. Most recently, some authors [2, 9] have also employed this procedure in cases of multiple-vessel disease, stenoses of saphenous vein grafts, and acute ischemic episodes. Initially, our experience – at the Department of Cardiovascular Surgery, 2nd Medical School University of Naples, Italy – was restricted to only single (rarely double) and proximal coronary artery narrowing and especially to patients with progressive myocardial ischemia.

Material and Method

From January 1982 to December 1984, 35 patients with signs of progressive myocardial ischemia underwent PTCA as an emergency procedure during the coronary angiography. Age ranged from 31 to 57 years (average, 39.5 years); 28 patients were male and 7 female.

Table 1. Results of PTCA related to coronary artery lesions in 35 patients (January 1982 – December 1984)

Coronary artery	No. of patients	%	Post-PTCA			
			Successful NYHA		Unsuccessful	
			I	II	Emergency	Elective
LAD	26	74.3%	19	6	1 CABG > no AMI	
Cx	5	14.3%	2	1	1 CABG >> AMI	1 CABG (2 days later)
RCA	2	5.7%				2 CABG
LAD + Cx	2	5.7%	2			(2 days later)
Total	35	100%	23	7	2 (5.7%)	3 (8.5%)

LAD, left anterior descending artery; RCA, right coronary artery; AMI, acute myocardial infarction; Cx, circumflex artery

All patients with progressive myocardial ischemia showed: (1) unstable angina not responsive to aggressive medical treatment (triple-drug therapy: beta-blockers, calcium antagonist, and nitrates), (2) transient modifications of "S-T" and "T" waves on ECG in 23 patients, (3) reversible alteration of the normal value of cardiac enzymes.

All patients had critical ($\geqq$90%) proximal narrowing in one or more major coronary arteries as shown in Table 1. PTCA was performed immediately after coronary angiography, with an open heart surgical team on standby.

Results

No deaths occurred in our series after PTCA. During PTCA there were some ischemic myocardial complications: (1) reversible in seven patients: because of coronary artery spasm improved by Ca antagonist and intracoronary nitroglycerine and (2) irreversible in two patients: because of an unresponsive vasospasm of LAD in one and dissection of circumflex artery in the other. The latter two patients immediately underwent emergency surgery with about 120 min from the onset of pain, and only the patient with dissection of Cx showed ECG signs of inferior myocardial infarction postoperatively.

In addition, three patients (8.5%) had no benefit from the procedure and underwent elective surgery later with no new signs of myocardial ischemia.

At follow-up, ranging from 6 to 30 months (average 18 months), 23 patients were in the 1st NYHA functional class and 7 in the 2nd NYHA class. Coronary angiography was performed in five patients after about 6 months post-PTCA and showed a complete resolution of the lesions. Furthermore, all patients underwent Tl-201-myocardial scintigraphy at rest and on exercise: good myocardial perfusion was demonstrated.

Discussion

The effectiveness of PTCA for treatment of coronary artery disease has been documented by many investigators [4, 5]. In addition, a PTCA registry was instituted by the National Heart Lung and Blood Institute to study extensively the patient population and results of PTCA [1, 7]. It is now established that PTCA offers a relatively safe and effective nonsurgical method of myocardial revascularization in selected patients [1–5]. In our series the indications for PTCA were restricted to patients with single and proximal lesions, rarely to those with double-vessel disease. In accordance with the NHLBI registry for PTCA, our primary success rate was around 85.7%. Only two patients (5.7%) required an emergency operation and one patient (2.8%) had a postoperative myocardial infarction. Reversible myocardial ischemia, observed also during and immediately after balloon inflation, improved through aggressive medical treatment. Finally, although no deaths occurred in our series, we agree entirely with some authors [6, 8] that a standby open heart service for PTCA is warranted, and that PTCA should be performed only in hospitals with a support staff of skilled cardiovascular surgeons.

References

1. Dorros G, Cowley MJ, Simpson J et al. (1983) PTCA. Report of complications from the NHLBI PTCA registry. Circulation 67:723–730
2. Ford WB, Wholey MH, Zikria EA et al. (1980) Percutaneous transluminal angioplasty in the management of occlusive disease involving the coronary artery and saphenous vein graft. J Thorac Cardiovasc Surg 79:1–11
3. Gruentzig AR, Myler R, Hanna E et al. (1977) Transluminal angioplasty of coronary artery stenosis. Circulation 56:84 (abstract)
4. Gruentzig AR (1982) Results from coronary angioplasty and implications for the future. Am Heart J 103:779–783
5. Hall RJ, Mathur VS, Massumi A et al. (1984) PTCA update. Tex Heart Inst J 11:10–16
6. Kabbani SS, Bashour TT, Jones R et al. (1984) Surgical experience following PTCA. Tex Heart Inst J 11:112–116
7. Kent KM, Bentivoglio LG, Block PC et al. (1982) PTCA. Report from the Registry of NHLBI. Am J Cardiol 49:2011–2020
8. Murphy DA, Graver GM, Jones EL et al. (1982) Surgical revascularization following unsuccessful PTCA. J Thorac Cardiovasc Surg 84:342–348
9. Vliestra RE, Holmes DR, Reeder GJ et al. (1983) Balloon angioplasty in multivessel coronary artery disease. Mayo Clinic Proc 58:563–567

Clinical, Angiographic, and Procedural Factors Presumably Related to Persistent Success After Percutaneous Transluminal Coronary Angioplasty*

A. ORIOL, P. GUITERAS, J. M. AUGÉ, M. MASOTTI, C. PERAZA, and C. CREXELLS

Introduction

Ever since the use of percutaneous transluminal coronary angioplasty (PTCA) was introduced to achieve coronary revascularization, comparison of its results with those of CABG has been of major concern to everybody. Morbidity [4, 6, 7], cost [2, 3, 10], return to work [9], etc. have all been analyzed, yet much remains to be said about lasting effects of successful PTCA. Why do some cases restenose? Are there some factors that one could relate to persistent success? Are such factors of clinical or angiographic nature? Could they simply be related to the technique?

To answer these questions we set up the present study. It is not yet finished; thus only some preliminary results will be presented.

Material and Methods

Percutaneous transluminal coronary angioplasty was successful in 87 patients out of 131 consecutive attempts at our institution between September 1981 and May 1985. The PTCA technique has already been published in detail [1]. Success was defined as the residual stenosis being 50% or less. Of these 87 patients, including only 6 women, 21 had multivessel disease, on which PTCA was attempted successfully in 6, while in the remaining 15 only one lesion was dilated. As a whole there were 100 dilated lesions: 73 in the anterior descending artery, 10 in the circumflex artery, 16 in the right coronary artery, and 1 in the main stem.

Clinical and angiographic follow-up had been set up for all patients since we started PTCA. Only four patients did not accept a second coronary angiogram at the 6th month post PTCA and in one patient neither clinical nor angiographic follow-up could be completed because he moved away from the area of the hospital.

In 17 cases the second hemodynamic study had to be performed before the established 6th month because of recurrence of symptoms, and in 30 cases it was delayed from 1 to 10 months for the patient's convenience.

* This study was in part supported by the ACARD association (Associació Catalana d'Ajut a la Cardiologia).

Clinical end points were established as: (1) a change in the level of angina equal or superior to two functional degrees, (2) when the patient underwent elective coronary artery bypass grafting (CABG), or (3) a second attempt at PTCA.

The angiographic end point was defined as the appearance of a restenosis equal or greater than 70% regardless of symptoms. Listed in Table 1 are the 50 variables analyzed for each patient. Eighteen were clinical, including past and present data on risk factors, and 21 were related to angiographic or hemodynamic parameters. The last 11 variables were related to the technique, including the angiographer's experience.

To assess the influence of factors more clearly related to a long-lasting success after an initially successful PTCA, all the variables listed were entered into a univariate analysis. Chi-square tests were used for discrete variables and Student *t*-tests and analysis of variance for continuous data.

Significant variables obtained from the above-mentioned tests were used to stratify the clinical follow-up data according to the Mantel-Haenszel actuarial model [8]. The log-rank test was used to assess differences among the groups. Significant grouping variables were fed into a Cox model [8] to determine covariables significantly related to clinical end points. BMDP software [5] was used for all statistical testing and an error of 0.05 was accepted as statistically significant for all tests. All statistics were carried out on a VAX 11 computer[1].

Results

Average clinical follow-up was 14.1 (range 1–49) months in 86 patients out of the 87 initially included in the study up to May 1985. Of the 86 patients, 25 reached the end point at an average 5.4 months (range 1–10), 12 because of going into a second PTCA, 4 into elective CABG and another 9 simply because they developed angina to a degree equal or greater than two functional classes over the existing level immediately after PTCA. This last group of patients went on medical treatment alone.

Figure 1 shows the baseline functional class of angina for all patients as well as their clinical situation immediately after PTCA and at the time of the second angiographic control. As a whole in 23 patients the angina level worsened to reach the end point during clinical follow-up; 56 patients remained asymptomatic and 3 developed functional class I angina.

In the univariate analysis only two variables showed to be significant: blood pressure level and geometry of the lesion.

Figure 2 shows actuarial curves in both cases through 24 months of follow-up.

Both the presence of hypertension and an initially eccentric lesion appear to favor angina reappearance some time between 3 and 6 months after PTCA.

---

[1] Kindly put at our disposal by the Institut de Cibernètica of the Universitat Politècnica de Catalunya.

Table 1. Variables entering univariate analysis

Clinical	Angiographic	Procedural
Age	Extent of CAD (one-, two-, three-vessel disease)	Translesional gradient: Pre-PTCA
Sex	Regional left ventricular wall motion	Post-PTCA
Smoking status	Left ventricular ejection fraction	Type of dilating catheter: Used first
Serum cholesterol (nmol/liter)	Stenosis:	Used after
Serum triglycerides (nmol/liter)	Number of lesions dilated	Number of balloon catheters used
Actual systemic hypertension	Number of vessels dilated	∅ of largest balloon used
Actual diabetes mellitus	Artery (LMT, LAD, RCA, LCX)	Number of inflations
Family history of CAD	Site (proximal, mid-distal)	Maximal inflation pressure (atmospheres)
History of:	Length (mm)	Ratio ∅ inflated balloon/∅ proximal artery
Prior MI	Geometry (concentric, eccentric)	
Prior CHF	Morphology (discrete, tubular, diffuse)	Ratio ∅ inflated balloon/ ∅ stenosis
Prior CABG	Calcification	Tension developed on lesion
Prior unstable angina	Involved branch	Coronary dissection (mild, moderate, occlusion)
Duration of angina	Severity pre-PTCA (%)	
Duration of actual level of angina	Severity post-PTCA (%)	Angiographer's experience
Actual angina: on effort[a]	Collaterals: Before PTCA	
Unstable, excluding variant	After PTCA	
Variant	∅ of proximal healthy artery (mm)	
	∅ of dilated stenosis (mm)	

CAD, coronary artery disease; CHF, congestive heart failure; CABG, coronary artery bypass grafting; LMT, left main trunk; LAD, left anterior descending; RCA, right coronary artery; LCX, left circumflex; PTCA, percutaneous transluminal coronary angioplasty; ∅ diameter

[a] Canadian Cardiovascular Society Angina Class

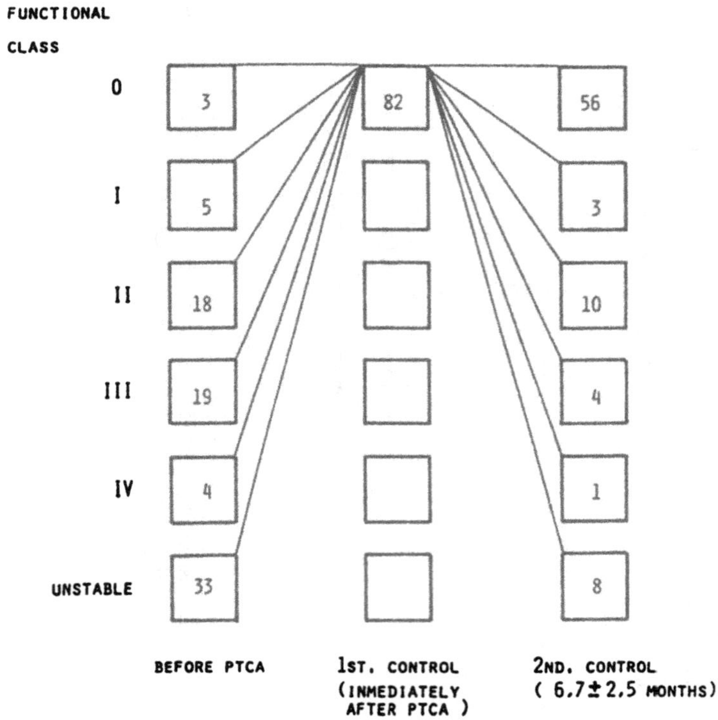

Fig. 1. Distribution of patients according to their level of angina before, immediately after, and at 6 months after PTCA

Table 2. Univariate analysis: factors influencing reappearance of angina and/or restenosis

Variable	*P*
Eccentric lesion	0.003
Systemic hypertension	0.014
Mid-distal lesion	0.022
Residual stenosis (40%)	0.03
Long stenosis	0.03
Ø of proximal healthy artery	0.048

Ø, diameter

Table 3. Logistic regression analysis of factors influencing a long-lasting success (Cox model)

	Covariable	β-coefficient	*P*
Clinical follow-up	Lesion eccentricity	1.382	0.0065
($n = 86$)	Systemic hypertension	1.028	0.0385
Angiographic follow-up	Systemic hypertension	1.297	0.0134
($n = 82$)	Residual stenosis	0.0303	0.0378

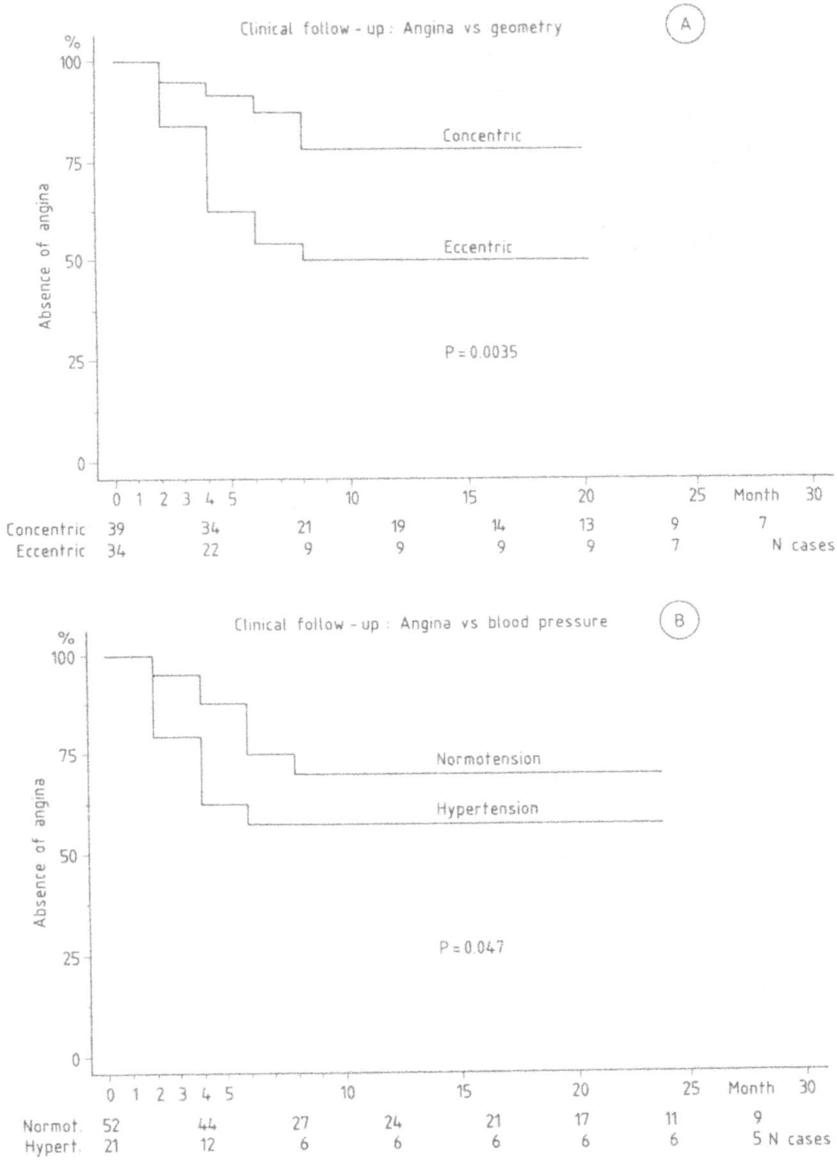

Fig. 2 A, B. Actuarial curves showing the percentage of patients that remain free of symptoms after 24 months with a successful PTCA in **A** when the dilated lesion was concentric or eccentric and in **B** with high or normal blood pressure

Average angiographic follow-up was 6.7±2.5 months in 82 patients. Four asymptomatic and 16 symptomatic patients of this group showed restenosis equal to or greater than 70% at the site of the previously dilated lesion.

Univariate analysis (Table 2) showed a significant correlation of hypertension, distal, longer, and eccentric lesions, narrower arteries and a more severe residual stenosis, to early reappearance of angina.

The results of applying the Cox model to relate clinical, angiographic, and procedural covariates to both clinical and angiographic end points are shown in Table 3. Only hypertension, residual stenosis, and eccentricity showed a highly significant *P* value.

Discussion

This preliminary report of our study does not allow for long discussion as more cases have to be analyzed and certainly a longer follow-up is needed. Yet the trend that our results suggest is logical as it goes along with common sense and is also encouraging since it points toward the possibility of better selection of patients (do not include eccentric lesions), better use of the technique (avoid leaving an important residual stenosis), and a better treatment after the procedure (management of hypertension).

References

1. Augé JM, Crexells C, Oriol A, Garcia J, Carreras F, Peraza C (1985) Angioplastias de las arterias coronarias por la técnica de Grüntzig. Evolución de la metodología y resultados iniciales en el Hospital de la Santa Creu i Sant Pau. Rev Esp Cardiol 38 [Suppl I]: 14–20
2. Bresco S, Oriol A, Garcia J, Augé JM, Crexells C (1985) Coste de la ACTP en un hospital terciario de nuestro medio. Rev Esp Cardiol 38 (Suppl I): 79–82
3. Cherrier F, Danchin N, Cherrier PH, Cullière M, Faivre G (1984) Coût d'une angioplastie transluminale coronaire comparé à celui du pontage aorto-coronaire unique. Incidènces économiques. Arch Mal Cœur 13: 1450–1455
4. Cowley MJ, Vetrovec WG, Wolfang TC (1981) Efficacy of percutaneous transluminal coronary angioplasty: technique, patient selection, salutary results, limitations and complications. Am Heart J 101: 272–280
5. Dixon WJ, Brown MB, Engelman L et al. (1983) BMPD statistical software. 1983 Printing with Additions. University of California Press, Berkeley
6. Dorros G, Cowley MJ, Simpson J et al. (1983) Percutaneous transluminal coronary angioplasty: report of complications from the National Heart, Lung, and Blood Institute PTCA registry. Circulation 63: 723–740
7. Dorros G, Cowley MJ, Janke L, Kelsey SF, Mullin SM, van Raden M (1984) In-hospital mortality rate in National Heart, Lung, and Blood Institute percutaneous transluminal angioplasty registry. Am J Cardiol 53: 17 C–21 C
8. Elandt-Johnson RC, Johnson NL (1980) Survival models and data analysis. Wiley, New York
9. Holmes DR, van Raden MJ, Reeder GS et al. (1984) Return to work after coronary angioplasty: a report from the National Lung, Heart, and Blood Institute. Transluminal Coronary Angioplasty Registry. Am J Cardiol 53: 48 C–51 C
10. Jang GC, Block PC, Cowley MJ et al. (1984) Relative cost of coronary angioplasty and bypass surgery in a one-vessel disease model. Am J Cardiol 53: 52 C–55 C

Determinants of Restenosis After Coronary Angioplasty*

P. GUITERAS, J. M. AUGÉ, M. MASOTTI, C. PERAZA, C. CREXELLS, and A. ORIOL

Introduction

The restenosis rate after successful percutaneous transluminal coronary angioplasty (PTCA) has been reported in the literature to be anywhere from 12% [5] up to 33.6% [4]. Such a large range suggests that many factors are probably involved in the development of restenosis. Differences in selection of patients, techniques used, or the angiographer's experience probably all play a role.

The present study was set up to investigate which of a wide selection of variables would correlate most with angiographic restenosis at a given time after PTCA, regardless of symptoms.

What we present here is in a way a complementary analysis of what has already been presented in this same Workshop on Persistent Success after PTCA [7].

Material and Methods

From November 1981 until May 1985, PTCA was attempted in 131 patients (12 women) at our catheterization laboratory. A successful PTCA, defined as an immediate post-PTCA stenosis equal to or less than 50%, was achieved in 87 patients and 100 lesions without procedure-related complications. This study is based upon 82 patients (5 women), with a mean age of 52 ± 9 years, who underwent repeat angiography 6.7 ± 2.5 months after PTCA. Four men and 1 woman (6%) refused control angiograms.

Table 1 describes the major baseline characteristics of the 82 patients.

The angioplasted lesion involved the left anterior descending artery in 69 cases, the right coronary artery in 15, the left circumflex artery in 10, and the ostium of the left main trunk in 1.

Hand drawings of the proximal healthy artery and the stenosis were obtained from end-diastolic frames in two orthogonal projections and digitized on magnetic cardboard using a hand-held sonic pen. Absolute measurements of the proximal healthy artery and stenosis were obtained with software implemented

* This study was in part supported by the ACARD association (Asociació Catalana d'Ajut a la Cardiologia).

Table 1. Baseline characteristics of 82 patients (95 stenoses)

Age: years (x ± SD) range	52 ± 9 (25–71)
Sex: men/women	77/5
Duration of angina: months (x ± SD)	12.7 ± 22.8
Duration of actual level of angina: months (x ± SD)	2.4 ± 3.3
Type and class of angina	
Effort, class I or II	23 (28%) [a]
Effort, class III or IV	23 (28%)
Unstable angina	33 (40%)
No angina (+ exercise test)	3 (4%)
Coronary stenosis ≧ 70% [b]	
One vessel	62 (76%)
Two vessels	15 (18%)
Three vessels	4 (5%)
Left main trunk	1 (1%)
Number of segments dilated: One	74 (90%)
Two	6 (7%)
Three	2 (2%)
Tandem	6 (7%)
Regional left ventricular wall motion	
Abnormal	52 (63%)
Characteristics of the distal lesion	
Mid-distal	42 (44%)
Eccentric	40 (42%)
Calcified stenosis	4 (4%)
Stenosis ≧ 90%	13 (14%)
Major branch involved	20 (21%)

[a] Percentage always referring to *n* patients
[b] Including total occlusions that were not dilated

in a Kontron P/M 2.2 computer, using the average of three measurements corrected for X-ray magnification with the shadows of the 7F coronary angiography catheter (2.3 mm). Left ventricular end-diastolic and end-systolic frames were drawn and used to determine global and regional left ventricular function with the above-mentioned facilities. These measurements were obtained from the angiograms performed before, immediately after, and at the 6-month check after PTCA. A coronary lesion was considered significant when there was a 70% or greater reduction in the internal diameter of the artery.

The severity of stenosis pre- and post-PTCA was obtained as the linear percentage of luminal narrowing of the diameter of the stenosis to the diameter of the proximal healthy artery. This estimated percentage was obtained as an average of two orthogonal views.

Percutaneous transluminal coronary angioplasty was performed as described previously [1].

Ratios of the diameter of the larger inflated balloon to the diameter of the proximal healthy artery and dilated stenosis were calculated. A rough assessment of the maximal tension endured by the coronary arterial wall was de-

Table 2. Variables entering univariate analysis

Clinical	Angiographic	Procedural
Age	Extent of CAD (one-, two-, three-vessel disease)	Translesional gradient: Pre-PTCA
Sex	Regional left ventricular wall motion	Post-PTCA
Smoking status	Left ventricular ejection fraction	Type of dilating catheter: Used first
Serum cholesterol (nmol/liter)	Stenosis:	Used after
Serum triglycerides (nmol/liter)	Number of lesions dilated	Number of balloon catheters used
Actual systemic hypertension	Number of vessels dilated	∅ of largest balloon used
Actual diabetes mellitus	Artery (LMT, LAD, RCA, LCX)	Number of inflations
Family history of CAD	Site (proximal, mid-distal)	Maximal inflation pressure (atmospheres)
History of:	Length (mm)	Ratio ∅ inflated balloon/∅ proximal artery
Prior MI	Geometry (concentric, eccentric)	
Prior CHF	Morphology (discrete, tubular, diffuse)	Ratio ∅ inflated balloon/ ∅ stenosis
Prior CABG	Calcification	Tension developed on lesion
Prior unstable angina	Involved branch	Coronary dissection (mild, moderate, occlusion)
Duration of angina	Severity pre-PTCA (%)	
Duration of actual level of angina	Severity post-PTCA (%)	Angiographer's experience
Actual angina: on effort[a]	Collaterals: Before PTCA	
Unstable, excluding variant	After PTCA	
Variant	∅ of proximal healthy artery (mm)	
	∅ of dilated stenosis (mm)	

CAD, coronary artery disease; CHF, congestive heart failure; CABG, coronary artery bypass grafting; LMT, left main trunk; LAD, left anterior descending; RCA, right coronary artery; LCX, left circumflex; PTCA, percutaneous transluminal coronary angioplasty; ∅ diameter

[a] Canadian Cardiovascular Society Angina Class

rived as the product of the larger inflated balloon to the proximal healthy arterial wall times the maximal inflation pressure.

Restenosis was defined as an increase to a 70% stenosis or more from an immediate post-PTCA stenosis of 50% or less.

Univariate analysis was applied to the 18 clinical, 19 angiographic, and 14 procedural variables listed in Table 2. Pearson's and maximal likelihood Chi squares were complemented with Fisher's exact test to analyze discrete variables. The unpaired *t*-test and one-way analysis of variance were used for continuous variables. Variables found to be significantly related to restenosis equal to or greater than 70% were further analyzed using multivariate logistic regression analysis according to the iterative method of Newton-Raphson's algorithm [6]. A 0.05 *P* value was accepted for all the analyses.

Results

The present series' restenosis rate was 28% for the patients and 24% for the arteries, respectively.

The average symptom-free interval from PTCA to the recurrence of angina was 6 ± 5.5 months, and angiographic restenosis equal or greater than 70% was documented 6.7 ± 2.5 months after PTCA. Although six patients were diagnosed after 6 months of PTCA, 74% of the angiographic restenoses were documented within the first 6 months post PTCA.

Univariate analysis related angiographic restenosis (Table 3) to persistent systemic hypertension and certain baseline characteristics of the lesion, such as mid-distal, eccentric longer stenoses, and narrower proximal healthy arteries. More severe post-PTCA stenoses were also measured in the lesions that later restenosed.

Table 3. Univariate analysis: factors influencing restenosis

Rate of restenosis:	Patients 23/82 (28%) Segments 23/95 (24%)	*P*
Clinical variables (82 patients)		
Actual systemic hypertension	11/21 (53%)	0.014
Angiographic and procedural variables (95 lesions)		
Mid-distal lesion	17/42 (40%)	0.022
Eccentric lesion	17/40 (42%)	0.003
Immediate post-PTCA stenosis		
Restenosis	31.9 ± 13.9	
VS long success	23 ± 14.7	0.03
Length of stenosis		
Restenosis	8.7 ± 3.6	
VS long success	6.9 ± 2.3	0.03
Ø of proximal healthy artery		
Restenosis	3.0 ± 0.7	
VS long success	3.5 ± 0.7	0.048

Ø, diameter, VS, versus

Table 4. Logistic regression analysis of factors determining restenosis ≧ 70%

	β-coefficient	*P*
Clinical variables		
Actual systemic hypertension	0.808	0.05
Angiographic and procedural variables		
Eccentric lesion	1.078	0.009
Immediate post-PTCA stenosis	0.053	0.044
Constant	−14.841	

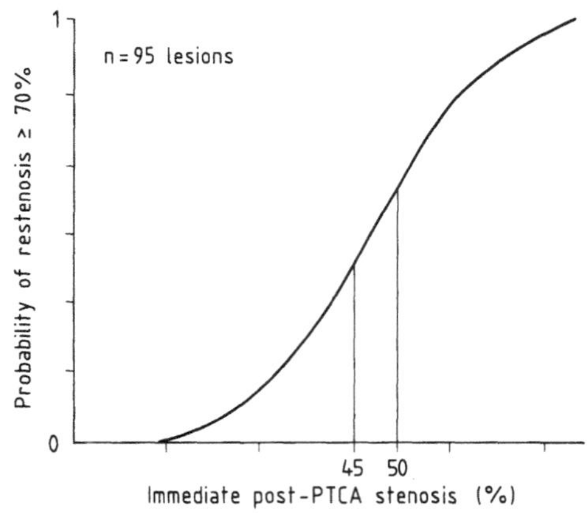

Fig. 1. Logistic curve relating residual stenosis after successful PTCA to probability of angiographic restenosis

Finally, the multivariate logistic model independently related angiographic restenosis to persistent systemic hypertension, eccentric lesions, and severity of the immediate post-PTCA stenosis (Table 4).

In Fig. 1, a logistic curve relates immediate post-PTCA stenosis on the x-axis to the probability of angiographic restenosis of up to 70% on the y-axis. Using the coefficient obtained from the logistic restenosis analysis, immediate post-PTCA stenoses of 40% or less show a weak probability of restenosis, but the curve rises steeply for 45% or more for immediate post-PTCA stenoses.

Discussion

Angiographic restenosis after successful PTCA is difficult to study because of the different definitions used and the lack of systematic angiographic follow-up on consecutive patients regardless of symptoms. Previous NHLBI (National Heart Lung and Blood Institute) reports from the PTCA registry use data from different sources that is clearly biased by symptoms [4, 5]. The present study, with a 94% angiographic follow-up regardless of symptoms, showed only asymptomatic angiographic restenosis in four patients (5%) and a restenosis rate of 28% for the patients and 24% for the lesions which is lower than that reported by the PTCA registry [4].

Kaltenbach, with an even lower restenosis rate (12%), considers this a consequence of better patient selection, longer inflation pressures, and long-term treatment with calcium antagonists and antiplatelet agents. Yet no long-term medical treatment has been proved to reduce restenosis rate after successful PTCA [3, 8].

Since the mechanism of angioplasty has been shown to be an aneurysm formation at the level of the lesion [2] with intima splitting and dilation of the media and adventitia, it seems sensible that any local factor that favors the slowing of flow may also favor restenosis. Therefore, a 50% or more residual stenosis in an eccentric lesion, submitted to the repeated microtrauma of persistent systemic hypertension, may well favor restenosis. Further research and especially a longer follow-up is needed to confirm the data presented, but certainly our results point toward what at first sight looks like a promising future.

References

1. Augé JM, Crexells C, Oriol A, Garcia J, Carreras F, Peraza C (1985) Angioplastia de las arterias coronarias por la técnica de Grüntzig. Evolución de la metodología y resultados iniciales en el Hospital de la Santa Creu i Sant Pau. Rev Esp Cardiol 38 (Suppl I): 14–20
2. Block PC (1984) Mechanism of transluminal angioplasty. Am J Cardiol 53:69C–71C
3. Corcos T, David PR, Guiteras P et al. (1985) Failure of Diltiazem to prevent restenosis after percutaneous coronary angioplasty. Am Heart J 109:926–931
4. Holmes DR, Vlietstra RE, Smith HC et al. (1984) Restenosis after percutaneous transluminal coronary angioplasty (PTCA): a report from the PTCA registry of the National Heart, Lung and Blood Institute. Am J Cardiol 53:77C–81C
5. Kaltenbach M, Kober G, Sherer D, Vallbracht C (1985) Recurrence rate after successful angioplasty. Eur Heart J 6:276–281
6. McCullagh P, Nelder A (1983) Generalized linear models. Chapman and Hall Ltd. Ed. University Press, Cambridge, Chapter 4, pp 72–99
7. Oriol A, Guiteras P, Augé JM, Masotti M, Peraza C, Crexells C (1985) Clinical, angiographic and procedural factors presumably related to persistent success after PTCA. Proceedings, Salzburg 1985
8. Thornton MA, Grüntzig AR, Hollman J, King SB, Douglas JS (1984) Coumadin and aspirin in prevention of recurrence after transluminal coronary angioplasty: a randomized study. Ther Prevent 69:721–727

Percutaneous Transluminal Coronary Angioplasty in the Management of Recurrent Angina Pectoris Following Coronary Bypass Grafting

PH. BETTENDORFF, J. M. HABICHT, M. OULHACI, P. VALENTI, J. MARCO, and E. HAUF

From July 1983 through April 1985, we performed 2929 coronary bypass operations, including 129 reoperations. The percentage of reoperations has increased each year, going from 3.5% in 1983 to 8.7% in 1985. Confirming the results reported in the literature [8], our reoperations had a nonnegligible mortality and morbidity rate.

Introduced in 1977, percutaneous transluminal coronary angioplasty (PTCA) has given a new approach to the treatment of coronary obstruction. Because of its reliability, we have proposed this alternative to 32 patients who have developed restenosis after CABP (Coronary Artery By-Pass).

Patients and Methods

Our series included 32 patients – 29 men (90%) and 3 women (10%) – with multivessel disease who had undergone myocardial revascularization (2.5 bypasses/patient) for angina pectoris, mainly postinfarction. The mean age was 53 years, ranging from 43 to 71 years. Each patient had one or several new lesions involving either the bypass, the distal segment of the bypassed vessel, or another coronary artery. The interval between operation and PTCA ranged from 3 months to 8 years, with a mean interval of 20.7 months. Thirty-five percent of the patients had angina pectoris NYHA class I or II, and 65% were in NYHA class II or IV.

The technique and protocol of transluminal angioplasty are now classical. After i.v. administration of 10000 U heparin and sublingual administration of 20 mg nifedipine, the infusion of 500 cc Rheomacrodex (dextran 40) is started. Coronary arteriography is performed using a guide catheter to locate the stenoses and assess their importance. An H-torque wire is then introduced, along which the dilatation catheter (Simpson-Robert or other) will be advanced. After intracoronary injection of 300 μg trinitrin, the dilatation catheter is pushed to the site of the stenosis and inflated successively and progressively with 3–9 atmospheres for 20–60 s.

In this series, we performed a total of 52 dilatations: 22 in bypasses and 30 in coronary arteries.

The stenoses were classified according to their location (Fig. 1) as follows:

- ST_1: lesion at the proximal anastomosis of a graft
- ST_2: lesion on the bypass graft itself
- ST_3: lesion at the distal anastomosis

- ST_4: lesion on the bypassed artery. Dilatation of the lesion of the previously bypassed vessel was performed in ten cases of total bypass occlusion (19% of all angioplasties).
- ST_5: distal lesion with regard to the implanted graft, including lesions having developed on nonbypassed vessels

Lesions of the diagonal artery were included with the lesions of LAD.

We observed that 50% of the patients in this series (16/32) underwent PTCA *within 12 months* following their bypass operation, and that the lesions were mainly in ST_1, ST_2, and ST_3 (18 of 28 lesions, i.e., 64%). On the other hand, after 1 year, we found mainly lesions related with progression of the disease (ST_5) (13 of 24 lesions, i.e., 54%).

Seventeen of 52 lesions (33%) were dilated *within 6 months* following the bypass operation. Eight lesions involved the LAD, four the RCA, and five the circumflex artery. Most of the lesions were located on the bypass graft itself (12%) or at the site of its distal anastomosis (52%).

Eleven lesions (21%) were treated by PTCA *6–12 months* after the operation. Ten dilatations were performed in LAD territory, one in RCA territory. Here again, most of the lesions involved the bypass: 9% the graft itself and 54% its distal anastomosis.

Twenty-four lesions (46%) were dilated *12 months or more* after the operation: ten in the LAD territory, four in the RCA territory, and ten in the circumflex territory. In this group, however, most of the lesions concerned the coronary arteries: 25% in ST_4 and 54% in ST_5 (Fig. 2).

Table 1 shows the number of stenoses in relation to the involved coronary territory and to location:

- Twenty-eight lesions affected the LAD territory.
- Stenoses of the proximal anastomosis or of the body of the graft (ST_1 and ST_2 respectively) were rare. Seventeen lesions were located at the site of the distal anastomosis (ST_3) and 19 lesions belonged to ST_5.
- Out of these 19 ST_5 lesions, 11 affected previously bypassed vessels, and 8 affected nonbypassed vessels. The appearance of lesions in nonbypassed vessels gives true information on the progress of the coronary disease with time. The mean interval between CABG and PTCA in this group was 34 months.

Table 1. Number of stenoses in relation to the involved coronary territory and to location

	ST_1	ST_2	ST_3	ST_4	ST_5	
Right		1	4	1	3	9
LAD	2	3	11	5	7	[28]
CX			2	4	9	15
	2	4	[17]	10	[19] (11 Grafted / 8 Ungrafted)	52

LAD, left anterior descending artery; Cx (Circumflex artery)

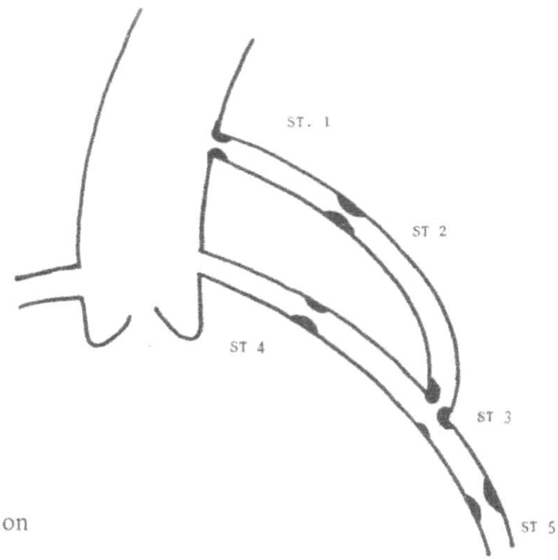

Fig. 1. Location of the stenosis: classification

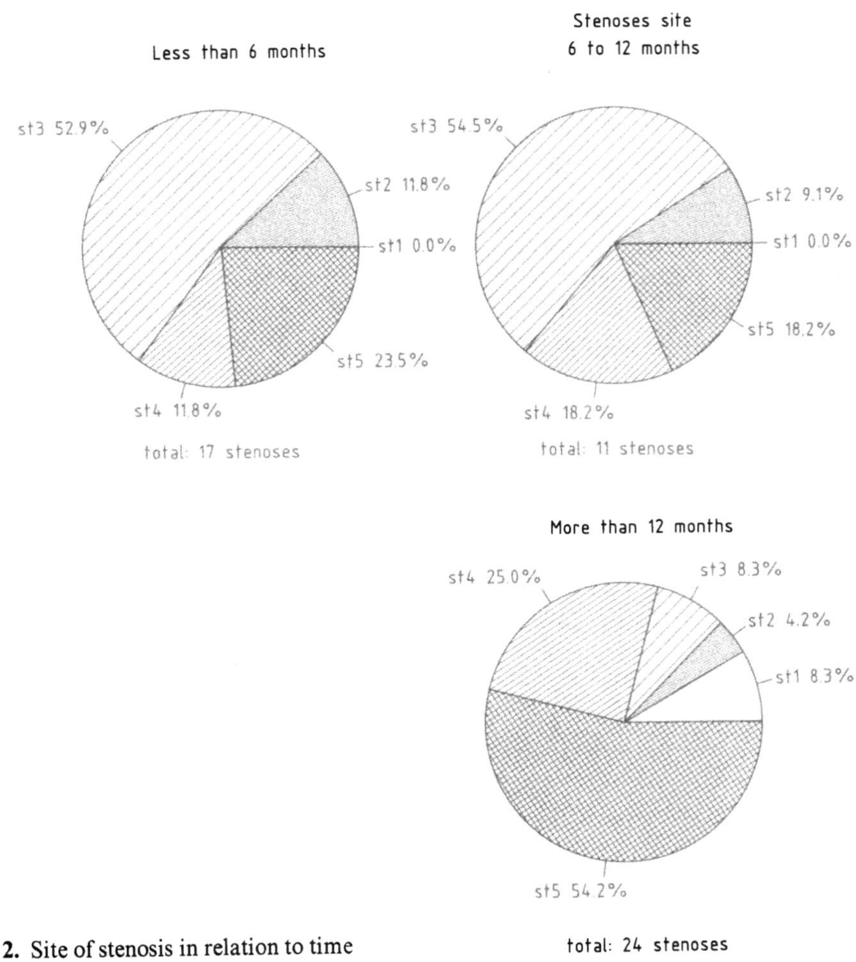

Fig. 2. Site of stenosis in relation to time

Results

Out of 52 dilatations, 46 were successful in 29 patients (91%). The mean gain with regard to the lumen at the site of the lesion was 66%, ranging from 20% to 85%. We had no death, no emergency operation, no ECG alterations to report. The enzymes were checked systematically after each dilatation; no significant increase of the CK-MB (Creatine Kinase-Myocardial Isoenzyme) was noted.

Analyzing the gain (Table 2) with regard to the location of the stenosis, we observed that:

- The number of dilatations in ST_1 and ST_2 is too small to be representative.
- There is no significant difference between the gain obtained in ST_2, ST_3, and ST_4 (69% – 72%), but the gain is significantly smaller in ST_5 (61%).
- Failure rate is identical no matter where PTCA was attempted.
- We had one case of peripheral embolism of stratified material inside the bypass. We noted transitory electric modification with angina pectoris, but no electrocardiographic or enzymatic signs of myocardial infarction were observed.

There is a homogenous distribution of the gain obtained in all coronary territories concerned (62% – 73%), but we note a 20% failure rate in the circumflex territory vs. 11% in the LAD territory. There were no failures in the RCA territory.

Analyzing our six failures, we note that the three complete failures in three patients were caused by the impossibility of reaching across and dilating the stenosis, and resulted in elective surgery. One totally unsuccessful dilatation concerned the stenosis of a proximal anastomosis, which was corrected by the implantation of a new bypass. The other two complete failures concerned stenosis of the distal anastomosis, which had to be corrected with patches.

With regard to the three partial failures, they were partial because we were dealing with multiple stenoses of which only one could be dilated. Two patients had additional distal lesions on the diagonal artery and on the circumflex artery, respectively; the dilated lesion, however, showed an 80% gain. PTCA improved these two patients' condition considerably. The third patient had had three bypasses 15 months earlier: the RCA bypass was still patent, but the LAD

Table 2. Gain with regard to the location of the stenosis

	Number of successes	Gain %	Number of failures	Failures
ST_1	1	50	1	
ST_2	4	69	0 (+1 embolism)	
ST_3	15	70	2	11
ST_4	9	72	1	10
ST_5	17	61	2	10
		66		

and circumflex bypasses were thrombosed. His ejection fraction was of less than 30%. The indication, therefore, was probably doubtful. In spite of the successful dilatation of the LAD stenosis, obtaining a 70% gain, the patient had a sudden blood pressure drop and had to be assisted with an aortic balloon for 3 days. Therefore, dilatation of the circumflex artery was not performed but in spite of that the patient improved from NYHA class III to NYHA class II. Unfortunately, he died 4 months later from progressive heart failure.

Follow-up

In our center as in many others, it is difficult to study the patient's follow-up, for we inevitably lose track of some of our patients who should have follow-up coronary angiographies even if they are asymptomatic. Only 20 of the 29 patients (69%) having had a successful PTCA could be followed-up regularly (Fig. 3). The mean follow-up was 11.8 months, ranging between 3 and 25 months.

Three patients (15%) had recurrent symptoms and needed a second dilatation after which they returned to their predilatation NYHA class, i.e. class I for 2 of them and class II for the other. Recheck angiography of these three patients prior to the second dilatation showed total recurrence of the stenosis at the site of dilatation. Redilatation resulted in a lasting gain of 80%.

Altogether, 13 patients of the followed-up group, who had had a total of 16 dilatations approximately 5 months earlier, had recheck coronary angiography either because of recurrent symptoms or in the course of a routine check-up. Five of the restenoses (32%) were total: three of them were redilated, and two were treated medically since the patients were asymptomatic. With regard to location, two stenoses recurred at the site of the distal anastomosis and three on the coronary arteries. These three restenoses of the coronary arteries were the ones to be redilated successfully with a lasting gain of 80%. The follow-up an-

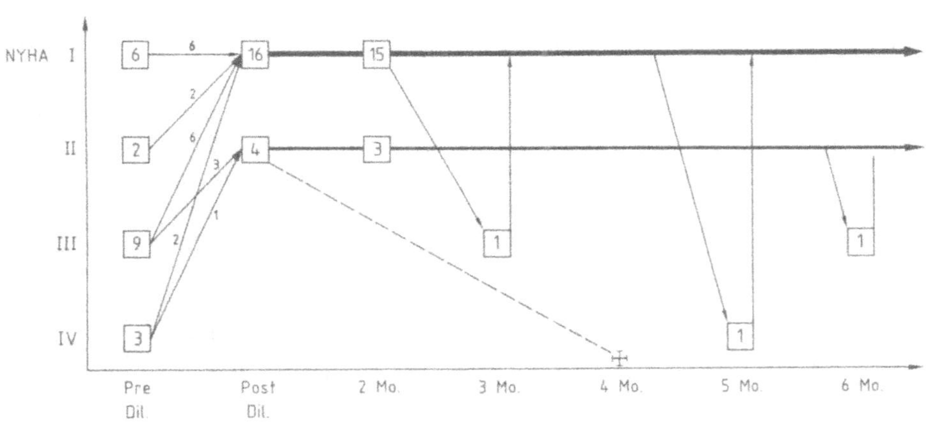

Fig. 3. Follow-up

giography revealed a mean gain loss of 11.5% for the other 11 dilated stenoses; the patients were totally asymptomatic, and the stenoses were equally distributed among groups ST_3 and ST_5.

All the patients with positive ergometry below 100 W (12 of 20) prior to PTCA improved significantly by an average of 50 W after dilatation. The other patients with ergometry performance of more than 100 W also improved, but less significantly.

Discussion

Following coronary artery surgery, recurrence or aggravation of the symptomatology occurs at a rate of 5%–10% a year [6]. Consequently, 7% of the patients operated on up to this date will probably need a reoperation in the next 10 years [11].

Redo-surgery is constantly improving [11], but it still has a nonnegligible mortality and morbidity rate. Even though redo-surgery represents a more radical solution with possibly better long-term results [12], the alternative of PTCA should not be forgotten and should be offered to patients with recurrent symptoms – type of lesions and hemodynamics permitting. Furthermore, PTCA will probably be more readily accepted by the patients.

When analyzing the gain obtained after dilatation, we did not always consider the transstenotic gradient. We may be criticized on this point, although other teams [10] deny the relevance of gradient measurements in peripheral arteries because of their nonnegligible margin of errors. The extent of the stenoses was assessed by studying the most severe lumen reduction in the photograms. Furthermore, the possibility of spasms [1] was eliminated by the intracoronary injection of either calcium channel blockers or trinitrin. Confirming the findings of other authors [6, 8], we observed that approximately 50% of the lesions in our series recur during the 1st year after bypass surgery. Of these lesions, 64% are located either at the site of the anastomoses or on the bypass graft itself. On the contrary, after these first 12 months, most of the recurrent lesions are found on the coronary arteries. Let us mention that in nonbypassed vessel, atheromatous lesions susceptible of being dilated develop within a period of approximately 4 years (33.9 months).

The mean gain of 66% which we obtained corresponds to the mean gain reported after PTCA by other teams [9]; our gain was significantly lower when the stenoses were located in the distal part of coronary arteries, and our failure rate was significantly higher when they involved the circumflex territory.

When attempting to assess the value of dilatation according to the site of the lesion, we noted that:

- The number of patients with lesions at the site of the proximal anastomoses was relatively small in our series. Therefore, we are not in a position to confirm the findings of other authors [6, 8] who reported difficulty in dilating this kind of stenotic lesions because of difficult catheterization and of frequently fibrotic and rigid vessels at the site of the lesions. The restenosis rate

is approximately 50% after 1 year and increases in a parallel direction with the age of the bypasses.
- Lesions located on the bypass itself run the risk of embolization if the graft has been in place for more than 12 months [2, 5]. Furthermore, the restenosis rate is 50%–60% at this location. Therefore, dilatation is best indicated in the case of lesions recurring early after bypass surgery.
- When dealing with lesions at the site of the distal anastomoses or on coronary arteries, PTCA is technically easy. These two sites represent good indications for dilatation, the more so as the recurrence rate (14%–40%) is lower than for dilatations at other locations [2, 4–6, 8].

The mortality rate for PTCA reported in the literature [3] is 0.9%. It may reach 2.5% for dilatation in previously bypassed territories, with preexistent impairment of the left ventricular function as it is often the case in multivessel disease. Our statistics show no early death and no incidence of myocardial infarction, but a failure rate of 11.5% (6 of 52 dilatations) requiring elective surgery in three patients.

Eighty percent of the patients were asymptomatic (NYHA I) after an average of 11.8 months. Other developed recurrent symptoms and needed redilatation, with good result. Redilatations often have a good prognosis and a longer-lasting effect than first dilatations [13] because restenoses are generally less severe and because the tissues show less mechanical resistance.

Some patients remained symptomatic even though their follow-up angiography revealed restenoses. This phenomenon is not uncommon since it is reported in 24% of the cases of the PTCA registry [7], and can be explained on the basis of the currently available data on the pathophysiology of angina. Actually, only functionally significant stenoses result in angina.

All patients, apart from the one who died later, are now in NYHA class I or II, and 70% (14 of 20) are event-free. Event-free patients are those who have had no symptoms, infarction, redilatation, or reoperation.

In spite of the nonnegligible percentage of restenosis, PTCA is to be considered in the case of recurrent symptomatology after CABG. It appears to be a very good indication when dealing with stenoses of the native arteries or of the distal anastomosis of bypasses, and a relatively good indication when dealing with stenosis of the bypass grafts themselves, of the proximal anastomosis, or in patients with low ejection fraction.

On the basis of these data, one must choose the solution most appropriate for each patient; however, patients will probably prefer PTCA to reoperation.

References

1. Atkinson JB, Forman MB, Perry JM, Virmani R (1985) Correlation of saphenous vein bypass graft angiograms with histologic changes at necropsy. Am J Cardiol 55:952–955
2. Dorros G, Johnson WD, Tector AJ, Schmahl TM, Kalush SL, Janke L (1984) Percutaneous transluminal coronary angioplasty in patients with prior coronary artery bypass grafting. J Thorac Cardiovasc Surg 87:17–26

3. Dorros G, Cowley MJ, Janke L, Kelsey MF, Mullin SM, van Raden M (1984) In-hospital mortality rate in the national heart, lung, and blood institute percutaneous transluminal coronary angioplasty registry. Am J Cardiol 53:17 C – 21 C
4. El Gamal M, Bonnier H, Michels R, Heijman J, Stassen E (1984) Percutaneous transluminal angioplasty of stenosed aortocoronary bypass grafts. Br Heart J 52:617 – 620
5. Ford WB, Wholey MH, Zikria EA et al. (1980) Percutaneous transluminal angioplasty in the management of occlusive disease involving the coronary arteries and saphenous vein bypass grafts. J Thorac Cardiovasc Surg 79:1 – 11
6. Hall D, Corzo O, Douglas J, Gruentzig ARC (1984) Percutaneous transluminal coronary angioplasty in patients with prior coronary bypass surgery. Int J Cardiol 6:645 – 650
7. Holmes DR Jr et al. (1984) Restenosis after percutaneous transluminal coronary angioplasty (PICA): a report from the PTCA registry of the National Heart, Lung, and Blood Institute. Am J Cardiol 53:77 C – 81 C
8. Jones EL, Douglas JS, Gruentzig AR, Craver JM, King SB, Guyton RA, Hatcher CR (1983) Percutaneous saphenous vein angioplasty to avoid reoperative bypass surgery. Ann Thorac Surg 36, 4:389 – 395
9. Kent KM, Bentivoglio LG, Block PC et al. (1982) Percutaneous transluminal coronary angioplasty: report from the Registry of the National Heart, Lung and Blood Institute. Am J Cardiol 49:2011 – 2019
10. Kornfeld J (1985) PTCA pressures are misleading. Cardiol News pp 12 – 15
11. Loop FD, Lytle BW, Gill CC, Golding LAR, Cosgrove DM, Taylor PC (1983) Trends in selection and results of coronary artery reoperations. Ann Thorac Surg 36, 4:380 – 388
12. Mills NL (1983) Reop or Not. Ann Thorac Surg 36:375 – 376
13. Williams DO, Gruentzig AR, Kent KM, Detre KM, Kelsey SF, To T (1984) Efficacy of repeat percutaneous transluminal coronary angioplasty for coronary restenosis. Am J Cardiol 53:32 C – 35 C

Percutaneous Transluminal Coronary Angioplasty with Dislocated Cardiac Surgery

G. Alber and O. Bosse

Since the introduction of the method by Andreas Grüntzig in 1977, percutaneous transluminal coronary angioplasty (PTCA) with balloon catheters has been developed into a third therapeutic method which is used worldwide in addition to medical and operative methods of treating coronary heart disease. Both pioneers of the method and present-day cardiologists have demanded the immediate availability of a cardiac surgical team on standby – if possible in the same setting – as one of the essential conditions for performing the method. But this demand has been fulfilled only by a *few* bigger cardiologic centers. The waiting times have approached those of bypass surgery. On the other hand, increased experience and advanced technique have improved the PTCA procedure and therefore numerous cardiologists, especially in the United States, have begun to perform balloon dilatations even without a directly available surgical unit. In the case of an emergency they transfer the patients by car or helicopter to the next cardiac surgery hospital. This procedure certainly is not without problems and especially Grüntzig and Kaltenbach have warned against it and have demanded additional precautions formulated by Hopf and Kunkel [5]. However, it has been shown by many authors, that PTCAs could be performed also in a hospital without cardiac surgery, given severe indications and an immediately available surgical standby, without any statistically provable additional hazards for the patient (J. Meyer, Mainz/T. Ischinger, Munich).

Methods and Results

The Department of Cardiology in the hospital of Traunstein (FRG) therefore after a 2-year experience in Munich (Stiftsklinik Augustinum/Herzchirurgische Klinik der Universität München) began to perform coronary angioplasties. Traunstein is a small town in southeast Bavaria and has a hospital with a modern, well-equipped cardiologic department and a wide admission area. The first 21 PTCAs (out of 162) were performed by the staff of our hospital in the operating theater of the cardiac surgery of the University of Munich (director Prof. Dr. W. Klinner). Since 1984 we have performed all PTCAs in Traunstein under good operative conditions but with a 100-km distant surgical standby in Munich and a ready helicopter at the hospital. During this period two patients had to be transferred to a emergency operation in Munich. The outcome of these cases is seen in Table 1.

Table 1. Patients given emergency cardiac surgery

Patient	Complication	Cardiac surgery	Transport time	Outcome
1. W. R. m. 55y.	Pericardial tamponade by vessel rupture	Munich	40 min Helicopter	OK
2. M. W. m. 58 y.	RCA occlusion by unsuccessful attempt	Munich	50 min Helicopter	Posterior infarction
3. N. F. m. 60 y.	LAD occlusion by dissection	Salzburg	22 min Helicopter	Nontransmural infarction
4. W. J. m. 47 y.	LAD occlusion by unsuccessful attempt	Salzburg	19 min Helicopter	No infarction
5. A. H. m. 49 y.	LAD stenosis increasing (thrombus)	Salzburg	16 min Helicopter	No infarction
6. St. D. m. 63 y.	Intermittent LAD occlusion by dissection	Salzburg	50 min	No infarction

The first patient had pericardial bleeding after rupture of a small diagonal branch after the balloon was inflated in the wrong vessel. After 40 min he was in the operation room. The bleeding had stopped spontaneously and he underwent bypass grafting.

The second patient had an occlusion of the right coronary artery in an unsuccessful attempt to pass a high-degree stenosis. He had reached the operation room after 50 min and in spite of patent bypass 90 min after occlusion of the RCA he suffered a posterior infarction.

From March 1985 the new Department of Cardiac Surgery of Salzburg (Prof. Dr. F. Unger) gave us a surgical standby at a distance of only 30 km and reachable by helicopter within 6–12 min. During PTCA the operation room is kept free and the surgical staff are ready. During the period March to September 1985 we have had a higher incidence of 4 emergency cases out of 55 PTCAs.

Two patients showed a total occlusion of the left anterior descending artery (LAD) by dissection or an unsuccessful attempt to pass the stenosis. Another patient had an incomplete occlusion by a growing thrombus and the last patient an intermittent occlusion by dissection (and spasm?). All four patients from the "Salzburg period" received a single graft; only the first one (patient No. 3 in Table 1) suffered an infarction. Finally, out of 162 PTCAs and out of 129 elective PTCAs, 6 patients (3.7% and 4.6% respectively) underwent an emergency bypass grafting in an external cardiac surgery center. All six patients survived, one suffered a transmural, another a nontransmural, infarction. The PTCA procedure was performed as previously described [8], by transfemoral approach with guiding and balloon catheters (Schneider). Initially, we used balloon catheters with fixed guide wire, later catheters with steerable and exchangeable long wire. The premedication was carried out with 100 ml low molecular weight

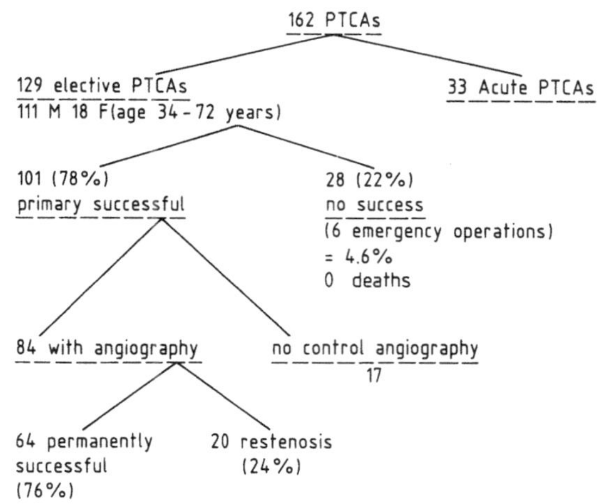

Fig. 1. Outcome of 162 PTCAs performed between 1 July 1983 and 30 September 1985 at the hospital in Traunstein

dextran, 10000 units i.v. heparin, 100 mg acetylsalicylic acid orally, and 3×10 mg nifedipin. During PTCA the patient received nitroglycerin only and/or nifedipin orally or directly into the coronaries. Thirty-three out of 162 PTCAs were "acute PTCAs" in acute infarctions with or without thrombolysis. In these cases surgical standby was not possible and not necessary (Fig. 1).

Discussion

The requirement for a surgical standby immediately available during elective coronary angioplasty can be of life-saving importance for the individual patient, but from a statistical viewpoint and from experience so far it is not justified.

Satter and Scherer [7] demonstrated (Table 2) that in spite of rapid emergency operation in the same hospital after vessel occlusion in PTCA an infarction mostly cannot be avoided. Murphy and Craver (Atlanta) came to similar results [6]. The times of ischemia between the occluding event and a working bypass were 40–240 min and 75–210 min respectively. These rather long times were

Table 2. Results of rapid emergency operations after vessel occlusion in PTCA [6, 7]

Frankfurt	
39 Emergency operations	31 infarctions 2 deaths
Ischemia time	40–240 min
Atlanta	
17 emergency operations	12 infarctions No deaths
Ischemia time	135 min (75–210 min)

presumably due to operation theaters not being kept free. For disposal only the next free room was available. The surviving time of myocardium is 20 min in the most unfavorable case, and therefore an infarction mostly cannot be avoided.

On the other hand, if all present-day working cardiologic centers without cardiac surgery dropped PTCA, the waiting times for PTCA would exceed those of bypass surgery, with the consequence of an increasing number of infarctions and deaths during the waiting time. Especially patients after thrombolysis in acute infarctions or with unstable angina must be revascularized as early as possible. In the light of our results (Table 3), we believe that coronary an-

Table 3. Results with PTCA

	n	Primary success	Restenosis	Emergency ACVBG	Deaths
Early NHLBI	1939	65%	25%	7.1%	0.8%
Recent results of:					
Atlanta			27%		
Richmond	1551	92%	25%	2.6%	0.12%
Piladelphia			12%		
(pooled)					
Frankfurt 1984	762	78%	17%	5.1%	0.26%
Own results 7/83–9/85	129 elective PTCA's	78%	24%	4.6%	0

ACVBG, aorto-coronar-venous-bypass-graft

Table 4. Indications for elective PTCA

1. Single-vessel proximal high-degree stenosis with documented ischemia and/or angina but *not* left main stem disease
2. Two-vessel disease of two *not* supplemental arteries
3. ACVB (aorto-coronary-venous-bypass) stenosis with angina
4. High-degree stenosis after thrombolysis in infarction-related artery:
   a) As in 1) or 2)
   b) With unstable postinfarction angina
5. Two-vessel disease with one vessel occluded and supplied by the other narrowed vessel
6. Short-time-short-distance-occluded vessels

Table 5. Indications for emergency operation after unsuccessful PTCA

1. Dissection with occlusion
2. Dissection with growing thrombus
3. Large dissection with ischemia signs
4. Unsuccessful attempt to bypass the stenosis with:
   a) Vessel occlusion } in spite of
   b) ECG signs of ischemia } nitroglycerin, nifedipine

gioplasty can be done and is justified also in cardiologic centers without cardiac surgery, if the following conditions are fulfilled:

1. A surgical standby must be available, because a bypass graft is sometimes of life-saving importance.
2. The operation room should be kept free and prepared for the arriving patient. The duration of ischemia than is no longer than in catheter labs with surgery (< 120 min).
3. There are severe indications for PTCA which are carefully considered, and there are no high-risk cases (Table 4).
4. An early decision for bypass is made in the case of an unsuccessful attempt (Table 5).
5. The PTCA team is experienced.

These requirements were recently confirmed at the third autumn session of the Gesellschaft für Herz-Kreislaufforschung in Vienna also by J. Meyer (Mainz) and T. Ischinger (Munich). The satisfaction of these requirements guarantees our patients an early date for PTCA without additional risks from the procedure itself or from a long waiting time, reducing the mortality and incidence of infarcts.

References

1. Baim DS (1985) Coronary angioplasty 1985: technical and clinical considerations. Herz 10:269–274
2. Bentivoglio LG (1985) Immediate and long-term results of percutaneous transluminal coronary angioplasty. Herz 10:275–280
3. Dorros G, Cowley MJ et al. (1983) Percutaneous transluminal coronary angioplasty. Report of complications from the NHLBI PTCA Registry. Circulation 67:723
4. Faxon D, Kelsey SF et al. (1984) Determinants of successful percutaneous transluminal coronary angioplasty: Report from the National Heart, Lung and Blood Institute Registry. Am Heart J 108:1019
5. Hopf R, Kunkel B et al. (1985) Koronarperfusion bei akutem Gefäßverschluß im Rahmen der transluminalen Koronarangioplastik (TCA). Z Kardiol 74:580–584
6. Murphy AD, Craver JM et al. (1982) Surgical revascularization following unsuccessful percutaneous transluminal coronary angioplasty. J Thorac Cardiovasc Surg 84:342–348
7. Satter P, Scherer D (1985) Der akute aorto-koronare Bypass bei Komplikationen nach Katheterdilatation der Koronararterien. Dtsch Med Wochenschr 110 [14]:540
8. Seidel F, Alber G et al. (1983) Transluminale Koronardilatation. Fortschr Med 101 [45]:2065

III. Surgical Techniques

Myocardial Revascularization in Septuagenarians and Beyond

A. Fletcher, C. Voleti, W. Brenner, H. Dajee, P. Sidhu, M. Singh, J. Livermore, and S. Khonsari

Myocardial revascularization began about 18 years ago. Over the years the results of coronary artery bypass graft surgery have been evaluated and reevaluated many times, and its role in the management of patients with coronary artery disease has now become well established. However, indications for its utilization continue to be refined.

Previous reports by Anderson and Rahimtoola [1] have introduced the concept of "time frame" and its influence on the results of revascularization surgery. Analysis of data collected over this 18-year period reveals an important qualitative improvement in the group of patients operated on since 1974 as the later time frame, as compared with the group operated on prior to 1974, the earlier time frame. The 8-year survival rate is 76±2% for the patients operated upon between 1968 and 1973, and 83±1.3% in the group operated on since 1974 [2].

The dramatic improvement in the later group is due to many important factors. An enormous increase in the frequency with which coronary artery bypass surgery is performed has naturally given rise to greater surgical expertise and superior operative technique. The number of coronary arteries grafted per patient has increased since 1974 in order to achieve maximal revascularization. The introduction of Prolene as a refined suture material has improved the quality of anastomoses. Hemodynamic monitoring in the postoperative period has facilitated the care of the critically ill patient, thus adding to the safety of the operation. Cardiovascular parameters can be manipulated for optimum cardiac function through the use of pharmacologic agents such as nitroglycerin, nitroprusside, beta blockers, and calcium antagonists. Intraaortic balloon counterpulsation has also been helpful in augmenting cardiac performance in selected groups of patients with poor left ventricular function [3].

Analyzing our data shows that patients in the current time frame are at higher risk than those in the earlier time frame due to age, number of diseased vessels, and incidence of wall motion abnormalities. Therefore, it seems clear that coronary artery bypass surgery since 1974 has become an entity quite different from the operation performed in the earlier time frame. For these reasons, a review and analysis of results obtained from only those patients operated on during the past year from the current time frame will reflect our true experience and current philosophy as to the management of patients with ischemic heart disease in the 1990s.

Table 1. Profile and parameters in the two age groups of patients ($n = 548$)

Age (years)	≦69	≧70
Number of patients	464	84
Average age	58.7	73.2
Sex		
Male	398	65
Female	66	19
% female	14.2	22.6
Unstable angina (%)	5	17
Left main disease (%)	7	11
Stay CSU (days)	3.46	3.92
Stay PO (days)	9.7	11.3
Deaths	10	7
Mortality (%)	2.2	8.3
Chronic hospitalization (> 30 days)	6	3
%	1.3	3.6

Materials and Methods

From 1 June 1984 through 31 July 1985, 548 adult patients who continued to be symptomatic on maximal medical management underwent isolated coronary artery bypass graft (CABG) surgery at the Kaiser Foundation Hospital of Los Angeles. This hospital is a regional referral center for an area of southern California encompassing nearly 2 million people. We compared patients 70 years and older with their younger counterparts (Table 1); 84 patients (15%) were 70 years or older (range 70–85 years). The remaining 464 patients (85%) were 69 years or younger (range 28–69 years). We divided the patients over 70 years of age into two subgroups, those who had isolated coronary artery bypass graft surgery and those who had coronary artery bypass graft surgery plus valve replacement (27 patients). All patients were kept intubated overnight following surgery. The endotracheal tubes were removed when patients were awake and their weaning criteria and continuous positive airway pressure (CPAP) blood gases were satisfactory. Pulmonary artery catheters were used in all patients. They were usually inserted preinduction of anesthesia and were removed when patients were hemodynamically stable and not requiring intravenous ionotropic agents or vasodilator therapy.

Results

The average age of patients over 70 was 73.2 years, compared with 58.7 years for the younger patients (Fig. 1). There were 19 (22.6%) females in the older age group and 66 (16.6%) females in the younger group, a slight increase in the ratio of females in the older group.

The operative mortality was 8.3% for the older group compared with 2.2% for the younger group, which is a 3.8-fold increase in mortality for the older group.

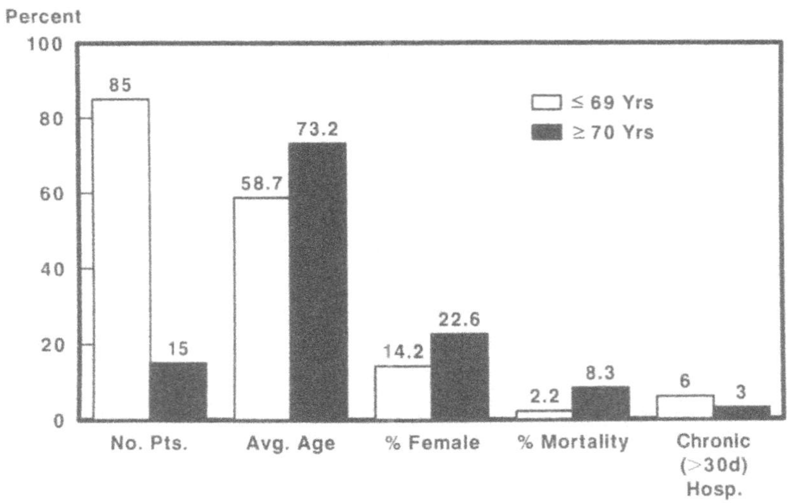

Fig. 1. Comparison of number of patients, age, sex, operative mortality and chronic morbidity in the two age groups of patients

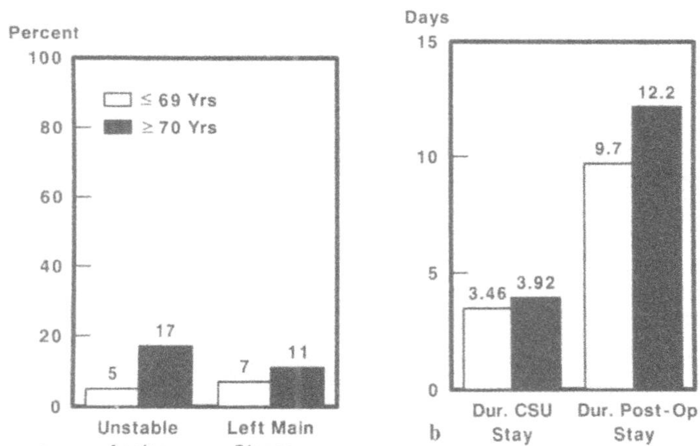

Fig. 2. a Incidence of unstable angina and left main disease in the two age groups of patients. **b** Duration of stay in cardiac surgery intensive care unit (CSU) and postoperative hospital stay in the two age groups of patients

There was a higher incidence of unstable angina (17% vs. 5%) and left main disease (11% vs. 7%) in the older group. Surgery on an emergency or urgent basis was also indicated more frequently (30% vs. 5%) in the older group, which probably contributes to their higher mortality rate.

The average duration of intubation was essentially the same for both groups and likewise there was no significant difference in the length of hemodynamic monitoring (Fig. 2).

The cardiac surgery intensive care unit (CSU) stay, which we considered the early recovery period, was 3.92 days for the older group and 3.46 days for the younger group. Total postsurgical hospital stay for the older patients was 1.6 days longer than for the younger ones, 11.3 days as compared with 9.7 days.

There were three patients (3.6%) in the older group and six patients (1.3%) in the younger group requiring prolonged hospitalization (> 30 days) due to postsurgical complications.

There was no significant difference in the average age between the two subgroups of older patients (Table 2). There was, however, a significant increase in the percentage of female patients requiring coronary artery bypass graft surgery plus valve replacement (30% vs. 22.6%). There was a higher mortality rate in the patients who had coronary artery bypass graft surgery plus valve replacement (14.8% vs. 8.3%).

Table 2. Profile and parameters in the older group of patients according to whether myocardial revascularization was performed in isolation or with concomitant valvular surgery

	CABG	CABG+valves
No. of patients	84	27
Average age	73.2	73.7
Sex		
Male	65	20
Female	19	8
% female	22.6	30
Duration intubation (h)	27	26.4
Duration PA catheter (h)	57	59.3
Stay CSU (days)	3.92	3.76
Stay PO (days)	11.3	12.2
Deaths	7	4
Mortality (%)	8.3	14.8

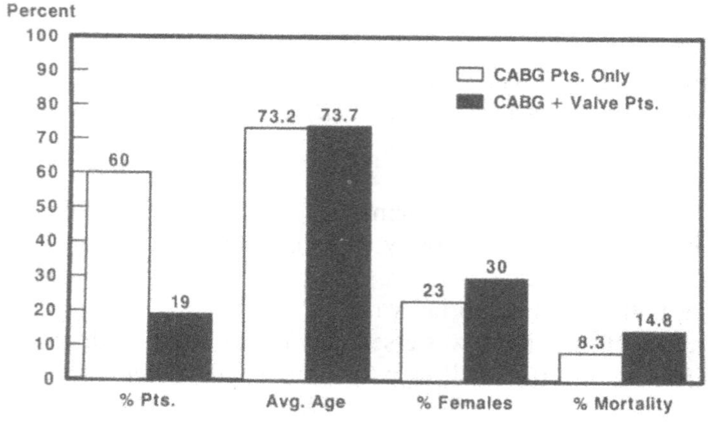

Fig. 3. Comparison of ratio, age, sex and operative mortality in the older group of patients with isolated myocardial revascularization and those with concomitant valvular surgery

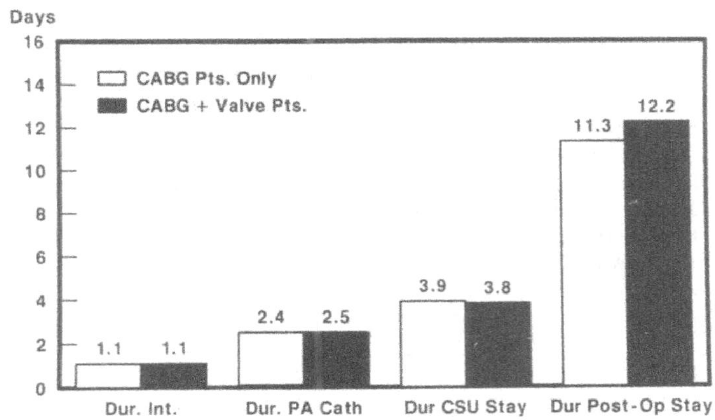

Fig. 4. Comparison of duration of intubation and PA catheterization, time in CSU and postoperative hospital stay in the older group of patients with isolated myocardial revascularization and those with concomitant valvular surgery

The average duration of intubation was 1.1 days for both groups. The duration of hemodynamic monitoring was also essentially the same for both groups (2.4 days vs. 2.5 days) (Fig. 3).

Six patients (6%) in the isolated coronary artery bypass graft surgery group and one patient (4%) in the combined procedure group required intraaortic balloon pump for stabilization in the postoperative period.

Although there was no significant difference in the early recovery period (CSU stay) between the two subgroups of patients over 70 years, there was, however, a 1-day increase in the length of postoperative stay for the patients who had coronary artery bypass graft surgery plus valve replacement (Fig. 4). These patients have been followed and are doing well.

Discussion

The development of advanced surgical technique has enabled us to operate on older patients to try to improve their quality of life, a trend which is likely to accelerate in the nineties.

We can probably expect to operate on an increasing number of female patients in the older age group because of their longer average life span. Combined procedures will become more common because calcific and degenerative valvular disease occur with increasing frequency with advancing age.

There may have been some reluctance in the past to operate on these older patients. Many have thus deteriorated in the interim, contributing to their higher mortality rates at surgery. Probably, these patients should be evaluated and refered for surgery earlier.

References

1. Anderson RP, Rahimtoola SH, Bronchek LI, Starr A (1974) The prognosis of patients with coronary artery disease after coronary bypass operations. Time-related progress of 532 patients with disabling angina pectoris. Circulation 50:274
2. Rahimtoola SH, Nunley D, Grunkemeier G, Teply J, Lambert L, Starr A (1983) Ten year survival after coronary bypass surgery for unstable angina. N Engl J Med 308:676
3. Khonsari S, Starr A (1984) Coronary artery bypass surgery: the total experience at the Oregon Health Sciences University. In: Hust JW (ed) Clinical essays on the heart, vol 2. McGraw Hill, New York, p 173

Abstract

Standardized Technique for Complete Revascularization in Diffuse Three-Vessel Disease

M. SCHMUZIGER

The best long-term results can be achieved by revascularization as complete as possible. Complete revascularization in diffuse three-vessel disease implies tactical and technical modifications of the standard revascularization routine. A standardized revascularization technique, using two sequential grafts and considering coronary flow capacities and the problems of postoperative scarring, mechanical graft stress, and even the possibility of late reoperation has been developed.

From December 1983 to August 1985, 149 patients with diffuse three-vessel disease have been revascularized with from five to nine peripheral anastomoses. Ventricular function was excellent or good in 69%, moderate in 25%, and bad in 6%. Aneurysmectomy, valve replacement, or supplementary vascular surgery occurred in 5%. Endarterectomy had to be done in 10% of all patients. Operative mortality was 1.3% (cardiac 0.7%). The perioperative infarction rate was 7%. Satisfactory clinical results in a group of patients often no longer considered as surgical candidates encourage continuation in this direction. The technical and tactical aspects need to be discussed.

Myocardial Revascularization Results in Women Compared with Body Surface Area and Bypassed Vessel Diameter

R. RAGUSA, G. GAMBA, R. RIZZOTTI, F. CONTI, E. TAPPAINER, F. PERANZONI, N. IVIC, and G. BESA

Introduction

It has often been reported in the literature [1–5, 7] that myocardial revascularization surgical results in women are less favorable than in men. This is supported by the fact that both in the operating theater and in postmortem studies [6], women's coronaries look thinner, more ramified, tortuous, with thin and fragile walls. These anatomical findings increase operative risk of both higher infarction and mortality rates. Further studies carried out by Loop et al. [5] pointed out that a small vascular diameter and body surface area involve a higher operative risk. Our aim was to investigate these findings in more detail by comparing bypassed vessel diameter (BVD) and body surface area (BSA) of the female population to surgical results.

Material and Methods

From 1971 to 1985, 2315 patients underwent coronary artery bypass operations at the Cardiovascular Dept. of Verona Hospital, Italy; 2130 were male, 185 female. Our study refers only to patients operated on from January 1979 up to October 1984 for myocardial revascularization only via coronary artery bypass grafting (CABG) representing a homogeneous group as far as surgical techniques and myocardial protection is concerned. The average age of the 132 female patients analyzed in the present study was 57.7 years, maximum 72, minimum 39; 3.8% of patients were asymptomatic, 25% were suffering from effort angina, and 70% from rest angina. Thirty-seven percent showed preoperative myocardial infarction, 38% hypertension, 24% obesity, and 15% diabetes.

According to EF (ejection fraction) impairment, patients were divided into subgroups as follows: 51.5% normal ventricular contraction, 15.7% moderate impairment, and 5.3% severe impairment. In 17.5% of cases EF was not calculated. Average BSA of the 132 operated patients was 1.72 m^2 (Table 3). BSA was divided into three sizes: small, medium, large, respectively, ranging from 1.25–1.45, 1.46–1.75, and 1.76–1.95 m^2 (Table 1). Six percent of patients were small in size, 80% medium, and 14% large. Vessel diameter was measured by probing the inside of the branch after the arteriotomy.

The heart was divided into three sectors, corresponding to the left anterior descending artery (LAD), circumflex artery (CX), and right coronary artery

Table 1. Comparison of BSA and BVD squared per LAD, CX, and RCA sector in 132 patients

Patients	8	106	18
BSA	Small 1.25– 1.45 m²	Medium 1.46– 1.75 m²	Large 1.76– 1.95 m²
BVD			
LAD (1.75 mm)	1.8 mm	1.7 mm	1.8 mm
CX (1.74 mm)	2.0 mm	1.7 mm	1.8 mm
RCA (1.9 mm)	2.0 mm	1.8 mm	2.0 mm

Table 2. Operative mortality and vasculopathy extension ratio

	Patients	Deaths
One-vessel disease	19	–
Two-vessels disease	38	1 (2.6%)
Three-vessel disease	70	4 (5.7%)

(RCA) blood supply areas. For each sector the average diameter of the incised vessels was calculated (Tables 1, 3, 4). Three hundred and fifty-seven bypasses were carried out; the LAD sector registered an average vessel diameter of 1.75 mm, the CX 1.74 mm, and the RCA 1.9 mm. In evaluating the extent of the coronary lesions, we considered only the three main coronary branches: LAD, CX, RCA, leaving aside the secondary ones (Table 2).

Results

The overall operative mortality was 3.7% (five patients), caused by myocardial infarction in four cases, three of them due to early bypass closing, while the fifth patient died from mesenteric thrombosis. One patient suffered from hypertension, one from diabetes, three registered preoperative infarction, and the last suffered from both diabetes and hypertension. Average BSA of the five patients who died was 1.6 m². Eighteen coronary artery bypass graft surgeries (CABGs) were performed; average vessel diameter was 1.43 mm for the LAD branch, 1.5 mm for the CX, and 1.37 for the RCA.

Long-term follow-up, 6 months – 5 years (mean 3.2 years), was based on 121 answers supplied by 127 patients who survived; 84% patients were asymptomatic, 8% showed effort angina, and 5% showed rest angina. Three deaths were reported, and two caused by acute myocardial infarction due to late graft closing, and one caused by pulmonary edema, with a total mortality rate of 3%. No reply to our questionnaires was received in 4.5% of cases.

Statistical correlations between the average BVD and BSA in long-term patients are given in Table 4.

Table 3. Comparison between average bypassed vessel diameter squared per LAD, CX, and RCA sector in the 132 operated patients and 5 deaths

132 operated patients Total bypassed vessels: 357	5 dead patients Total bypassed vessels: 18
LAD 1.75 mm ($P<0.05$)	1.43 mm ($P<0.05$)
CX 1.74 mm (NS)	1.5 mm (NS)
RCA 1.9 mm (NS)	1.37 mm (NS)
Average BSA 1.72 m^2	Average BSA 1.6 m^2

Table 4. Long-term results of BSA and BVD

Patients	Clinical findings	BVD squared per sector (mm)			Average BSA
		LAD	CX	RCA	
102 (84%)	Asymptomatic	1.8	1.8	1.9	1.73 m^2
10 (8%)	Effort angina	1.6	1.8	2.1	1.59 m^2
6 (5%)	Rest angina	1.6	1.5	2.0	1.66 m^2
3 (3%)	Deaths	1.7	1.7	1.5	1.60 m^2
121					

$P=$ NS

Discussion

As already mentioned, few authors [5] emphasize the importance of the BSA related to operative risk, a small BSA producing a higher risk. As far as we are concerned, we have not observed the same results in our female population since the operative and long-term deaths occurred in medium-size patients (BSA ranging between 1.46 and 1.75 m^2) and not in the small ones as expected (Table 3). The accurate study on coronary diameter squared per LAD, CX, RCA sectors gave clear-cut results as for early mortality: in fact death occurred in those patients who had a notably narrower average vessel diameter in the LAD, CX, and RCA sectors (1.43, 1.5, 1.3 mm) than all the other operated ones (1.75, 1.74, 1.9 mm) (Table 3). Such results have shown a statistical significance for the LAD sector only ($P<0.05$), but not for both the CX and RCA sectors (NS). The high vasculopathic severity of two-vessel or three-vessel disease has shown a high operative mortality with double percentage (5.7%) in women with three-vessel disease compared with those with two-vessel disease (2.6%) (Table 2). The correlation between coronary diameter and BSA in asymptomatic, symptomatic, and dead patients at long-term follow-up is meaningless, the figures being almost the same (Table 4): the asymptomatic group patients reported a medium-size BSA, with an average coronary diameter of 1.8 mm for the LAD and CX and 1.9 mm for the RCA; the symptomatic ones have an average BSA which is still within the medium-size range with a large coronary diameter (see Table 1); the three patients who died showed average BSA and a coronary diameter similar to the two previous groups also suffering from three- vessel disease.

Conclusion

The results of the present study are as follows:

1. Operative mortality is significantly higher in patients with a smaller LAD diameter ($P < 0.05$).
2. Operative and long-term mortality is not influenced by the body surface area.
3. Operative mortality is definitely higher in patients suffering from three-vessel disease.

References

1. Barboso G, Fragnito C, Beghi C, Fesani F (1985) Il bypass aorta coronarico nella donna risulati immediati ed a distanza. Chir Toracica 3:134–138
2. Cooley DA, Wukasch DC, Bruno F, Reul GJ Jr, Sandiford FM, Zillgitt SL, Hall RJ (1978) Direct myocardial revascularization: experience with 9364 operations. Thorax 33:411–417
3. Killen DA, Reed WA, Arnold M, MacAllister BD, Bell HH (1982) Coronary artery bypass in women: long-term survival. Ann Thorac Surg 34 [5]:559–563
4. Douglas JS Jr, King SB III, Jones EL, Craver JM, Bradford JM, Hatcher CR (1981) Reduced efficacy of coronary bypass surgery in women. Circulation 64 [Suppl II):11–16
5. Loop FD, Golding LR, Macmillan JP, Cosgrove DM, Lytle BW, Sheldon WC (1983) Coronary artery surgery in women compared with men: analyses of risks and long-term results. J Am Coll Cardiol 2:383–390
6. Spray TL, Roberts WC (1977) Status of the grafts and native coronary arteries proximal and distal to coronary anastomotic sites of aortocoronary bypass grafts. Circulation 55 [5]:741–749
7. Tyras DH, Barner HB, Kaiser GC, Codd JE, Laks H, Wilman VL (1978) Myocardial revascularization in women. Ann Thorac Surg 25 [5]:449–453

Aortocoronary Bypass Procedures Without Cross-Clamping the Aorta

P. SATTER, L. ECKEL, S. KHURI, and E. KRAUSE

Induced ventricular fibrillation is an old method of cardiac arrest still used in aortocoronary bypass surgery mostly combined with intermittent aortic cross-clamping. In our own clinical practice ventricular fibrillation without cross-clamping combined with hypothermia and left ventricular venting yields favorable results. With a continuously perfused myocardium we are theoretically not limited in our operation time. However, opinions about the safety of the method concerning myocardial preservation are still controversial [4, 5].

Method

Aortocoronary bypass grafting (ACBG) is performed in hypothermic ventricular fibrillation without cross-clamping of the aorta including the following conditions:

1. Venting of the left vntricle
2. Hypothermic fibrillation (arterial blood temperature, 25° C)
3. Perfusion pressure, 60 mm Hg
4. Control of bleeding (anastomosis)
   a) Air-water blower
   b) Intraluminal occluder

Distal anastomoses are carried out: first left anterior descending, then right, and finally circumflex coronary artery. After completion of the anastomosis every graft is immediately perfused by a side line from the arterial line with oxygenated blood. Rewarming starts when all the distal anastomoses are finished. After defibrillation, the aortic anastomoses are performed sequentially with the heart beating.

Results

Since August 1983 850 operations have been performed. The first 155 patients with 402 bypasses have been investigated.

Mortality was 0.6% (one patient). Perioperative myocardial infarction occurred in six patients (4%).

Myocardial biopsies ($n = 11$) were studied by electron microscopy and scored according to Flameng [7]: 0, normal structure; 1, granules absent; 2, swollen

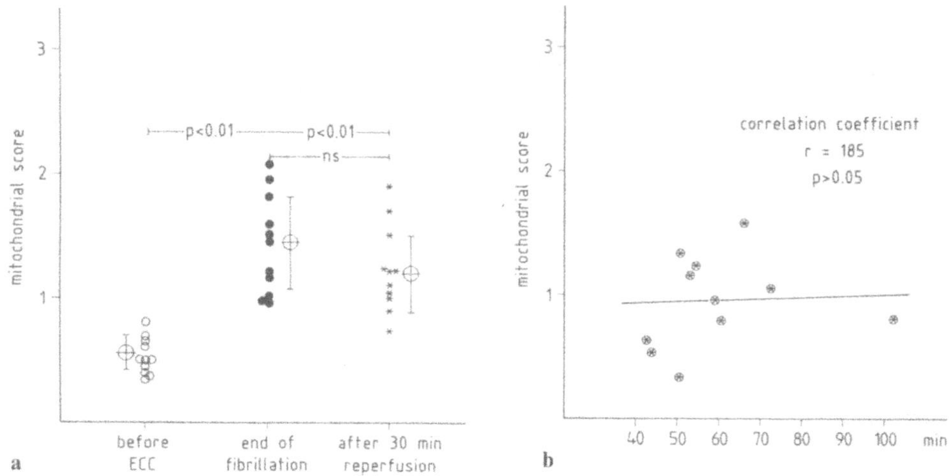

Fig. 1. **a** Mitochondrial score of CABG patients in hypothermic fibrillation. **b** Relationship of mitochondrial score and bypass time

mitochondria; 3, disruption of mitochondrial crests (irreversible damage); and 4, disruption of the crests and inner and outer membrane. The mitochondria are well preserved (score 1–2) and the damage is unrelated to bypass time (Fig. 1).

Experimental Study

To assess the effects of hypothermic ventricular fibrillation on the myocardium, interstitial myocardial pH measuring and estimation of myocardial edema as metabolic parameters were related to global left ventricular function curves. Eighteen dogs were evaluated in a study period of 100 min under extracorporeal circulation, with vented left ventricle and general hypothermia. The dogs were randomly assigned to three study groups. In seven dogs (group I) the heart was kept empty and beating for the period of the study. In five dogs, group II heart was electrically fibrillated at the beginning of the study period and electrically defibrillated at its completion. In six dogs (group III) the heart was fibrillated and the aorta cross-clamped intermittently for periods of 15 min alternating with periods of reperfusion of 5 min duration. At the completion of the study period, the heart was electrically defibrillated.

Myocardial Temperature

The integrated mean myocardial temperatures for the study period, 27.2° (I), 28.1° (II), and 27.1° (III), were not statistically different.

Intramyocardial pH of Left Ventricle

Intramyocardial pH was monitored continuously (Fig. 2).

The mean integrated pH for the study period and the drop of pH (ΔpH) from baseline to study period were not significantly different between groups I (−0.09) and II (−0.06). In contrast endomyocardial pH was significantly lower and the pH was much greater in group III (−0.34) than in both groups I and II.

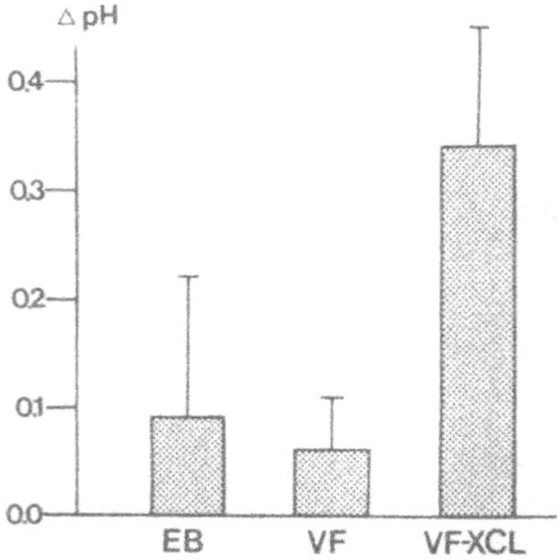

Fig. 2. Quantification of the myocardial acidosis during the study period of empty beating (*EB*), fibrillation (*VF*), and fibrillation with intermittent aortic cross-clamping (*XCL*). *ΔpH*, difference between the baseline pH and the mean integrated pH of the study period

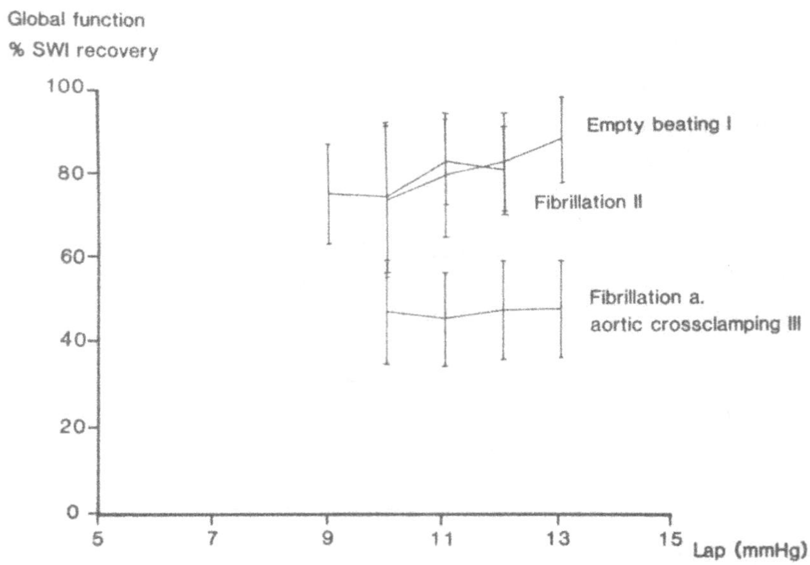

Fig. 3. Global left ventricular function after the study period. Percentage stroke work index recovery

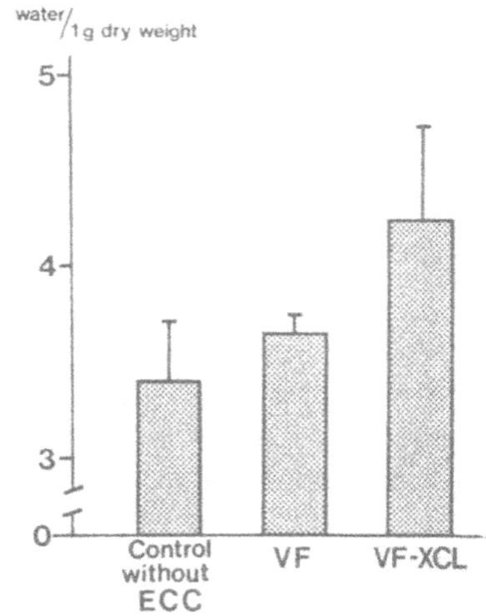

Fig. 4. Myocardial edema after fibrillation (*VF*) and fibrillation with aortic cross-clamping (*VF-XCL*) during extracorporeal circulation (*ECC*)

Global Left Ventricular Function

Function curves were obtained just prior to and soon after cardiopulmonary bypass (Fig. 3).

Function was depressed after the study period in all the groups. The recovery of function as measured by the comparison between pre- and post-bypass function curves was similar in groups I and II (81.5%; 78.6%). In contrast the percentage recovery of function in group III (56.9%) was significantly depressed when compared with groups I and II.

Myocardial Edema

Myocardial edema at the end of the study period was measured in the right and left ventricles in groups II and III. The results (mean $\pm$ SD) are detailed in Fig. 4. The water content of the left ventricle in the group with fibrillation (II) was slightly increased (+7%) compared with a control group without ECC. However, in the group fibrillating with intermittent aortic cross-clamping (III), water content was significantly raised (+24%).

Discussion

The goal of our investigation was to answer the question how safe is myocardial protection with the technique of hypothermic ventricular fibrillation in the continuously perfused and vented heart.

Our experimental results show that ventricular fibrillation under the above-mentioned conditions is a safe method of cardiac arrest, not harmful to the myocardium. This corresponds to the results of many other authors [1, 6, 10, 11]. Grover [8] in contrast found a rise of myocardial lactate in the fibrillating heart but the temperature was 37° C.

After a series of experiments, Buckberg and Hottenrott [5] summarized the conditions under which subendocardial ischemia develops in fibrillating hearts:

1. When the normal ventricle is fibrillated with a sustained electrical stimulus.
2. The hypertrophied ventricle is allowed to fibrillate spontaneously.
3. The fibrillating heart becomes distended or the perfusion pressure is reduced to approximately 50 mm Hg.

With the conditions of hypothermic ventricular fibrillation and an adequate perfusion pressure [2], myocardial ischemia can be avoided.

Perfusion pressure distal to a critical coronary stenosis may be reduced. This problem also plagues the technique of hypothermic potassium cardioplegia. It has been clearly demonstrated that the distribution of cardioplegic solutions in severely diseased coronary systems may be nonuniform, leading to differential cooling and marginal or inadequate protection of some segments of myocardium [3, 9].

Our clinical practice when handling the problem of hypoperfusion in the poststenotic area is:

1. Hypothermia to about 25° C to reduce fibrillation and oxygen consumption
2. Immediately after completion of the distal anastomosis perfusion of each graft by oxygenated blood from a side line of the arterial line.

The washout of acid metabolites is another advantage of continuous perfusion with blood during ventricular fibrillation.

Conclusion

Eight hundred and thirty ACBG operations in hypothermic ventricular fibrillation have been performed. The first 155 patients with 402 bypasses (2.6/patient) have been investigated. Mortality was 0.6%; myocardial infarction, rate 40%). Hypothermic ventricular fibrillation at 28° C during continuous coronary perfusion with a vent in the normal dog heart under ECG causes a slight pH decrease (ΔpH = −0.06) and myocardial function (78%) is well preserved. Intermittent aortic cross-clamping during ventricular fibrillation, however, causes a myocardial acidosis (ΔpH = −0.34), a worse left ventricular function (54%), and a significant myocardial edema. Hypothermic ventricular fibrillation is an effective method of myocardial protection for an almost unlimited time. Intermittent aortic cross-clamping during ventricular fibrillation, however, leads to significant myocardial acidosis deterioration of ventricular function and should be avoided.

References

1. Baird RJ (1975) Ventricular fibrillation. J Thorac Cardiovasc Surg 70:1027
2. Baird RJ, Dietka F, Okumori M, de la Rocha A, Goldblach MM, Hill TJ, Mac Gregor DC (1975) Surgical aspects on regional myocardial blood flow and myocardial pressure. J Thorac Cardiovasc Surg 69:17

3. Becker H, Vinten-Johansen J, Buckberg GD, Follette DM, Robertson JM (1981) Critical importance of ensuring cardioplegic delivery with coronary stenosis. J Thorac Cardiovasc Surg 81:507
4. Brazier J, McConnell D, Cooper N, DeLand E, Buckberg G (1974) The effects of temperature, time and perfusion pressure on the adequacy and distribution of coronary flow during ventricular fibrillation. Surg Forum 25:172
5. Buckberg GD, Hottenrott C (1975) Ventricular fibrillation. Ann Thorac Surg 20:76
6. Cox JL, Anderson RW, Pass HI, Curie WD, Roe CR, Mikat E, Wechsler AS, Sabiston DC (1977) The safety of induced ventricular fibrillation during cardiopulmonary bypass in nonhypertrophied hearts. J Thorac Cardiovasc Surg 74:423
7. Flameng W, Borgers M, Daenen W, Stalpaert G (1980) Ultrastructural and cytochemical correlates of myocardial protection by cardiac hypothermia in man. J Thorac Cardiovasc Surg 79:413
8. Grover FL, Fewel JG, Ghidoni JJ, Norton JB, Arom KV, Trincle JK (1976) Effects of ventricular fibrillation on coronary blood flow and myocardial metabolism. J Thorac Cardiovasc Surg 73:616
9. Hilton CJ, Tenbl W, Acker M, Levinson HJ, Millard RW, Riddle R, McEnany MT (1979) Inadequate cardioplegic protection with obstructed coronary arteries. Ann Thorac Surg 28:323
10. Martino RA, Kissack AS, Stuckey JH, Kavaler F, Fisher VJ (1969) Myocardial function after electrically induced ventricular fibrillation. Am J Cardiol 24:537
11. Rudolph W, Sebening F, Klinner W (1967) Der Stoffwechsel des flimmernden menschlichen Herzens bei erhaltener Koronarzirkulation. Z Kreislaufforsch 56:646

Risk Factors for Perioperative Complications in Coronary Artery Surgery

G. S. Kobinia, P. Hartl, and P. Brücke

Introduction

Decreasing morbidity and mortality in primary myocardial revascularization has been documented in recent studies [1, 4]. Changes have occurred in surgical techniques, risk factors, and cause of death. This study was carried out to evaluate the occurrence of morbidity and mortality for patients undergoing coronary artery bypass graft operations in a non-university-associated city hospital. In addition, patient data were examined statistically for identification of risk factors.

Patients and Methods

Between January 1978 and May 1985, 1000 open heart procedures were performed at the First Surgical Department of the City Hospital, Linz. During this period 794 patients underwent aortocoronary bypass grafting (CABG). The data from these 794 patients were retrieved and analyzed in a microcomputer system. There was a male preponderance of 671 (84%) versus 123 females. Except for rare cases the saphenous vein was used for grafting. The mean number of distal anastomoses was 2.4 over the total period; this number increased from 1.3 in 1978 to 2.9 in 1985 ($P > 0.000$). Mean age of the patients was 57.1 years; mean age had increased from 55.4 years in 1978 to 62.2 years in 1985 ($P > 0.000$). The following events were listed as complications in this study: (1) mortality, (2) need for reoperation, (3) a problem that would result in mortality without immediate and adequate therapy, and (4) problems that require prolonged stay in hospital for more than 2 weeks. Thus mortality is included under the term complication but it has also been listed separately as the most severe complication.

The following patient data were examined for their possible association with increased frequency of complications: age, gender, number of bypasses, performance of a snake graft, number of snake anastomoses, emergency, and reoperation (for mortality only). Analysis was performed using a multivariate logistic regression analysis. In addition, for intergroup comparison of frequencies the chi-square test was used. Cardiac function data were recently examined by our cardiology group [4].

Table 1. Annual frequency of coronary artery bypass grafts, mortality, and complications

Year	Number CABG	Mortality		Complications	
		N	%	*N*	%
1978	26	1	3.8%	9	34%
1979	40	2	5%	10	25%
1980	61	0	0%	17	27%
1981	100	3	3.3%	16	16%
1982	121	2	1.6%	17	14%
1983	166	1	0.6%	15	9%
1984	212	3	1.4%	29	13%
1985	(68)	1	1.4%	16	23%
	794	13		129	

Results

Table 1 shows the annual frequency of CABG operations between 1978 and May 1985. Also listed are the mortality and frequency of complications. There were 129 major complications recorded including a total of 13 deaths.

The different complications are listed in Table 2. Cardiac complications have been observed in a total of 32 patients (4% of all patients, 24% of all complications) with seven patients not surviving their cardiac problem. Mediastinal bleeding requiring reoperation was observed in a total of 30 patients (3.7% of all patients, 23% of all complications) and was the major reason for reoperations among a total of 66 reoperations. Sternal problems occurred in 33 patients and were the second most frequent reason for reoperation (28 reoperations). Neurological deficiency was observed postoperatively in seven patients (0.9% of all patients, 5.5% of all complications), with one death. Major technical problems were recorded in three instances, among them a patient whose coronary arteries seemed to be inaccessible during an operation in 1978 and who was reoperated on successfully in 1984 with two grafts. In addition to these typical complications we have observed complications that are not directly related to the cardiac disease and surgical intervention. In three patients, gastroduodenal ulcers requiring operative repair occurred postoperatively and more ulcers responding to early conservative treatment have been observed since [3]. In one patient with previous laparotomies the stab incision for placement of the mediastinal drainage perforated the transverse colon and resulted in mediastinal phlegmon with death. Drugs have been the source of complications in three instances. Twice anaphylactic shock occurred after routine i.v. administration of dipyrone (one death) and in one patient xylocaine was given in an overdose, resulting in temporary paresis of the legs. Bilateral pneumothorax was the cause of death in one patient and unilateral spontaneous pneumothorax was treated successfully in another patient at the Cardiac Care Unit. Alertness of the problem has helped us to identify the event of tension pneumothorax before closure of the chest more frequently in patients with emphysematous lungs.

Table 2. List of complications resulting in morbidity or mortality. Numbers of subdiagnoses resulting in death are in parenthesis

		Morbidity	Mortality
Cardiac		25	7
Infarction	11 (6)		
Pump failure	5 (1)		
Fibrillation	6		
Arrest	3		
Hemorrhage		28	2
Sternal dehiscence		33	
Wound complication		12	
Neurological deficit		6	1
Apoplexia	6		
Subdural hematoma	(1)		
GI tract		4	1
Duodenal ulcer	3		
Ileus	1		
Perforated colon	(1)		
Technical		3	
Aortic tear			
Coronaries not found			
Twisting of BP to RC			
Drugs		2	1
Anaphylaxis to dipyrone	1 (1)		
Overdosage of xylocaine	1		
Sepsis		1	
Renal embolus		1	
Pneumothorax		1	1
		116	13

Table 3. Risk factors for perioperative complications as determined by multivariate logistic regression analysis

Dependent variable *Complications*	
Emergency	$P<0.01$
Age	$P<0.01$
Dependent variable *Mortality*	
Emergency	$P<0.001$
Reoperation	$P<0.05$

Although the annual rate of frequency of complications has changed over the period observed (Table 1), this finding is not associated with a major change of any specific type of complication. It might, however, be noted that death due to cardiac failure occurred five times during the period 1978–1982 (348 cases) and only twice during the period 1983–1985 (446 cases, $P=0.1$).

Table 4. Rate of mortality and complications by sex

	Number CABG	Mortality		Complications	
		n	%	*n*	%
Male	671	11	1.6%	102	15%
Female	123	2	1.6%	27	21%
		NS		$P = 0.05$	

Risk factors for perioperative mortality and complications are demonstrated in Table 3. Appearance of perioperative complications was associated with the need for an emergency operation ($P < 0.001$) and increased age ($P < 0.01$). Mortality was associated with performance of an emergency operation and the need for reoperation ($P < 0.05$). Thus performance of an emergency operation was associated with higher morbidity and higher mortality when compared with elective operations.

The rate of mortality and complications by gender is demonstrated in Table 4.

Discussion

Identification of risk factors makes it possible to focus attention on these problems in an effort further to minimize surgical risks and accurately to assess the risk if an operation is undertaken. Multivariate logistic regression analysis identified increased age and need for emergency operation as risk factors for perioperative complications. Indeed after a low in mortality in 1980 (0%), 1981 showed a slightly increased death rate (Table 1) when operations for acute myocardial ischemia became more frequent. The number of complications, which had decreased to a low of 9% in 1983, increased in 1984 and 1985, when we started to operate on older patients more routinely (mean age 58 years in 1983 vs. 62 years in 1984 and 1985). Thus inclusion of new candidates for the bypass operation obviously resulted in an increased number of complications. The number of bypasses performed as a measure of the number of diseased vessels was not predictive for morbidity or mortality [2].

Female gender has been considered as a risk factor previously [2]. In our study (Table 4) female sex is not associated with higher mortality; however, for the presence of complications a marginal significance can be found ($P = 0.05$).

It is of interest to note that cardiac problems constitute only about one-fourth of all the complications observed and about one-half of all the mortalities observed. Advances made in the field of cardioplegic arrest of the heart have made ischemic damage a rare event. Consequently, however, factors other than cardiac injury emerge as increasingly significant contributors to perioperative complications. Factors related to surgery are mediastinal hemorrhage, sternal dehiscence, and wound problems at the site of the harvesting of the saphenous vein. Factors not related to surgery are neurovascular thrombosis or bleeding,

GI tract complications, drug side effects, and pulmonary problems. Further enhancements might be expected from better control of coagulation after extracorporeal circulation, improved techniques of sternal closure, and early recognition of systemic complications as GI and pulmonary problems.

The Cleveland group has recently published an extensive study of risk factors during coronary artery bypass surgery [1]. In their experience of 24672 patients operated on between 1970 and 1982, persistent and changing risk patterns are identified over the period. Persistent risk factors are emergency operation, increased age, female sex, and previous congestive heart failure. Emerging risk factors are incomplete revascularization and abnormal preoperative electrocardiogram. Cardiac causes of death decreased from 75% in 1974–1976 to 59% in 1980–1982. Left main disease, number of grafts, and poor ventricular function have been neutralized as risk factors. Our study is not based on as many parameters as the Cleveland study; however, for comparable data (age, emergency, number of grafts, gender) similar results are obtained.

Morbidity and mortality have been decreased for myocardial revascularization due to achievements in myocardial protection over the past decade. In consequence, system failures come to emerge as major contributors of complications.

References

1. Cosgrove DM, Loop FD, Lytle BW, Baillot R, Gill CC, Golding LAR, Tailor PC, Goormastic M (1984) Primary myocardial revascularization. Trends in surgical mortality. J Thorac Cardiovasc Surg 88:673–684
2. Hall RJ, Elayda MA, Gray A, Mathur VS, Garcia E, Castro CM, Maasumi A, Cooley DA (1983) Coronary artery bypass: long term follow up of 22284 consecutive patients. Circulation 68 (suppl II):II-20–27
3. Hanks JB, Curtis SE, Hanks BB, Andersen DK, Cox JL, Jones RS (1982) Gastrointestinal complications after cardiopulmonary bypass. Surgery 92, 2:394–400
4. Leisch F, Kerschner K, Schützenberger W, Hartl P, Gross C, Brücke P, Herbinger W (1985) Hauptstammstenose: Bedeutung des klinischen Stadiums für das angiographische und operative Risiko. Dtsch Med Wochenschr 110:1559–1563

An Alternative Route for Sequential Venous Grafts of the Lateral Aspect of the Heart

H. Vanermen, H. P. Wynant, and F. Wellens

Introduction

Sequential venous grafts on the lateral aspect of the heart are currently used in myocardial revascularization [1, 5–7]. With a side-to-side anastomosis constructed near to the base of the heart, the risk of kinking and consequent thrombosis is high when the vein graft has to be guided over the anterior aspect of the PA (Pulmonary Artery) or via the transverse sinus. In these cases an alternative nonanatomic route has been used in ±10% of our coronary artery bypass graft (CABG) procedures. The description of this technique forms the basis of this report.

Technique

Besides the routine CABG with the IMA (Internal Mammary Artery) as a preferential conduit to the anterior wall of the heart and several separate venous grafts to large coronaries, extensive myocardial revascularization of small vessels is sometimes mandatory. The use of the IMA (Internal Mammary Artery) as a single, double, or even triple graft in diffuse disease of the anterior wall is a routine procedure in our institution [3, 6, 9]. In a high percentage of the cases, multiple branches on the lateral and posterior aspect of the left ventricle have to be bypassed.

In these cases sequential grafts can be constructed in several ways. It is well known that the sequential graft has to be performed with a very precise and exacting technique to avoid kinking or tension along its course [4, 5, 8]. A few aspects of the construction of sequential grafts have to be emphasized. Major rules should be:

1. That the end-to-side anastomosis is made on the largest vessel to avoid a flow-drop in a distal segment of the graft
2. That the side-to-side anastomoses are made on the smaller vessels, but on their largest diameter and therefore as proximally as possible
3. That retrograde anastomoses are avoided for hemodynamic reasons

The different technical solutions are presented in Fig. 1A–C. Graft C is probably the best solution for several reasons:

1. The smaller vessels are bypassed in:
   a) A side-to-side fashion (better flow pattern)

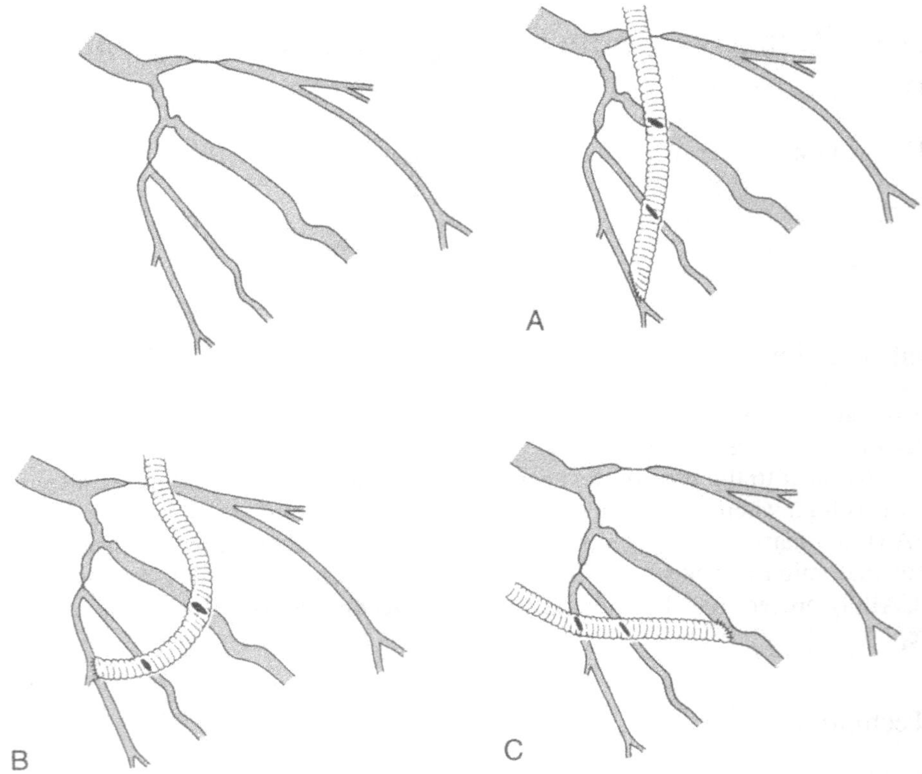

Fig. 1. Different technical solutions for a definite pattern of marginal branches

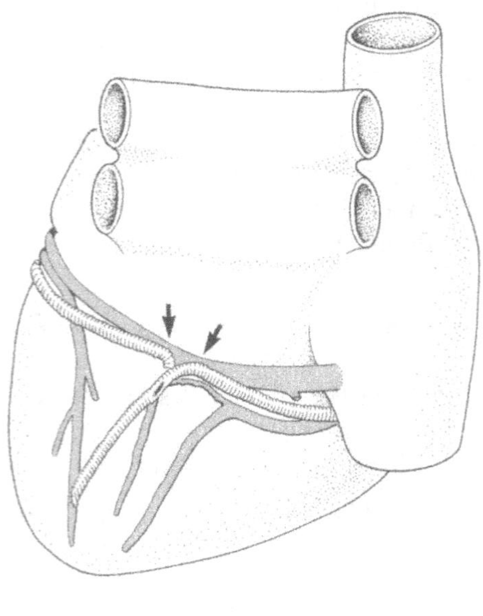

Fig. 2. Kinking of the graft proximal to the side-to-side anastomosis

b) Very proximally (larger diameter)
c) Longitudinally (easier in very small diameters)
2. The end-to-side anastomosis is made on the largest vessel.

Nevertheless, problems can be encountered in solution C proximally from the first suture at the base of the heart (Fig. 2), when the graft is passed either to the right or to the left side [2, 10]. The alternative route will avoid kinking of the graft site and will also shorten the length of the conduit to the ascending aorta.

After construction of all the distal anastomoses, the sequential graft of the lateral aspect has to run toward the sinus of Haller and pass behind the pos-

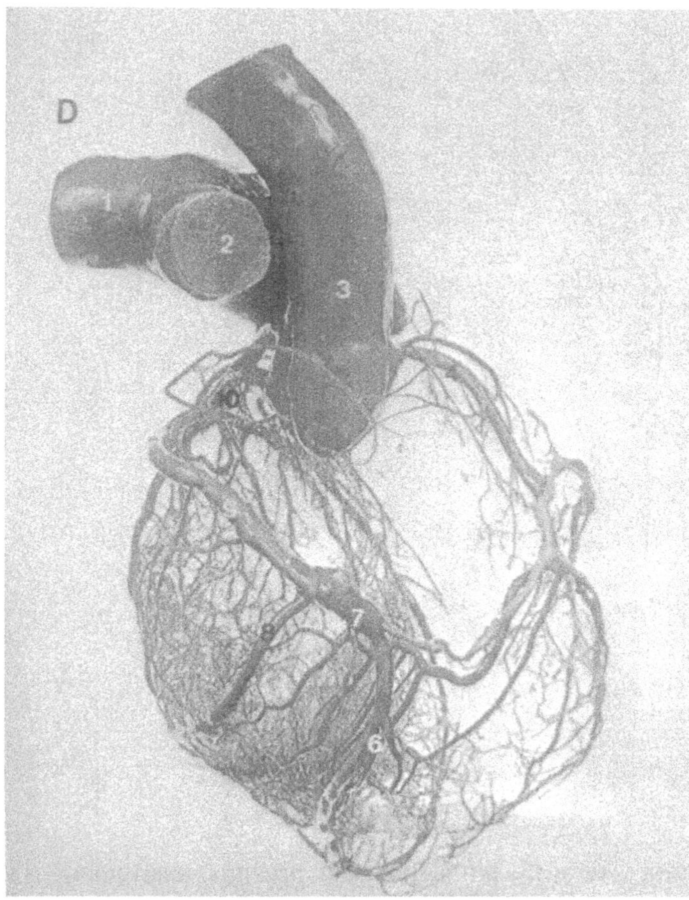

a

Fig. 3 a, b. Anatomical models. **a** D. Cast of cardiac vessels, from the right, below and behind. Sinus coronarius. 1. A. pulmonalis sinistra; 2. A. pulmonalis dextra; 3. Aorta ascendens; 4. A. coronaria dextra; 5. Marginal branch of a. coronaria dextra and v. cordis parva; 6. Ramus interventricularis posterior and v. cordis media; 7. Sinus coronarius; 8. V. posterior ventriculi sinistri; 9. V. cordis magna; 10. Ramus circumflexus a. coronariae sinistrae

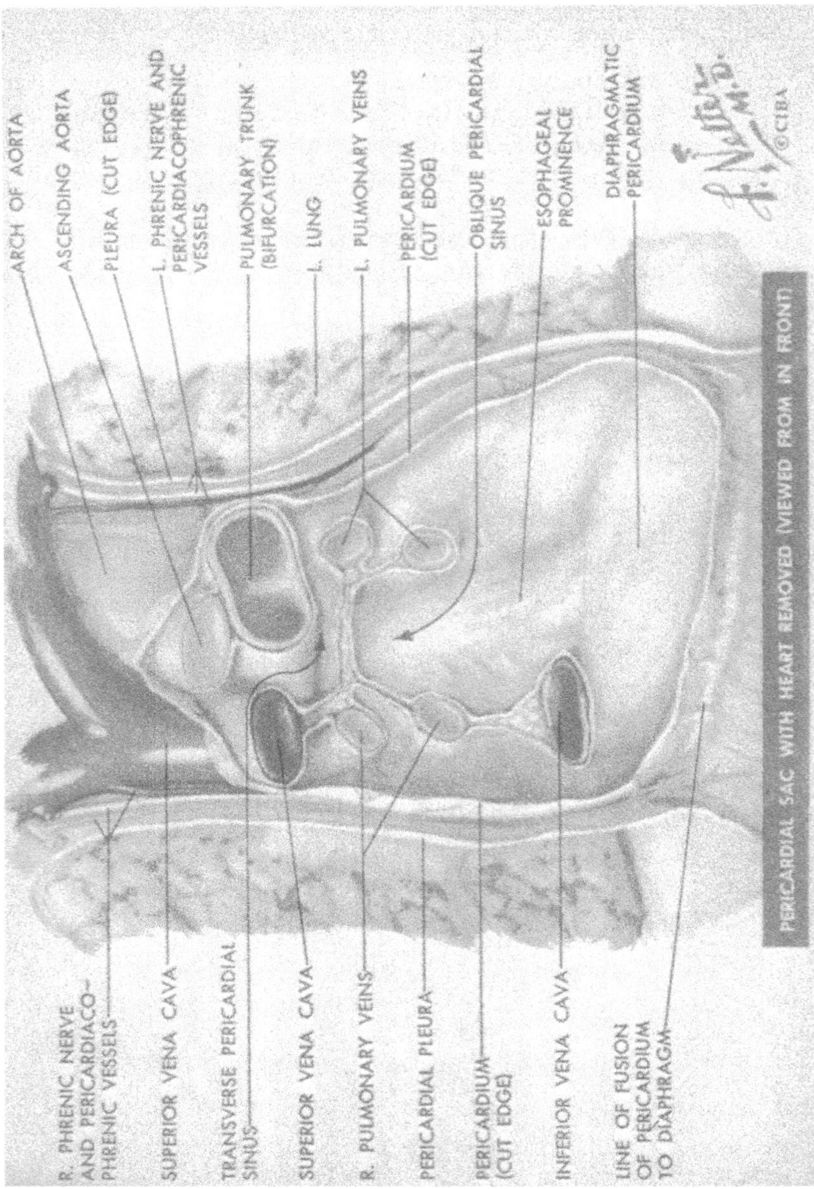

Fig. 3b

terior wall of the left atrium. The proximal anastomosis is then constructed on the right and posterior side of the ascending aorta.

With the right hand a long somewhat curved vascular clamp has to be passed between the right pulmonary vein and artery, medially of the VCS (Vena cava superior) in the direction of the spine and then guided to the sinus of Haller, while the heart is lifted with the left hand. The two pericardial reflections have to be perforated in the sinus of Haller. Care has to be taken in this manoeuver to avoid perforation of the posterior left atrial wall. Perfect hemostasis of the vein graft has to be achieved before pulling it through the new route. On an anatomical model it is obvious that this route is shorter and more direct (Fig. 3).

Patient Group

In 750 consecutive CABG (Fig. 3) operations performed in our institute this alternative route was used in 63 patients. The average number of distal anastomoses was 3.02. In our series 9.34% of the grafts to the posterolateral aspect were passed through the oblique sinus. There was no technique-related morbidity or mortality. Angiographic controls of several grafts showed excellent patency and a straight and short conduit between the coronary vessels and ascending aorta.

Conclusion

The oblique pericardial sinus is a safe and interesting route for both single and sequential grafts of the posterolateral aspect of the heart, especially when anastomoses are to be constructed on the very base of the heart. It also reduces the need for excess vein length and protects the bypass in a very elegant way in the case of resternotomy.

References

1. Bigelow JC, Bartley TD, Oage US et al. (1976) Long-term follow-up of sequential aortocoronary venous grafts. Ann Thorac Surg 22:507
2. Effler DB (1976) Revascularization with little coronary arteries (editorial). Ann Thorac Surg 21:83
3. Green GE (1978) Mammary coronary artery anastomosis for myocardial revascularization. Postgrad Med 63:153
4. Grondin CM, Limet R (1977) Sequential anastomoses in coronary artery grafting. Technical aspects and early and late angiographic results. Ann Thorac Surg 23:1
5. Grondin CM, Vouhé P, Bourassa MG, et al. (1978) Optimal patency rates obtained in coronary artery grafting with circular vein grafts. J Thorac Cardiovasc Surg 75:161
6. Johnson WD, Shore RT, Kamath ML (1986) Nine years observation of mammary coronary bypass grafts. J Thorac Cardiovasc Surg (in press)
7. Sewell WH (1974) Improved coronary vein patency rates with side to side anastomoses. Ann Thorac Surg 17:538
8. Spray TL, Roberts WC (1976) Tension on coronary bypass conduits: a neglected cause of real or potential obstruction of saphenous vein grafts. J Thorac Cardiovasc Surg 72:282
9. Tyras DH, Barner HB, Kaiser GC et al. (1980) Bypass grafts to the left anterior descending coronary artery: saphenous vein versus internal mammary artery. J Thorac Cardiovasc Surg 80:237
10. Ullyot DJ (1980) Current controversies in the conduct of the coronary bypass operation. Soc Thorac Surg vol 30 no. 2, August, pp 192–203

Abstract

Intraoperative Visualisation of Coronary Vessels

W. R. DIMITRI, R. SAPSFORD, R. STANBRIDGE, and A. NICHOLAIDES

Because of the serious limitations of coronary angiography and in order to provide additional multidimensional information, real-time high-resolution scanning was used intraoperatively to define coronary arteries, atherosclerotic lesions and saphenous vein graft anastomosis. A 12-mHz/2-cm probe was used in 30 patients undergoing myocardial revascularisation. The findings are detailed and scanning techniques described, emphasising the unique value of postreconstruction and endarterectomy imaging. The findings were compared with angiography and whenever possible with the surgical findings.

B-mode ultrasound is safe, repeatable and reproducible. It produces an accurate, multidimensional and anatomical image which accurately quantifies atherosclerotic lesions and precisely localises obscure coronary arteries. Postreconstruction imaging defines technical defects, allows immediate correction of errors if, when and where indicated, and may in the long term improve the quality of vascular reconstruction.

The integration of a pulse Doppler should provide comprehensive functional and anatomical information for the effective management of vascular pathology.

New Trends in Myocardial Protection

B. H. Walpoth

Despite major progress in the field of myocardial protection in recent years it is still suboptimal for a small number of high-risk patients. Several questions relating to the basic understanding of myocardial ischemia and its clinical implications remain open. Thus optimization of myocardial protection for cardiac surgery and myocardial preservation for cardiac transplantation is foreseeable.

Continuous or intermittent coronary (ante or retro) perfusion is cumbersome and sometimes hazardous and will not be discussed in this paper.

First we must consider the sequence of events during induction of global myocardial ischemia by aortic cross-clamping. The ensuing changes relate to the following problems:

1. *Ischemia* – with changes in function, energy reserves, and finally homeostasis, leading to acidosis, free radicals, ionic pump deficiency, membrane damage, and finally irreversible structural changes [1],
2. *Reperfusion* – with its detrimental effects on preexisting cellular alterations will enhance the ischemic damage and lead to severe ionic shifts (calcium overload/paradox), edema, vascular changes, and often further metabolic depletion, also called reperfusion injury [2].
3. *Myocardial energetics* – Probably the main principle to respect in order to avoid irreversible damage (contracture or the "stoneheart") is myocardial energetics [3, 4], which safe for a short initial period are entirely anaerobic and directly dependent on:
   a) *Myocardial reserves* – high-energy phosphate stores as adenosine-triphosphate (ATP), creatinine phosphate (PCr), and glycogen
   b) *Energy demands* of the ischemic myocardium
   c) *Energy production* (glycolysis) during ischemia

All the above-mentioned points can be challenged in order to avoid biodegradation of energy-rich phosphate compounds to the critical point (about 70% ATP reduction from the starting level) at which irreversible damage occurs due to lack of energy for the maintenance of cellular homeostasis.

Myocardial Energy Reserves – Optimal Starting Point

Patients undergoing cardiac surgery cannot be compared to healthy and well-fed animals. Patients may be stressed by their disease and the impeding operation and may show signs of malnutrition and/or require inotropic support, all of which are detrimental for myocardial reserves. We have recently shown that preischemic changes such as transient hypovolemia (removal of 25% of the rabbit's blood volume, followed by reinfusion after 5 min) will, even with complete restitution of hemodynamic parameters, lead to a marked decrease of the ischemic myocardial tolerance as assessed by time-resolved phosphorous nuclear magnetic resonance (^{31}P NMR), despite minor changes in the initial spectrum after the onset of ischemia. Similar alterations could be demonstrated with small doses of catecholamines in the preischemic period (adrenaline 1 : 1000 0.01 mg/kg and isoproterenol 1 mcg/kg).

In addition, a marked global myocardial acidosis can be observed as compared with the control hearts (pH 7.2 vs. 6.9 for shock and 6.7 for catecholamines) [5].

Figure 1 depicts pooled NMR spectra from freshly excised and stored hearts showing a reduction of beta ATP of 70% after 24 h. After induction of preischemic shock, or catecholamine administration, an identical decrease of energy is reached after 7.5 h and 4 h, respectively; this means that ischemic tolerance is six times shorter.

A major clinical problem is that correct preoperative assessment of myocardial energy reserves in patients was only possible, until now, with invasive tests. More recently, the whole body nuclear magnetic resonance (^{31}P NMR) has permitted noninvasive continuous monitoring of the high-energy phosphate stores and the internal cellular pH accurately [6]; this is why this new technique is so promising.

Several groups have demonstrated the possibility of increasing energy reserves before ischemia (starting point) [7], of preventing excessive biodegradation by selectively blocking breakdown pathways [8], or of refuelling the myocardium during or immediately after ischemia [9].

Myocardial Energy Demands

This point can be challenged most actively by a combination of the following principles:

1. Reduction of the level of metabolic turnover by hypothermia (systemic and local), which is temperature dependent and follows, more or less, the Q10 rule [10]
2. Rapid and complete cardiac arrest by induction of depolarization (hyperkalemia) as well as decreasing the physiologic cellular activity (reduction of extracellular sodium) and electromechanical decoupling (calcium removal or hypermagnesemia)
3. Prevention of marked cellular acidosis (high buffering capacity of the cardioplegic solution) to avoid interruption of glycolitic phosphorylation which would lead to further degradation, membrane pump inactivation, and thus to ionic shifts and, finally, structural damage
4. Enhancement of membrane stability and reduction of the ionic pumpwork by blocking specific channels as for calcium [11]

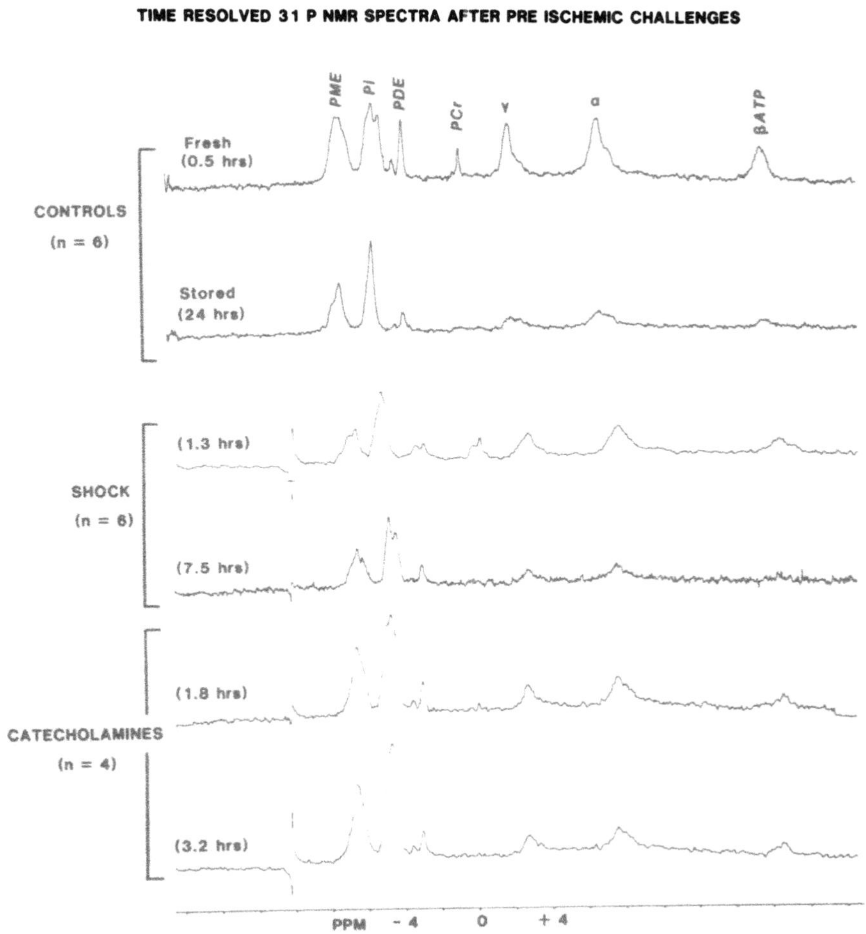

Fig. 1. Time resolved (h) ^{31}P NMR spectra of fresh and stored control hearts as well as after preischemic shock and catecholamine administration (pooled NMR data for each group). The zero of the *PPM* (parts per million) scale is adjusted on the phosphocreatine (*PCr*). The other peaks are: *PME,* phosphomonoester; *Pi,* inorganic phosphorous; *PDE,* phosphodiesters; *ATP,* adenosine triphosphate

Probably one of the main parameters to consider is the reduction of biodegradation by hypothermia. We have shown that even at very low temperatures there is a significant difference between 0° C and 8° C after 24 h of cardioplegic hypothermic storage (Fig. 2). Hearts preserved at 8° C were all below the critical ATP level (reduction of beta ATP by 88% of its preischemic value) whereas hearts preserved at 0° C showed less reduction, better function, and recovery [12].

More recently several groups have worked with calcium channel blockers to reduce calcium inflow and thus the ionic pump work during ischemia. These also produce coronary dilation, making better postischemic reperfusion possible and they avoid calcium overload (paradox) during reperfusion.

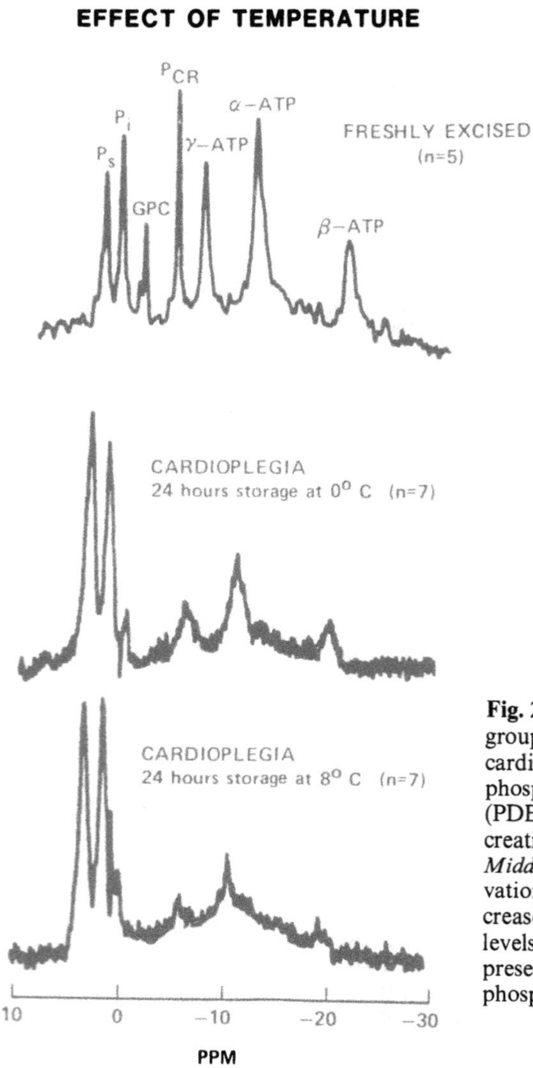

Fig. 2. Pooled ^{31}P NMR spectra of each group: *Top spectrum* Freshly excised myocardium, labeled as follows: *Ps*, (PME) sugar phosphate; *Pi*, inorganic phosphate; *GPC*, (PDE) glycerophosphocholine; *Pcr*, phosphocreatine; *ATP*, adenosine triphosphate peaks. *Middle spectrum* Hearts after 24 h preservation at 0° C (cardioplegia) showing increased *Pi*, absence of *Pcr*, and lowered ATP levels. *Bottom spectrum* Same as above, but preserved at 8° C. Note that energy-rich phosphate preservation is better at 0° C

We could demonstrate all three effects in an experimental model which assessed ischemic and reperfusion damage separately. The results are summarized in Table 1 and show a significant change in "coronary vascular resistance" and intramyocardial calcium content as well as preservation and resynthesis of high-energy phosphate compounds in the group of animals pretreated with verapamil (0.2 mg/kg) after 24 h hypothermic storage in Euro-Collins solution, followed by reperfusion (cross-circulation) (Fig. 3) [13].

It is also important to remember that several pharmaceutical agents will have no action if applied during deep hypothermia, due to their lack of binding capacity under those conditions. This is especially true for all calcium channel blockers [14].

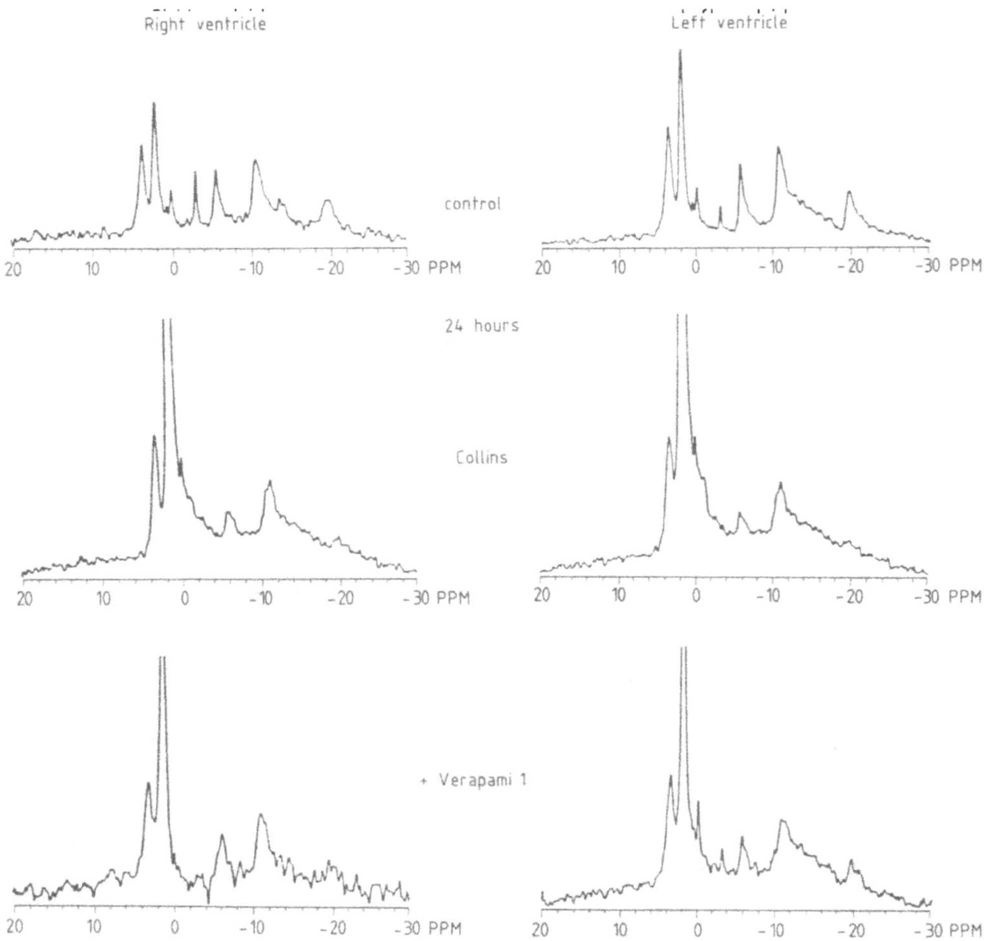

Fig. 3. ^{31}P NMR spectra of rabbit hearts: *right,* ventricle ischemia alone; *left,* ventricle after reperfusion for 30 min. Spectra represent computer-pooled data from five rabbits in each group. Peaks are as for other figures

Myocardial Energy Production

Energy production also depends on the level of energy, but mainly on myocardial glycogen reserves. Other factors are aerobiosis or anaerobiosis, internal pH, and sufficient levels of ATP to permit chemical steps such as phosphorylation. The drawback is concomitant lactate production which may produce a marked acidosis and, in turn, inhibit further glycolisis [15].

Recently, much attention has been given to oxygen-derived free radicals in tissue ischemia. Several drugs such as dismutase, katalase, and allopurinol have been used to protect the heart from oxygen-free radical production; these will reduce the detrimental membrane effect during reperfusion [16, 17].

Table 1. Hemodynamic and intramyocardial calcium content after storage and reperfusion

	"CVR" AOP (mm Hg)	LVP Isovolumic (mm Hg)	Max dP/dT (mm Hg/s)	Total Ca^{++} (mmol/ kg ww)	Mitochondrial Ca^{++} (nmol/mg protein)
Controls	67±13	102±39	1500±359	2.2±0.1	15.7± 1
		*	*	*	*
Euro-Collins 24 h, 0 °C	91±31	39±20	380±249	6.8±1.4	45.6± 7.6
	*			*	
Verapamil (0.2 mg/kg) + Euro-Collins 24 h, 0 °C	54±21	58±34	660±488	4.9±1.2	41.8±21.3

$\bar{x} \pm SD$; *, $P<0.05$; $N=6$; CVR, coronary vascular resistance as assessed by aortic perfusion pressure; *LVP*, isovolumic left ventricular pressure; max dP/dt, index of contractility; Ca^{++}, calcium

In conclusion, several innovations have shown promising results but still need to be confirmed by clinical studies.

In addition, the clinical application of the myocardial protection is of paramount importance including cardiopulmonary bypass, hypothermia, myocardial emptying (venting), injection and reinfusion of cardioplegia to counteract the noncoronary collateral blood flow and rise in temperature and to cleanse the breakdown products away. Special attention should be given to severely ischemic hearts during the reperfusion period.

Most importantly, no direct conclusions may be drawn from animal studies with different starting points (healthy and with a normal heart) to patients undergoing cardiac surgery. Thus, the clinical safe ischemic tolerance lies around 3 h, whereas our experimental data and work from other authors show good function and energy resynthesis after 24 h of preservation.

References

1. Kirklin JW, Conti VR, Blackstone EH (1979) Prevention of myocardial damage during cardiac operations. N Engl J Med 301:135
2. Reitz BA (1982) Myocardial protection during cardiac surgery. Ann Rev Med 33:1515–1562
3. Opie LH (1983) In: Drake-Holland AJ, Noble MIM (eds) High energy phosphate compounds in cardiac metabolism. Wiley & Sons, p 279–307
4. Jennings RB, Hawkins HK, Lowe JE, Hill ML, Kotman S, Reimer KA (1978) Relation between high energy phosphate and lethal injury in myocardial ischemia in the dog. Am J Pathol 92:187–207
5. Walpoth B, Schweizer A, Barbalat-Rey F, Faidutti B, Preischemic conditions affecting myocardial ischemic tolerance – a nuclear magnetic resonance study (^{31}P NMR), proceedings of the ESAO, 1985, Life Support Systems (Suppl.). Saunders, London (in print)
6. Flaherty JT, Weisfeldt ML, Bulkley BH, Gardner TJ, Gott VL, Jacobus WE (1982) Mechanisms of ischemic myocardial cell damage assessed by phosphorus-31 nuclear magnetic resonance. Circulation 65 (3):561

7. Cunningham Jr JN, Lashinger JC, Krieger KH, Knopp EA, Isom OW, Spencer FC (1983) Clinical use of preischemic enhancement replenishment of myocardial adenosine triphosphate stores in hypertrophied right ventricles. Surg Forum XXXIV, p 279–282
8. Rosenkranz ER, Okamoto F, Vinten-Johansen J, Buckberg GD, Bugyi HI, Leaf J (1983) Improved adenosine triphosphate recovery in energy-depleted hearts treated with 5-amino-4-imidazone carboxamide riboside (AICAR). Surg Forum XXXIV, p 330–331
9. Rousou JH, Engelman RM, Dobbs WA, Anisimowicz L (1983) Metabolic enhancement of myocardial preservation during cardioplegic arrest; Surg Forum XXXIV, p 332–334
10. Tyers GF, Williams EH, Hughes HC, Todd GH (1977) Effect of perfusate temperature on myocardial protection from ischemia. J Thorac Cardiovasc Surg 73 (5):766
11. Clark RE, Ferguson TB, West PN, Shuchleib RC, Henry PD (1977) Pharmacological preservation of the ischemic heart. Ann Thorac Surg 24 (4):307–314
12. Walpoth B, Zhao H, Jardetzky N, Jardetzky O, Jamieson S, Shumway N (1985) Time resolved assessment of ischemic myocardial tolerance in normothermia and hypothermia by ^{31}P nuclear magnetic resonance (NMR). Curr Surg 42:198–201
13. Walpoth B, Bleese N, Zhao Hong-xu, Kashara K, Billingham ME, Jardetzky N, Jardetzky O, Jamieson SW, Shumway NE (1984) Assessment of rabbit hearts during reperfusion after hypothermic long-term storage: the role of verapamil and its effect on myocardial calcium. Surg Forum, p 288–291
14. Hearse D, Yamamoto F, Fukunami H, et al. (1984) The apparent temperature-dependency of calcium-antagonists. Circulation 68 (III): 184
15. Bretschneider J, Hubner G, Knoll D (1975) Myocardial resistance and tolerance to ischemia: physiological and biochemical basis. J Cardiovasc Surg 16:241
16. McCord JM (1985) Oxygen-derived free radicals in postischemic tissue injury. N Engl J Med 159 (312):3
17. Shlafer M, Kane PF, Kirsh MM (1982) Superoxide dismutase plus catalase enhances the efficacy of hypothermic cardioplegia to protect the globally ischemic, reperfused heart. J Thorac Cardiovasc Surg 83:830–839

The Role of Endarterectomy in Coronary Surgery

H. H. SCHELD, F. W. HEHRLEIN, G. GÖRLACH, R. HÖGE, and J. MULCH

Introduction

In diffuse coronary artery disease, complete revascularization is often not feasible without performing endarterectomy. But due to an increased risk of perioperative myocardial infarction and a reduced patency rate the role of this method in coronary surgery is still a matter of discussion [1, 3, 4, 7]. The purpose of our study was to demonstrate that proper technical performance and completeness of endarterectomy prevent the above-mentioned draw-backs.

Method

Between January 1980 and December 1984, 239 patients underwent coronary artery bypass grafting combined with endarterectomy of the left and right coronary artery system. They constituted 11.8% (239/2002) of all our patients undergoing myocardial revascularization. Thirty patients were female and 209 were male. The mean age of the patients was 55.67 ± 8.64 (SD) years (range 42−71 years). Seventy-two percent (172/239) had one or more myocardial infarctions prior to surgery. Mean ejection fraction (EF) was measured as 61.46 ± 16.51 (SD)% and a mean left ventricular end-diastolic pressure of 14.79 ± 9.17 (SD) mm Hg was recorded.

The surgical management was standardized. In all cases extracorporeal circulation was performed using a bubble oxygenator (BOS 10, Bentley Laboratories, D-4000 Düsseldorf 30, FRG) with a priming volume of 2 liters crystalloid solution. The right atrium and left ventricle were vented routinely.

Cardioplegic arrest of the heart was always induced using Bretschneider HTK (Fa. Köhler Chemie, D-Alsbach, FRG) solution. During a single cross-clamping period the endarterectomy and all distal anastomoses were performed. Following an initial infusion of 2000 ml additional cardioplegia solution was administered after each distal anastomosis through the already been performed anastomoses. During heart arrest moderate hypothermia (28 °C) was used.

The mean ischemic period was 85.6 ± 25.29 (SD) min (Table 1); the number of grafts varied from 3 to 10 and the number of endarterectomies per patient from 1 to 4. In 29.7% (71/239), endarterectomy of the left coronary artery system was performed, while in 70% (168/239) right-sided endarterectomies were performed. We performed endarterectomy whenever the common revasculari-

Table 1. Coronary endarterectomy: perioperative data

Aortic cross-clamping time (min)	85.66±25.59 (SD)
Number of CABGs per patient	Mean 4.1 (range 3–10)
Number of EAs per patient	Mean 1.5 (range 1–4)
Perioperative myocardial infarction	8.35% (20/239)
Perioperative mortality	3.34% (8/239) (4 MI, 2 LCO, 2 VD)

MI, myocardial infarction; LCO, low cardiac output; VD, ventricular dysrhythmia; EA, endarterectomy; CABG, coronary artery bypass graft

zation using conventional bypass grafting techniques was not feasible due to diffuse coronary disease. For the past 5 years we have not refused surgical therapy because of diffuse disease or nonvisualization of the distal segment beyond complete obstruction.

The endarterectomy starts with a short incision in the most calcified area of the coronary artery, dissecting the atheromatous core using a Holle intestinal clamp. By smooth traction and step-by-step dissection the extraction of the atheromatous core including all side branches is possible. We always control the completeness of the specimen by looking for tapering ends of the terminal branches and inject Cardiogreen (Paese GmbH u. Co., Frankfurt a. Main, FRG) into the endarterectomized vessels to exclude remaining parts of the specimen. If the core breaks or remaining parts of the specimen are visualized by this solution a distal arteriotomy is performed to obtain the remaining part of the core.

Results

The overall early mortality rate was 3.34% (8/239). There were four cases of myocardial infarction, two patients with low cardiac output failure, and two patients died because of intractable ventricular dysrhythmia. During the follow-up period of 6–54 months (mean, 36 months) there were 5.4% (13/339) late deaths. The perioperative myocardial infarction rate was 8.3% (20/239), assessed by both electrocardiogram (epicardial leads) and enzyme surveillance (Table 1). During the observation period graft reinvestigation by coronary angiography could be done in 85 patients, who gave informed consent (Table 2).

Table 2. Coronary endarterectomy: patency rate

Coronary artery	LCA	RCA	Total
Number of restudied grafts	26	59	85
Patent grafts	22	50	72[a]
Patency rate	84.6%	84.7%	84.7%

[a] Including PTFE grafts ($n = 8$).
LCA, left coronary artery; RCA, right coronary artery

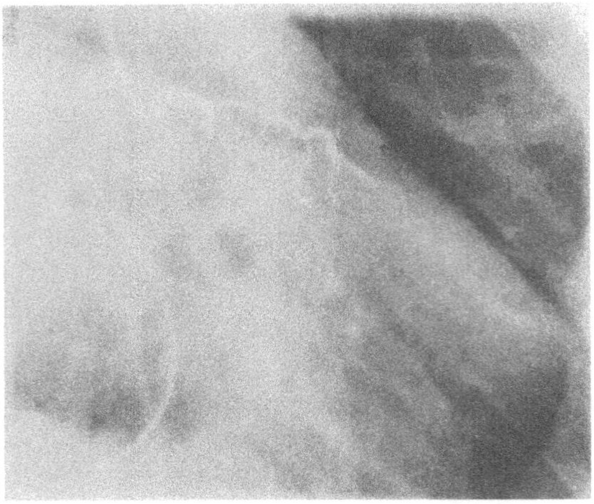

a

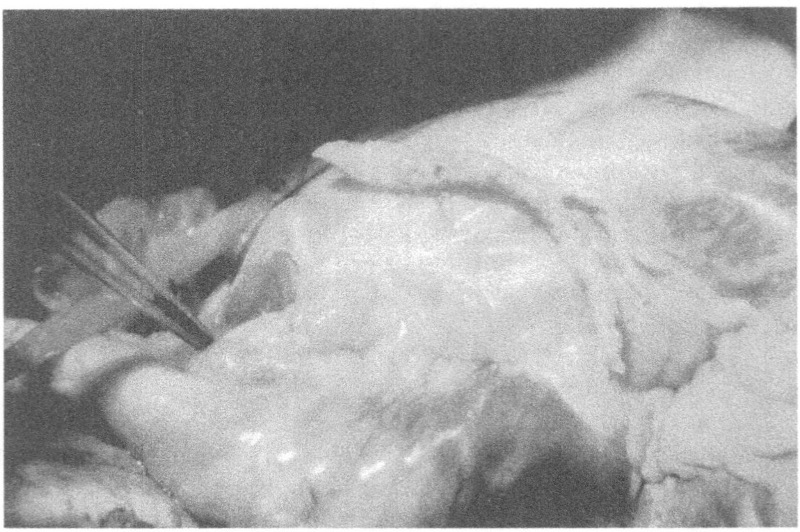

b

Fig. 1. **a** Preoperative coronary angiography: complete obstruction in the proximal circumflex and proximal left anterior descending artery. **b** Endarterectomy specimen: left anterior descending artery with major side branches. **c** Endarterectomy specimen: circumflex artery. **d** Postoperative coronary angiography 4 years after operation: aortocoronary ypsiloid saphenous vein bypass graft to the endarterectomized circumflex and left anterior descending artery with good distal runoff

The patency rate for all endarterectomized vessels was 84.7% (72/85), 84.6% (22/26) for the left coronary artery system, and 84.7% (50/59) for the right coronary artery system (Fig. 1a–d) including eight PTFE (polytetrafluoroethylene) grafts. Vein grafts to arteries non endarterectomized in the same group of patients were patent in 88.5% (269/304).

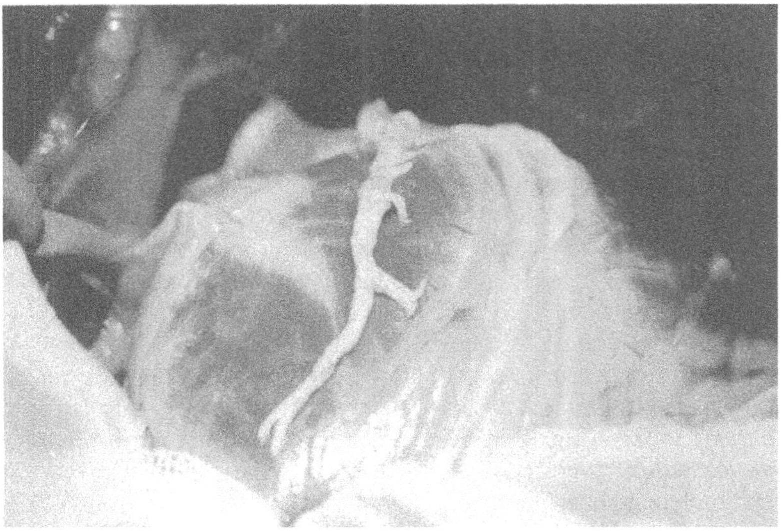

c

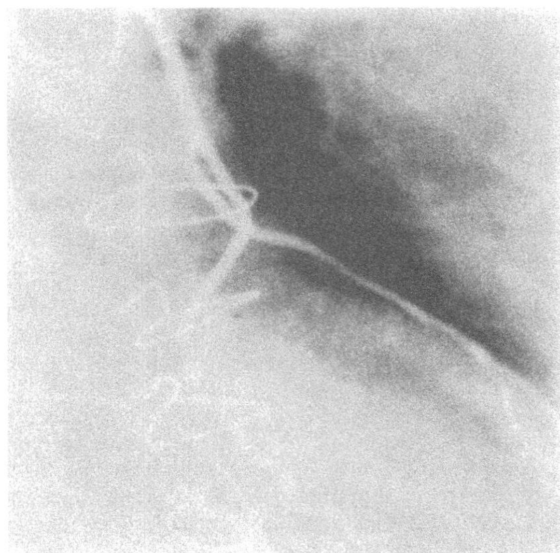

Fig. 1 c, d d

Discussion

Maximal relief of ischemia and optimal improvement of function are the aim of coronary surgery. Only complete revascularization can provide these results and is known to increase the life expectancy of the patients [2, 5, 6].

In diffuse coronary disease the performance of conventional bypass grafting is often not feasible. Vessels with diffuse atheromatous changes throughout the extracardiac course are unsuitable for grafting alone. Only combined endarterectomy allows complete revascularization in these cases [2, 8, 9]. However, this surgical method is known to have a higher perioperative infarction rate and limited patency rate [4, 6, 7].

In contrast to previous widely held opinions our results demonstrate that coronary endarterectomy could be performed with an acceptable perioperative infarction rate and mortality. According to our experience the results of endarterectomy are mainly determined by meticulous performance of this method: (1) Use one plane of separation throughout the procedure, (2) avoid distal breakage of the core by sustained tension, and (3) if breakage occurs or if the specimen has no thin tapering ends including the side branches, control the endarterectomized vessel with Cardiogreen and obtain the remaining part of the specimen by distal arteriotomy. The patency rate after coronary endarterectomy in our study group seems to support our opinion. Therefore we see no reason to restrict surgical therapy in diffuse coronary artery disease to incomplete myocardial revascularization.

References

1. Diethrich EB, Barmada B, Goldfarb D, Kaplitt MJ (1975) The role of endarterectomy in current myocardial revascularization. In: Norman JC (ed) Coronary artery medicine and surgery. Concepts and controversies. Appleton-Century-Crofts, New York, p 598–606
2. Hehrlein FW, Scheld HH, Mulch J, Görlach G (1985) Totalrevaskularisation des Myokards als Behandlungsprinzip der diffusen koronaren Herzerkrankung. Med Welt 36:1216–1219
3. Hochberg MS, Merrill WH, Michaelis LL, McIntosh CL (1978) Results of combined coronary endarterectomy and coronary bypass for diffuse coronary artery disease. J Thorac Cardiovasc Surg 75:38–46
4. Miller DC, Stinson EB, Oyer PE, Reitz BA, Jamieson SW, Moreno-Cabral RJ, Shumway NE (1981) Long-term clinical assessment of the efficacy of adjunctive coronary endarterectomy. J Thorac Cardiovasc Surg 81:21–29
5. Mulch J, Scheld HH, Hehrlein FW (1985) Koronare Endarterektomie heute. Med Welt 36:1287–1291
6. Qureshi SA, Halim MA, Pillai R, Smith P, Yacoub MH (1985) Endarterectomy of the left coronary system. Analysis of a 10 year experience. J Thorac Cardiovasc Surg 89:852–859
7. Schulte HD, Bircks W, Loogen F, Rivas-Martin J, Spiller P (1978) Resultate der Endarteriektomie im Rahmen der Koronarchirurgie. Thoraxchirurgie 26:266–269
8. Urschel HC, Razzuk MA (1979) Indications for distal coronary artery endarterectomy and proximal coronary artery bypass graft. In: Roskamm H, Schmuziger M (eds) Coronary heart surgery. A rehabilitation measure. Springer, Berlin Heidelberg New York, pp 108–111
9. Wallsh E, Weinstein G, Franzone AJ, Sterzer SH (1975) The use of distal right coronary endarterectomy and saphenous coronary bypass to decrease total grafts and extend operability in patients with coronary artery disease. In: Norman JC (ed) Coronary artery medicine and surgery. Concepts and controversies. Appleton-Century-Crofts, New York, pp 590–597

Repair of Mitral Insufficiency on an Ischemic Basis

O. ALFIERI, L. DESEINS, T. BIANCHI, J. BRONZWAER, and F. VERMEULEN

The operative risk in patients with severe mitral insufficiency on an ischemic basis who receive a mitral prosthesis in addition to coronary bypass grafting is not negligible. Furthermore, the long-term results of surgery in this group of patients are rather poor when compared with those obtained in patients who only undergo myocardial revascularization procedures [1–3]. In order to improve the overall surgical results in this subset of patients we adopted a policy including, whenever possible, preservation of the native mitral valve and correction of its insufficiency with a variety of techniques. The rationale of this approach is based on the assumption that mitral valve repair preserves left ventricular (LV) function by retaining the tethering effect of chordal attachments, thus preventing postoperative LV dilatation and moderating LV wall stress [4].

Moreover, the late complications related to the presence of an implanted prosthesis are obviously prevented when the natural valve is preserved. Mechanisms of mitral regurgitation secondary to coronary heart disease are different [5] and not always can mitral competence be adequately restored. The present study reports our experience with a selected group of patients in whom the incompetence of the mitral valve, although severe, was considered to be correctable without valve replacement.

The Patients

From 1981 to 1984, 19 patients underwent an intervention on the anulus, leaflets, and/or subvalvular apparatus to correct a hemodynamically important chronic mitral insufficiency on an ischemic basis. During the same period another 18 patients with chronic mitral insufficiency due to coronary heart disease were treated with valve replacement, as well as 3 additional patients who developed mitral insufficiency acutely after a myocardial infarction.

All the 19 patients who constitute the study group had at least one previous myocardial infarction and most of them were affected by diffuse coronary artery disease (Table 1). The age ranged from 44 to 73 years (mean, 60 years). Thirteen patients were in preoperative NYHA class III or IV. Angina pectoris was present in 16. In eight patients the ejection fraction was less than 0.40. Pulmonary artery pressure was elevated (mean $\pm$ SD = 42 $\pm$ 8.5 mm Hg). In all patients the left ventriculogram revealed a massive regurgitation of the contrast medium into the left atrium. By two-dimensional echo, the mechanism

Table 1. Repair of mitral insufficiency on an ischemic basis (19 patients)

Previous infarctions	*N*	Coronary involvement	*N*
Posterolateral	11	Main stem	1
Inferior	3	Three-vessel disease	12
Anterior	3	Two-vessel disease	4
Combined	2	One-vessel disease	2

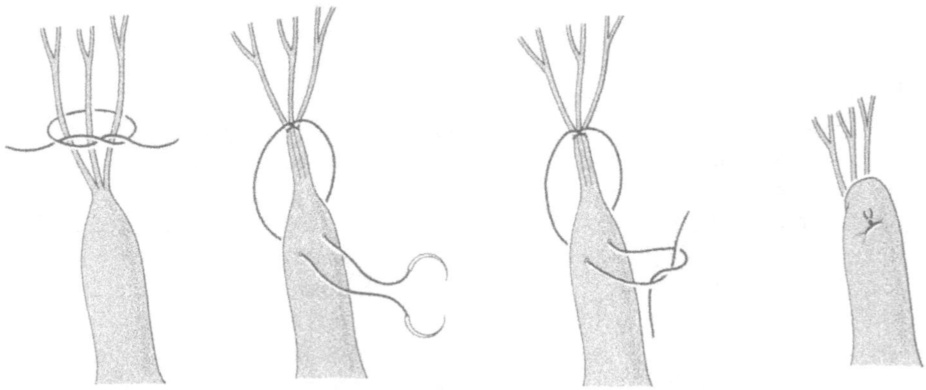

Fig. 1. Technique of chordae shortening

of the insufficiency of the mitral valve was anular dilatation and/or prolapse of the leaflets due to elongation or rupture of the subvalvular apparatus. In no patient was severely impeded elevation of the leaflets detected as the cause of the insufficiency.

The Operation

Most of the techniques used were developed by Carpentier [6], although we have also been using some modifications of the techniques originally described. In Fig. 1 our preferred method of chordae shortening is shown; in Fig. 2 the plication of an elongated fibrous papillary muscle is presented, and Fig. 3 shows

Table 2. Repair of mitral insufficiency on an ischemic basis (19 patients)

Type of mitral repair	*N*
Pure anular remodeling and reduction [a]	3
Correction of subvalvular apparatus	12
Quadrangular resection of posterior leaflet	8
Anulus remodeling [a] in combination	16

[a] With a Carpentier ring

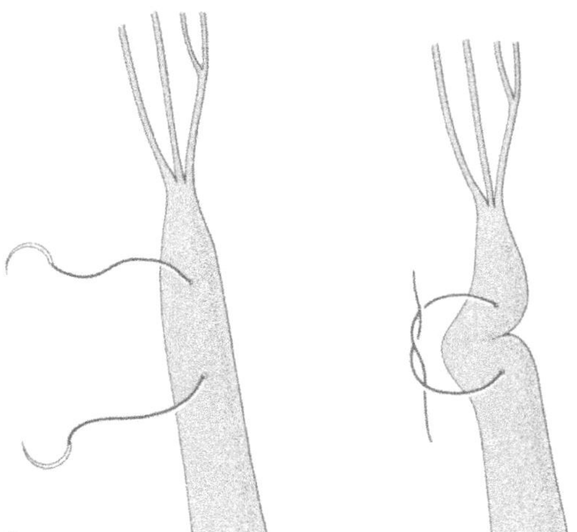

2

Fig. 2. Plications of an elongated fibrous papillary muscle

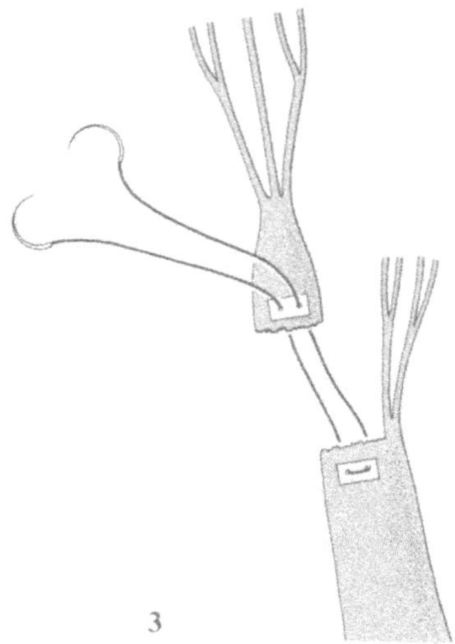

3

Fig. 3. Repair of a ruptured papillary muscle

the repair of a ruptured papillary muscle. The procedures which were carried out to restore the competence of the mitral valve are listed in Table 2. In all patients myocardial revascularization was carried out in addition (from 1 to 6 distal anastomoses per patient; mean $\pm$ SD $= 3 \pm 1.2$).

Results

The operative results are presented in Table 3. There was no hospital mortality and the postoperative course of the majority of the patients was rather smooth. Only three patients had a low cardiac output syndrome which was easily controlled with inotropic support and vasodilating agents. The events recorded during the follow-up period (range, 12–49 months; mean; 26 months) are listed in Table 4. There was a late death, 23 months postoperatively, due to persistent congestive heart failure without evidence of residual mitral incompetence. All

Table 3. Repair of mitral insufficiency on an ischemic basis (19 patients)

Operative results	*N*	%	70% CL
Mortality	0	0	0– 3.6
LCO	3	15	7–23
Other complications	3[a]	15	7–23

[a] One patient, diabetic, had mediastinitis; one had a VT episode; one had a small myocardial infarction. CL, confidence limits; LCO, low cardiac output; VT, ventricular tachycardia.

Table 4. Repair of mitral insufficiency on an ischemic basis (19 patients). Follow-up, mean 26 months (range, 12–49 months)

Events	*N*
Deaths	1[a]
Thromboembolism	0
Hemorrhage	1
Endocarditis	0
Reoperation	0

[a] Due to heart failure with no evidence of residual mitral insufficiency

the survivors are in NYHA class I or II. A murmur of mitral insufficiency is audible in four patients who are clinically well.

Comment

The study group consists only of patients with chronic mitral insufficiency on an ischemic basis, in whom the mechanisms of the incompetence of the valve were anular dilatation and/or prolapse of the leaflets. However, although our indication for mitral repair has been limited and restricted to the above-mentioned mechanisms of mitral incompetence, a considerable proportion (about half) of the patients with ischemic heart disease leading to severe mitral incompetence, according to our observations, could benefit from reconstructive procedures.

Carpentier has preserved the native valve also in patients with impeded leaflet elevation due to paradoxical ventricular wall motion [7]. This type of mitral incompetence should be treated by muscular wall resection and papillary muscle reimplantation. We have no experience with this procedure and have replaced the mitral valve in this type of patient, as well as in patients who developed mitral insufficiency acutely after a myocardial infarction.

Within the limits of our indications, we can conclude that the techniques of reconstruction used are reliable and the short-to medium-term results are encouraging.

References

1. Czer LSC, Gray RJ, De Robertis RA, Bateman TM, Stewart ME, Chaux AS, Maltoff JM (1984) Mitral valve replacement: impact of coronary artery disease and determinants of prognosis after revascularization. Circulation 70 (Suppl I):I-198
2. Pinson CW, Cobanoglu AD, Metzorff MT, Grunkemeier GL, Lay PH, Starr A (1984) Late surgical results for ischemic mitral regurgitation. J Thorac Cardiovasc Surg 88:663
3. Christakis GT, Weisel RD, Fremes SE, Scully HE, Baird RG, Goldman BS (1984) Morbidity and mortality in mitral valve surgery. Circulation 70 (Suppl II): abstracts

4. Bonchek LI, Olinger GN, Siegel R, Tresch DD, Keelan MH (1984) Left ventricular performance after mitral reconstruction for mitral regurgitation. J Thorac Cardiovasc Surg 88:112
5. Ballester M, Tasca R, Marin L, Rees S, Richards A, McDonald L (1983) Different mechanisms of mitral regurgitation in acute and chronic forms of coronary heart disease. Eur Heart J 4:557
6. Carpentier A (1983) Cardiac valve surgery – the "French correction". J Thorac Cardiovasc Surg 86:323
7. Carpentier A (1985) Discussion to the paper. "Experience with the Carpentier techniques of mitral valve reconstruction in 103 patients (1980–1985)" by F.C. Spencer et al. J Thorac Cardiovasc Surg 90:341

Myocardial Protection in Combined Coronary Bypass and Valve Procedure

T. K. KAUL, M. LLEWELLYN, R. A. KHADIMI, D. RAMSDALE, and J. B. MEADE

Introduction

In an attempt to reduce perioperative myocardial ischaemia and improve the long-term results of valve replacement in the presence of significant coronary artery disease, many cardiac units advocate combined valve replacement and myocardial revascularisation even in patients without angina. We have reviewed our experience with 138 patients undergoing combined procedures between 1975 and 1985, relating the results to the different methods of myocardial protection used during surgery.

Patients and Methods

One hundred and thirty-eight patients underwent coronary artery bypass surgery combined with valve replacement. The aortic valve was replaced in 70 (group A), the mitral in 53 (group B); 4 patients had an open mitral valvotomy (group B); and 11 underwent multivalvular procedures (group C). The age range of the series was 42 – 77 years (mean 59 ± 18 years); 63% were male. Cardiac catheterisation was performed in all patients, including coronary and left ventricular angiography. Lesions decreasing the luminal diameter by more than 60% were considered significant. Left ventricular function was classified as good (ejection fraction, 50%), moderately impaired (30% – 50%) and poor (< 30%): on the basis of angiographic assessment in RAO (right anterior oblique) projection.

Methods of Myocardial Protection

Between 1975 and 1978, 22 patients (20 group A, 1 group B and 1 group C) underwent surgery during one period of ischaemic cardiac arrest (group I). Between September 1978 and September 1982, 55 patients (27 group A, 24 group B and 4 group C) underwent systemic cooling (25° – 28° C) with aortic root injection of St. Thomas' Cardioplegic solution (4° C) and continuous irrigation of pericardial cavity with cold Hartmann's solution (8° C) (group II). Between September 1982 and May 1985, 61 patients (25 group A, 30 group B and 6 group C) underwent systemic hypothermia (25° – 27° C) with retrograde perfusion following distal coronary anastomoses and topical cooling as in group II

Table 1. Clinical details

	Group A $n = 70$	Group B $n = 57$	Group C $n = 11$
Angina	74% (77% with AS gradient 50)	21.7%	36%
Dyspnoea			
NHYA I + II	–	–	–
III + IV	47%	50%	38%
AS	58.5%	–	2
AI	12.8%	–	4
AS/AI	28.5%	–	6
MS	–	24.5%	5
MI	–	14%	–
MS + MI	–	61.4%	2
No. of patients with poor LV	11	7	–
Single CABG	40	34	5
Multiple CABG	30	23	6
Bjork-Shiley	68	43	15 (2 Bjork-Shiley aortic grafts)
Hancock	2	2	–
MMI prosthesis	–	1	1

n, number; NYHA, New York Heart Association; AS, aortic stenosis; AI, aortic incompetence; MS, mitral stenosis; MI, mitral incompetence; LV, left ventricle; CABG, coronary artery bypass graft

(group III). Serum lactate dehydrogenase (LDH) aspartate aminotransferase (AST) levels were recorded daily for the postoperative week. A diagnosis of perioperative ischaemia or myocardial infarction was made on standard electrocardiographic criteria.

Results

Early Mortality

Early mortality was 22% in group I, 18% in group II and 8.6% in group III. Early mortality was reduced in group III, but did not achieve statistical significance.

Release of LDH and AST (Summarised in Table 2)

The release of LDH was significantly reduced in group III compared with group II ($P<0.05$), which in turn was significantly less than in group I ($P<0.02$). The release of AST was significantly less in group III than in group I ($P<0.001$) and group II ($P<0.05$).

Table 2. Maximum release of LDH and AST

	LDH±SEM (U/litre)	AST±SEM (U/litre)
Group I	902±93	189 ±26.8
Group II	684±39	180 ±24.8
Group III	591±32.3	113.8± 9.5

Table 3. Recurrence of angina

	No. of survivors	Follow-up (months)	Incidence (% per patient year)
Group I	17	1445	0.14
Group II	45	2244	0.09
Group III	55	896	0.07

Postoperative Ischaemia

Electrocardiographic evidence of persistence of postoperative ischaemia in anterior and inferior leads was 21% in group I; and was significantly less ($P < 0.05$) in group II (12%) and in group III (8%).

Postoperative Angina

Seventy-eight percent of the survivors were free of angina and 22% had anginal symptoms on maximum exertion only (Canadian Cardiovascular Society Class I). The rate of recurrence of angina is summarised in Table 3.

Late Survival

The actuarial survival of the patients was improved in group II and group III (Fig. 1) and no late deaths occurred in 11 patients with poor left ventricular function in group III.

Discussion

There is a high incidence of coronary artery disease in patients with valvular disease who complain of angina pectoris; in addition, a high proportion of patients with valve disease without angina have significant silent occult coronary artery disease. The presence of coronary artery disease may increase early and late postoperative mortality. In this group of patients angina was more frequently associated with aortic valve disease than with mitral valve disease. Seventy-seven percent of patients with aortic s-enosis (gradient > 50 mm Hg) presented with angina. Earlier studies have shown an increased mortality in

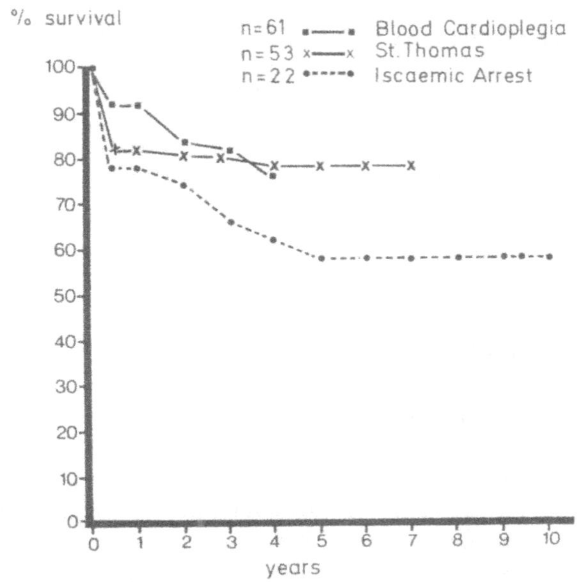

Fig. 1. Actuarial survival in relation to myocardial protection in combined coronary bypass and valve procedures

these complex combined procedures. However, improvement in myocardial protection and surgical technique in recent years has reduced the risk of this form of surgery.

In this series early mortality was not influenced by age, sex, number of grafts, or the valves replaced. We have recorded a marked reduction in the early mortality in the last 61 patients who underwent surgery with cold blood cardioplegic protection, despite the increasing complexity of the procedures in patients of higher operative risk. There was a significant reduction in the postoperative release of LDH and AST with cold blood cardioplegic protection; in addition, there has been a significant reduction in the incidence of postoperative ischaemia. Seventy-eight percent of survivors were free of angina and the rate of recurrence was reduced in group III. Cold blood cardioplegic protection also reduces late mortality, and the long-term survival of patients with poor left ventricular function was improved with cold blood cardioplegic protection.

We have observed an overall improvement in patient survival and well-being since the introduction of cold blood cardioplegic protection for patients undergoing combined valve and coronary bypass procedures.

Antidiuretic Hormone Levels During Cardiopulmonary Bypass

P. Mastroroberto, P. Pepino, L. di Tommaso, M. Chello, G. Jannelli, D. Pantaleo, F. di Lello, M. Monaco, V. de Amicis, and A. R. Marchese

Introduction

Cardiopulmonary bypass (CPB) has been referred to as "controlled shock" [2–4]. Marked increase in antidiuretic hormone (ADH) serum levels has been reported during CPB by other investigators [2–5]. The regulatory mechanisms of ADH plasma levels are shown in Fig. 1 and Table 1. Our purpose is to investigate the changes in serum levels of vasopressin before, during, and after CPB as correlated with the anesthetic management and the low-flow–low-pressure CPB.

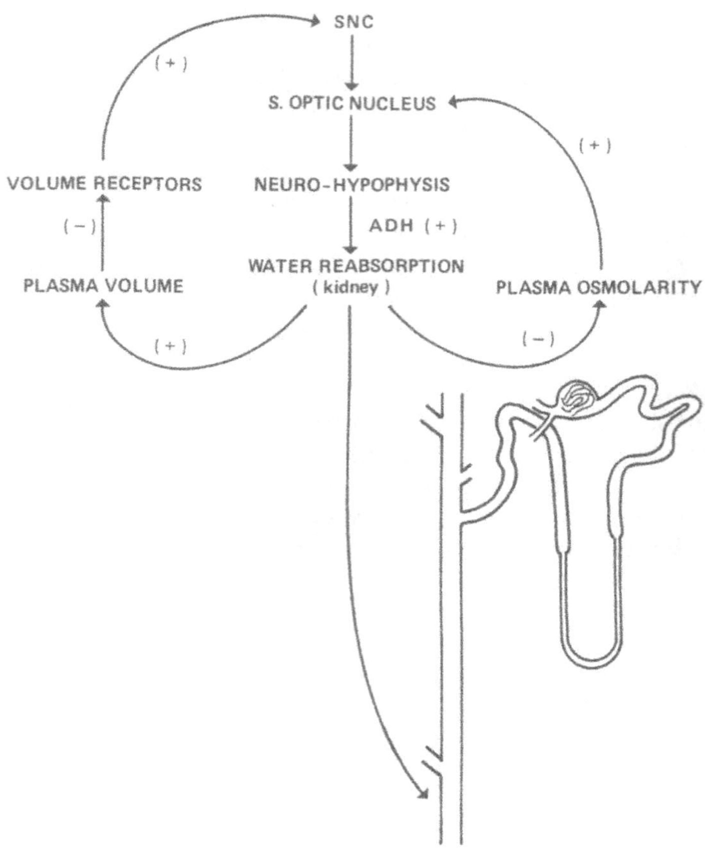

Fig. 1. Regulatory mechanism of antidiuretic hormone

Table 1. Control of ADH plasma levels

Increase in ADH	Decrease in ADH
> Plasma osmotic pressure < Extracellular volume < Arterial pressure	< Plasma osmotic pressure > Extracellular volume > Calcium plasma levels
Stress – pain	
Morphine, barbiturate, nicotine, beta-adrenergic, and colinergic drugs	Atropine Clorpromazine Alpha-adrenergic drugs, Difenilidantoin
Angiotensin	Alcohol

Patients and Method

Subjects

Forty-five adult patients, age ranging from 26 to 62 years (mean 43.3 years), 18 female (40%) and 27 male (60%), who underwent open-heart surgery under extracorporeal circulation, were the subjects of our study. Three operations (6.7%) were closure of an atrial septal defect, 7 (15.5%) mitral valve replacement (MVR), 8 (17.8%) aortic valve replacement (AVR), 4 (8.9% MVR + AVR, 18 (40%) coronary artery bypass graft (CABG), 2 (4.4%) left ventricular aneurysmectomy (LVA), and 3 (6.7%) CABG + LVA (Table 2).

Anesthesia

All patients were anesthetized by the same physician to ensure a consistent anesthetic approach. The anesthetic management (Table 2) consisted of a combination of diazepam, morphine, pancuronium, barbiturate, nitrous oxide + oxygen, and halothane. Morphine and pancuronium bromide were administered at the onset of CPB; in addition, for anesthetic maintainance a combination of pancuronium, halothane, and nitrous oxide + oxygen were administered (Table 3).

Table 2. Operations

– Atrial septal closure	3 (6.7%)
– Aortic valve replacement (AVR)	8 (17.8%)
– Mitral valve replacement (MVR)	7 (15.5%)
– Coronary artery bypass graft (CABG)	18 (40%)
– AVR + MVR	4 (8.9%)
– Left ventricular aneurysmectomy (LVA)	2 (4.4%)
– CABG + LVA	3 (6.7%)
Total patients	45
Male	27 (60%)
Female	18 (40%)

Table 3. Anesthetic management

Preanesthesia	Diazepam Morphine
Anesthetic induction	Pancuronium Barbituric
Anesthetic maintainance	Pancuronium Nitrous oxide Oxygen Halothane
At the onset of CPB	Morphine Pancuronium

Extracorporeal Circulation (Cardiopulmonary Bypass)

The CPB pump oxygenator (Harvey 1700) was primed with lactate Ringer's solution and 5% glucose. The arterial mean pressure was maintained at 50–60 mm Hg; the temperature of the patients was monitored from the nasopharynx (26°–28°C during CPB). The mean duration of CPB was 74.1±5.2 min.

Sampling

Eight milliliters of whole blood was drawn from the arterial line at nine sampling times. These were as follows: S1, anesthetic induction; S2, heparinization (3 mg/kg); S3, CPB on; S4, aortic cross-clamping; S5, lowest body temperature; S6, end of aortic cross-clamping; S7, CPB off; S8, protamine in; S9, second postoperative hour. The samples were centrifuged immediately and successively three more times. Serum levels of ADH were determined by radioimmunoassay (RIA) (normal value of ADH, 1–4 pg/ml) (Table 4).

Table 4. Antidiuretic hormone serum levels during CPB

Stage	Mean	±	SD	Median
1. Anesthetic induction	7.86		4.97	7.85
2. Heparinisation (3 mg/kg)	6.28		2.32	6.30
3. CPB on	4.71		1.25	4.78
4. Aortic cross-clamp	6.36		3.38	6.30
5. Highest hypothermy	5.11		2.54	4.98
6. End of aortic cross-clamp	7.16		2.43	7.16
7. CPB off	6.43		1.54	6.46
8. Administer protamine 1.5 mg/100 IU heparin	2.58		0.56	2.58
9. Second postoperative hour	3.05		2.52	3.00

Normal value of ADH plasma levels by radioimmunologic assay 1–4 pg/ml

Results

The serum level of ADH at S1 (Table 3) was 7.86 ± 4.97 pg/ml, and this increase was observed also at S2, S3, S4, S5, and S6. From the end of aortic cross-clamping we observed a progressive decrease of ADH serum levels; at the second postoperative hour (S9) the vasopressin concentration was in the normal range (3.05 ± 2.52 pg/ml).

Discussion

The peak increase in serum levels of ADH occurred from anesthetic induction to the end of aortic cross-clamping. The ADH level increases correlated well with the administration of morphine (at S3); other authors [4–7] reported a correlation also with the administration of halothane, enflurane, and high-dose fentanyl.

Our results are similar to those of other investigators who compared vasopressin during open-heart surgery under halothane anesthesia and under morphine anesthesia [1, 4, 5, 7]. The increase in serum levels of ADH is pronounced when we use high-dose morphine (preanesthesia, at the onset of CPB, and often during anesthetic maintenance). Besides we prefer a low arterial mean pressure during CPB (50–60 mm Hg), with consequent increase in vasopressin secretion (Table 1).

In conclusion we confirmed a marked rise in serum levels of vasopressin during CPB in adult subjects. These high levels are correlated with the low arterial mean pressure in the pump and the pharmacological influence of anesthetic drugs.

References

1. Brabdt MR, Korshin J, Prange Hansen A et al. (1978) Influence of morphine anaesthesia on the endocrine-metabolic response to open-heart surgery. Acta Anaesthesiol Scand 22:400–412
2. Matsuky A, Ishihara H, Tsubo T et al. (1979) Plasma levels of ADH and catecholamine during cardiopulmonary bypass. Jap J Anaesth 28:1549–1555
3. Oka Y, Nakayama S, Oyama T, Orkin LR et al. (1981) Cortisol and antidiuretic hormone responses to stress in cardiac surgical patients. Canad Anaesth Soc J 28 [4]:334–338
4. Philbin DM, Coggins CH, Emerson CW et al. (1979) Plasma vasopressin levels during cardiopulmonary by-pass. Comparison of halothane and morphine anaesthesia. J Thorac Cardiovasc Surg 77:582–585
5. Philbin DM, Coggins CH, Wilson N, Sokoloski J (1977) Antidiuretic hormone levels during cardiopulmonary by-pass. J Thorac Cardiovasc Surg 73:145–148
6. Wu W, Zbuzek VK, Bellevue C (1980) Vasopressin release during cardiac operation. J Thorac Cardiovasc Surg 79:83–90
7. Yamashita M, Ishihara H, Kudo M, Matsuki A, Oyama T (1984) Plasma vasopressin response to extracorporeal circulation in children. Acta Anaesthesiol Scan 28:331–333

Methods for Blood Usage Reduction During Cardiac Surgery

A. IATRIDIS and J. D. HILL

Introduction

Historically, blood transfusion requirements during cardiac surgery have been related to problems involving the usage of heart-lung bypass. Heat exchangers caused viscosity changes and slugging which resulted in denaturization of proteins and severe coagulopathy. The effect of generating particulate matter emboli caused pump lung syndrome. Early design concepts of heart-lung machines required large volumes of fresh heparinized blood.

Blood transfusions were not seen as major cause for concern until blood and material incompatibility, as well as design concepts, improved. In addition, the growth of cardiac procedures increased the number of transfusions resulting in rising incidence of disease transmission via transfusions. Viral diseases such as hepatitis A and B, non-A and non-B hepatitis, CMV, EBV, and HTLV III originated the caution we now experience regarding transfusions.

There are several programs in progress to reduce, eliminate, or make blood transfusions safer. Avoiding such transfusions if possible is most desirable; however, if needed, choice of donor bank site is desirable. Commercial banks have a higher risk compared with voluntary ones. Quality of a blood bank is determined by donor screening and selection methods. Some geographic locations are known to be safer than others.

In open heart surgery, large volumes of blood transfusions mandated additional methods to decrease transfusion usage. Routine practice such as control of anemia prior to surgery, treatment of bleeding disorders, donation of blood for autologus transfusion, use of frozen blood, and maintenance of careful surgical hemostasis are more stringently adhered to. This focus has occurred since AIDS.

Reduction of blood usage can be augmented via the extracorporeal circuit. Low prime volumes, hemodilution, pre-bleeding patients before bypass, use of membrane oxygenators, system integration for even lower prime, use of diuretics, and use of hemoconcentrators are some methods of conservation. Finally, when appropriate the circuit can be emptied back to the patient at the bypass end. Acceptance of lower postoperative hematocrit is an element, as well as autotransfusion.

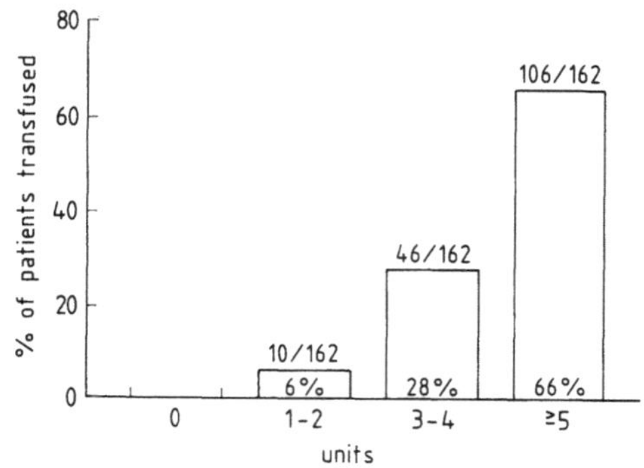

Fig. 1. Distribution of blood requirements in 162 consecutive patients during 1981. Average utilization was 6.1 units/patient

Methods

At the Pacific Presbyterian Medical Center in 1981, average blood utilization was 6.2 units per open heart procedure. Prior to this point, the importance of bloodless surgery was not as acute. In fact, 66% of adult operations were transfused with 5 or more units of blood (Fig. 1). A program was proposed to examine possible conservation techniques. The objectives were to reduce disease transmission, to reduce community blood requirements, and to reduce medical costs.

Three methods were introduced to study approaches best suited for blood conservation during cardiac surgery. Method 1 included cell saving, which offers leukocyte-poor washed red cells (LPWRC) at 50–85 hematocrit. During perioperative and immediate postoperative periods hematocrits were maintained at 20%–24%. Also incorporated was collection and autotransfusion of chest drainage. The guideline for this practice stated that up to 400 cc drainage or whatever was obtained in the first 4 postoperative hours and was available for transfusion. The final element was harassment of every team member as reinforced strict discipline at every step of the process. Method 2 simply required a hematocrit maintained at 30%, and method 3 combined methods for cell saving plus maintenance of hematocrit at 30%.

Results

Months later encouraging results were becoming apparent as noted in Fig. 2. Method 1 demonstrated that 27% of adults with primary procedures received no blood transfusions. Results for method 2 were 9% and 17% with method 3.

Since 1984 adult primary surgical procedures not requiring donor blood increased to 21%. As noted in Fig. 3, 37% required 1–2 units. Bloodless redo operations also increased from 12% in 1983 to 14% in 1984. However, there remained a large category requiring 5 units as shown in Fig. 4. In examining this category a relationship between weight and blood usage was plotted as seen in Fig. 5. As expected, heavier patients required fewer transfused units. In the case

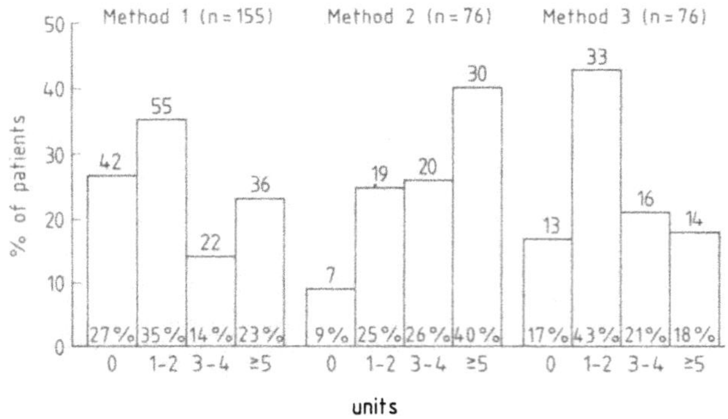

Fig. 2. Distribution of blood requirements in 307 consecutive patients using three different methods during 1983

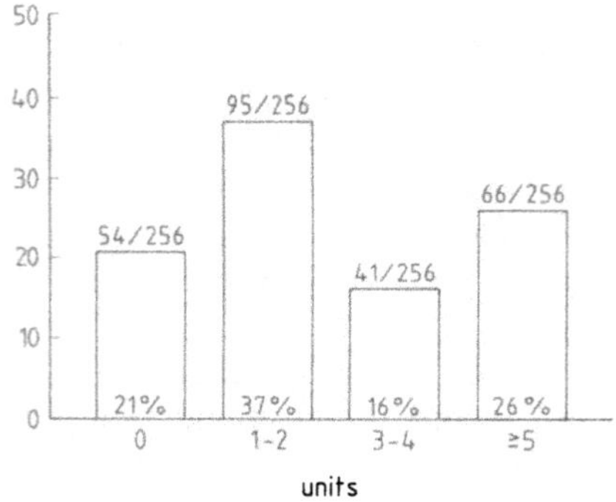

Fig. 3. Distribution of blood requirements in 256 consecutive patients during 1984

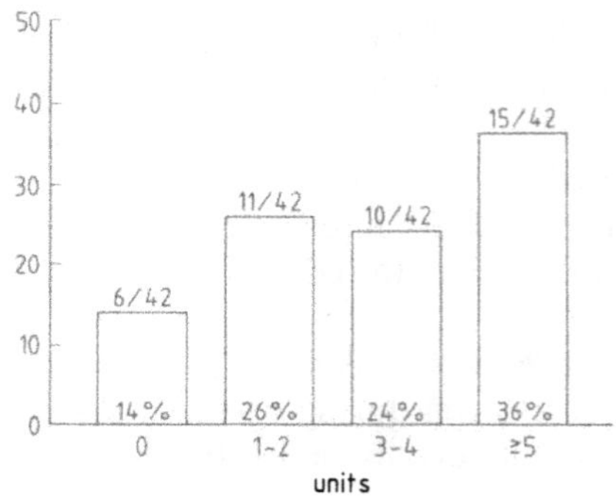

Fig. 4. Distribution of blood requirements in 42 consecutive Redo operations in 1984

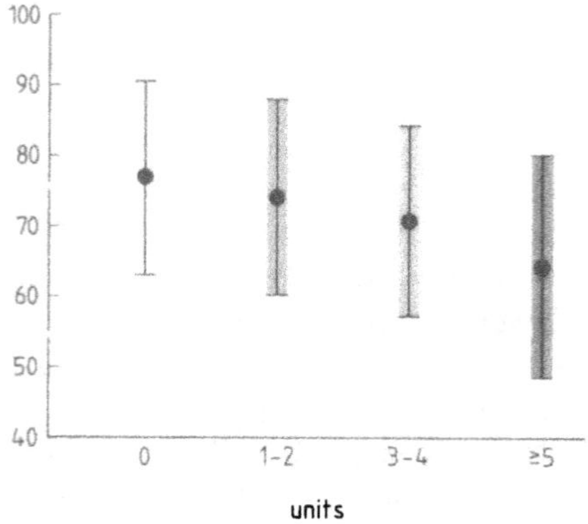

Fig. 5. Relationship of body weight to blood requirements during 1984

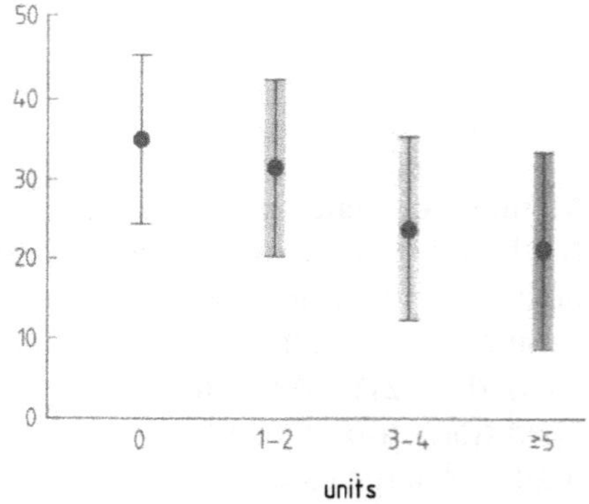

Fig. 6. Relationship of preoperative hematocrit to blood requirements during 1984

Table 1. Blood transfusion requirements: discharge hematocrit (all adult patients)

Transfusion units	1981 Mean (%)	1983 Mean (%)	1984 Mean (%)
0	–	30	31
1–2	32	30	31
3–4	34	32	31
≧5	34	31	31

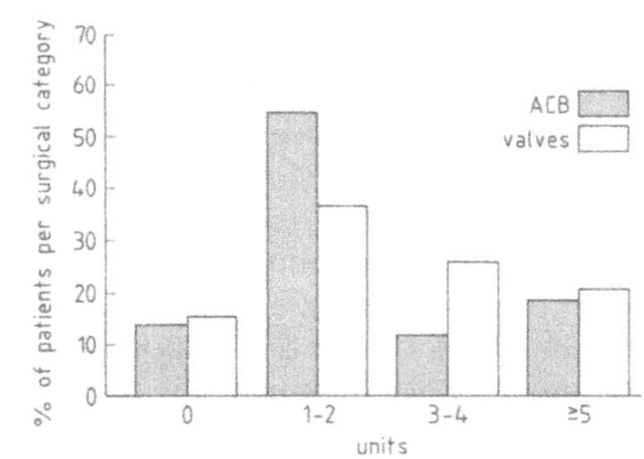

Fig. 7. Relationship of blood requirements to preoperative diagnosis using method I. There is no significant difference

of hematocrit versus blood usage, Fig. 6 demonstrates that patients with higher preoperative hematocrits required less blood.

Average discharge hematocrits for bloodless adult procedures were 31% in 1984 as seen in Table 1. In 1981 there were no bloodless procedure data available. The number of cases where 5 or more units of transfused blood were required has decreased since 1981, when conservation methods were implemented.

Method 1 was most effective in reducing blood usage. Therefore, a comparison was drawn between aortocoronary bypass grafts and valve procedures (Fig. 7). As indicated the number of bloodless cases in coronary artery bypass graft procedures is about equal to that of valves. However, the number of cases requiring 1–2 units of blood were greater in grafts than valves. Hypotheses have been developed to explain this, but time does not permit exploring them.

Complications

Institution of these conservation methods has been very successful during this crucial AIDS period. This is especially true since San Francisco has a large gay population and is seen as the "gay capital of the world." However, there are some complications worth mentioning. Postoperatively, patients recovering with low hemoglobins experience weakness and fatigue easily. This may prolong postoperative recovery and hospital stay. Wound healing may be prolonged. O_2-carrying capacity in patients with low hematocrits will be decreased as well as O_2 delivery, 2.3 DPG. This occurs until reconstitution when normal O_2 release from hemoglobin to tissues occurs. Patients with cardiac disorders and low hematocrit concentrations demonstrate tissue hypoxia and some pulmonary complications due to hemodilution and fluid accumulation. Cell-saving methods do remove most blood activators and platelets; thus coagulopathy and excessive bleeding may occur. With slow healing and other abnormalities, infection may set in. With all the complications mentioned medical costs increase.

Analysis of reoperations for postoperative bleeding showed that the rate was 3% in 1981 and 2.1% for 1982, 1983, and 1984. Method 1 patients bleed 1.2%, method 2 4.1%, and method 3 1.3%. The lower percentage in method 2 was associated with shorter pump times and faster surgery. In all, methods 1 and 3 have applied surgical hemostasis more carefully at the expense of longer pump runs. Infection rates since blood conservation methods were begun have not changed. In 1980 our infection rate was 2.0%, in 1981 2.6%, in 1982 1,0%, in 1983 1.6%, and in 1984 1.2%. The reduction from 1980 to the present may be attributed to better techniques and overall practice.

There are some contraindications to blood conservation. Patients who are infected should not be part of blood-saving and other methods. Contaminated autotransfused blood should not be reinfused. Patients with cardiac disease with hypertrophy, incomplete revascularization, and low cardiac output should not be treated with low hematocrit and blood with 2.3 DPG elevation. Pulmonary air leak cases are also contraindicated for blood preservation methods since the lungs will act as a bubble oxygenator in the area where the pulmonary air leak exists.

Blood conservation can be accomplished via autotransfusion, low hematocrit, pleural drainage autotransfusion, and strict adherence to technique for prevention of blood loss. Reasons for conservation include decreased transmission of disease and prevention of allergic reaction.

Blood quality with autotransfusion is good. 2.3 DPG is elevated. Cell fragility remains the same. The blood does not have to be cooled or rewarmed. There is a natural resistance to infection.

Autotransfused blood eliminates transfusion reaction resulting from clerical error that occurs with handling and processing of heterologous blood. This technique also permits surgeries on religious groups refusing transfusions. Surgical cancellation resulting from donor blood shortages is decreased. Lastly overall cost of cardiac surgical procedures is reduced.

In discussing this study there are a few experiences that should be shared. Perhaps every study offers some lessons that result from the protocol but are not part of it. For example, we found that every time a cell-processing device was in the immediate area conservation methods were more effective even though the machine may not have been utilized. Thus, the device served as a reminder of protocol, as a memorial statute would.

Beneficial effects were noted in method 2 where the protocol only called for maintenance of hematocrit at 30. It was noted that within this method surgeons were taking more time to obtain good hemostasis. Finally, not one element has resulted in noticeable change. However, the accumulation of all steps did result in significant differences.

Abstract

Intraarterial DSA for Postoperative Determination of ACBG Patency

B. URBANYI, K. H. HAUENSTEIN, G. NOELDGE, and V. SCHLOSSER

None of the noninvasive methods (CT, sonography, myocardial scintigraphy) developed over the past years have led to satisfactory results in determining bypass patency following ACBG (aorto-coronary bypass graft); the same is true for intravenous DSA (digital subtraction angiography).

In contrast, intraarterial DSA, with a bolus injection of 30 ml 30% contrast medium through a thin 5-F catheter into the aortic root bypass patency, may be demonstrated accurately; moreover, anastomotic width, stenoses or torsion in the graft, and patency of the anastomosed coronary arteries can be shown.

Over a 7-month period 90 patients were examined within the 5th and 14th postoperative days. Early graft patency was demonstrated in 92.5% of the grafts. In 80% the peripheral anastomoses and the anastomosed coronary vessels were visualized, showing that this method may be of early prognostic value.

Abstract

Experimental UV Laser Coronary Angioplasty: Initial Results

G. Laufer, G. Wollenek, G. Stangl, M. Deutsch, and E. Wolner

In the surgical management of coronary artery disease laser angioplasty has become a new therapeutic aspect for the future. Of the many types of medical lasers now in use (Nd-YAG, argon, CO_2 laser), removal or separation of tissue rely on a common mechanism: light absorption by the irradiated tissue, conversion of that light energy into heat energy, and subsequent vaporization of the tissue or plaque. In cases of coronary plaque irradiation photothermic tissue decomposition results in heat damage to the surrounding vessel wall.

In contrast the UV Excimer laser provides athermic ablative tissue decomposition. We used wavelengths 193 and 248 nm at 5 – 15 Hz and investigated laser effects on healthy and atherosclerotic coronary arteries of human and animal origin. The UV laser produced well-defined incisions with micrometer precision and no evidence of thermal damage. These observations were confirmed by temperature registration and histology.

Abstract

Eicosapentaenoic Acid, Persantine, and Aspirin for the Prevention of Vein Graft Intimal Hyperplasia

R. W. LANDYMORE, M. A. MACAULAY, B. SHERIDAN, and C. CAMERON

Antiplatelet drug regimens are currently used to reduce intimal hyperplasia (IH) and improve long-term vein graft patency following arterial reconstruction. Ninety-six autologous external jugular vein grafts were implanted between bilaterally divided femoral arteries in 48 dogs. The animals received a 2% cholesterol diet and antiplatelet drug regimens 1 week before and for 6 weeks following operation. Ten control animals (CON) received the diet alone, 10 dogs received Persantine (dipyridamole), 2.5 mg/kg, and 325 g aspirin (P-ASA), 11 dogs received cod-liver oil containing 1.8 g eicosapentaenoic acid (EPA) daily, and a further 17 dogs received 1.8 g EPA and 2.5 mg/kg Persantine daily (EPA-P). Prothrombin time (PT), partial thromboplastin time (PTT), bleeding times (BTS), and platelet counts (PTLS) were measured before operation and during antiplatelet therapy. Vein grafts were havested at 6 weeks and intimal thickness was measured with a Zeiss computerized microscope. The intima measured 6.1 ± 0.2 µm prior to implantation and increased to 78 ± 8 µm in the CON. P-ASA decreased IH to 33 ± 3 µm ($P < 0.001$), EPA decreased IH to 27 ± 3 µm ($P < 0.001$), and EPA-P reduced IH to 17 ± 1 µm ($P < 0.001$). PTL decreased in the P-ASA group ($P < 0.05$) and BT decreased in the EPA-P group ($P < 0.05$) but all other coagulation parameters were unchanged. Although all antiplatelet regimes reduced IH, EPA-P was the most effective ($P < 0.009$).

Further Studies of Graft Stenosis Following Aortocoronary Bypass: II. State of Vein Interstitium, Preliminary Report

J. H. KENNEDY and C. P. WINLOVE

Introduction

Myocardial revascularization using the autogenous saphenous vein for occlusive coronary artery disease has become a recognized treatment and is carried out in cardiac surgical centres worldwide with an acceptable mortality and relief of angina. However, some patients develop concentric subintimal fibrous stenosis of the graft and recurrence of symptoms.

A number of experimental and clinical studies have emphasized the importance of mural ischaemia by interruption of the vasa vasora [6], aortovenous anastomotic angle [11], elevated intraluminal pressure and endothelial damage [5] and reduced flow velocity [2] in the development of venous subintimal hyperplasia. Bonchek et al. [5] and Landymore et al. [12] have suggested platelet aggregation as an aetiological factor and reported prevention in experimental animals by anti-activation agents. A number of other technical reasons for graft occlusion exist; poor distal runoff, kinking, and suture compromise of the anastomosis, to name a few. As in other surgical grafts, its quality is an essential factor in success.

Histological findings in an earlier report [11] suggest trauma to venous endothelium and interstitium. This may be caused by hycraulic overdistension of the vein, which is frequently used during preparation. We describe a preliminary study designed to test the response of the interstitium to changes in pressure in which the umbilical cord is used as a simple model of vascular interstitium in order to measure [^{125}I] albumin and [^{51}Cr] ethylene diaminetetra-acetic acid (EDTA) spaces as a function of applied intraluminal pressure. These two probes were selected as the mobility and distribution of albumin, a relatively large molecule, is influenced by the steric exclusion by the extracellular matrix, and is therefore affected by state of hydration of the tissue, while EDTA, a small molecule, has access to almost all the extracellular water space, and therefore acts as a reference material for the investigation of changes in the interstitium.

Materials and Method

Fresh (less than 24-h postpartum) human umbilical cords from the same maternity unit were collected under sterile conditions and kept in 0.9% saline-moistened gauze in closed containers at 4° C until study as described by Meyer

[13]. Cord blood samples were screened for hepatitis B antigen for laboratory safety. All experiments were carried out at 4° C.

The diffusion of [^{125}I]serum albumin labelled by the chloramine-T method [3] and complexed with Evans Blue Dye and [^{51}Cr]EDTA (Amersham International, UK) was studied into 10-cm segments of umbilical cord under 60 mm Hg pressure through the cannulated umbilical vein, compared with cannulated, unpressured cord segments. All specimens were perfused with, and immersed in, 4% bovine serum albumin in phosphate-buffered saline (pH 7.0±0.1), which was found in preliminary experiments to be approximately iso-osmolar, in a covered aluminium perfusion chamber of 82 ml volume at 4° C for 3–168 h. The time period was chosen on the basis of albumin diffusivity in the tissue [13]. Label was added to the bath.

After the chosen time interval, 1-mm slices were taken from a central and distal (away from the pressure source) portion of each specimen, each of which were weighed, counted for ^{125}I and ^{51}Cr (Packard Autogamma Counter) and dehydrated to a constant weight at 94° C in order to determine water content. Bath samples were also collected at various times during the incubation period. The data were analyzed to provide the [^{125}I]albumin distribution space (ml/g tissue), the [^{51}Cr]EDTA distribution space, [^{125}I]SA/EDTA ratios, [^{125}I]SA counts/g dry wt., [^{51}Cr]EDTA counts/g dry wt. and weight change.

The calculations were carried out electronically using a program written for the purpose (VEINCTS), correcting for the crossover of specific activity from ^{51}Cr to ^{125}I counts. Statistical analysis was based on Wetherhill [15] by a program written for the purpose (T-Test) for both equal and unequal population variance.

Serial measurements of the supernatant fluid after final bath samples had been treated with 10 μl trichloroacetic acid revealed 0.02%–0.03% free radioiodine.

Results

A total of 8 paired experiments were carried out on 16 samples.

The weight gain by pressured cords was greater than unpressured cords, both incubated 3–168 h (0.52, SD = 0.4 vs. 0.3, SD = 0.2) (not significant).

As shown in Fig. 1, the dry weight albumin distribution space was greater (23.7, SD = 11.5 vs. 19, SD = 11) (NS). The water/dry wt. content was slightly greater in pressured cords (Fig. 2), 14.06 ml/gm (SD = 4.91) vs. 12.64 (SD = 2.90). As cord specimens varied in state of hydration, if each specimen served as its own control, the ratio pressured cord to unpressured cord was greater than one in weight gain, albumin distribution space and dry wt. water content. There was a significant difference ($P < 0.5$) in the ratio of dry wt. albumin distribution space to dry wt. EDTA distribution space in pressured, as opposed to unpressured, samples from the same specimen (Fig. 3); 0.82 (SD = 0.2) vs. 0.65 (SD = 0.15).

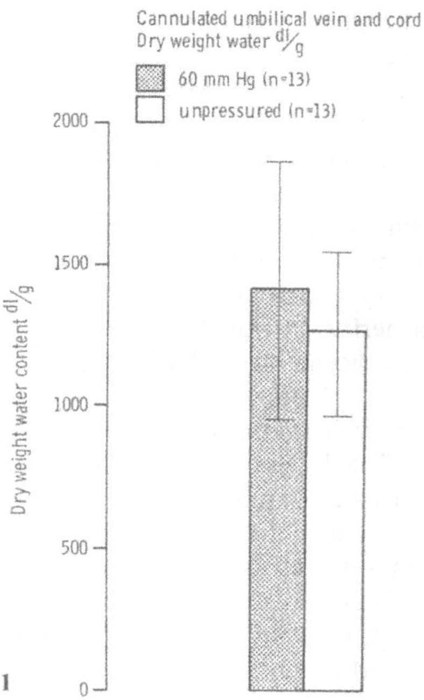

1

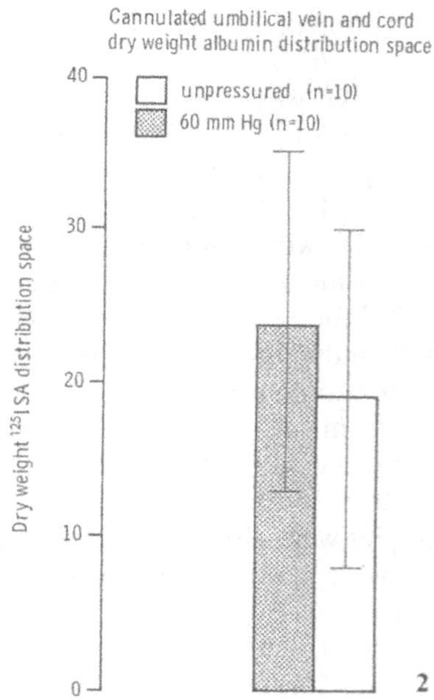

2

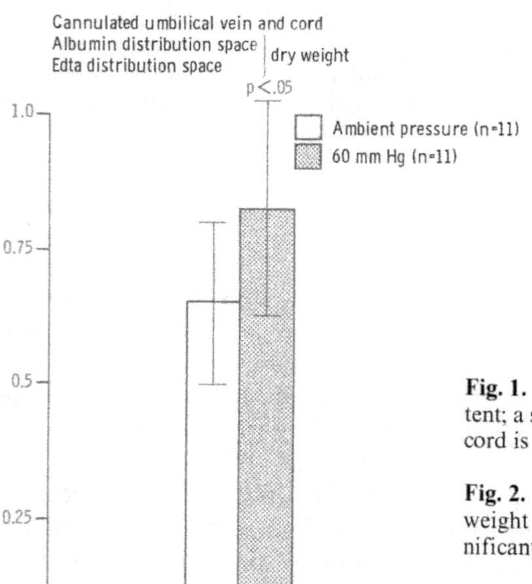

Fig. 1. Histogram of dry weight water content; a slight difference in favor of pressured cord is not significant

Fig. 2. Histogram: the slight increase in dry weight albumin distribution space is not significant

Fig. 3. Ratio albumin/EDTA distribution spaces: there is a statistically significant difference favoring pressured cord (*dark bars*)

Discussion

Reports by others suggest that transport through the blood vessel wall is influenced by intraluminal pressure [7, 8, 10] or by removal of the endothelium [9, 14]; the latter in turn is brought about by collapse of the vessel wall [1]. It is also possible that the physical state of the interstitium per se is an important factor. The goal of this project was demonstration of exclusion/entrapment of a labelled diffusible natural macromolecule in comparison with movement of a labelled small molecule in pressured, as opposed to unpressured, fresh human umbilical cord.

Entrapment of [^{125}I]SA in comparison to [^{51}Cr]EDTA from pressured, as opposed to unpressured, umbilical cord has been demonstrated in 3- to 168-h experiments. In addition to the technical limitations of in vitro incubated tissue as a model for SA flux in living mammals and doubts about the similarities of venous and umbilical cord interstitium, the nature of the entrapment/exclusion of labelled SA in the present study also remains unexplained. The mechanism may be mechanical entanglement in the amorphous phase of the interstitium, concentrated by water loss.

Conclusions

1. The results of a study of movement of fluid relative to labelled albumin pressured and unpressured umbilical cord, cannulated in vitro through the umbilical vein, have been reported.
2. As cord specimens varied in state of hydration, if each cord served as its own control, the ratio pressured cord to unpressured cord was greater than one in weight gain, albumin distribution space and dry wt. water content.
3. There were significant differences in the ratio albumin distribution space to EDTA distribution space ($P < 0.05$) in pressured, as opposed to cannulated, cord.
4. These findings suggest that umbilical vein intraluminal pressure has an effect on transmural transport in human umbilical cord, and add weight to the evidence of others that fibrous intimal hyperplasia following aortocoronary bypass grafting may be due to peroperative hydraulic overdistension.

References

1. Baldwin AL, Caro CG, Davis J, Winlove CP (1978) Structural and mechanical effects of vascular collapse. Physiol 278:14–15p
2. Berguer R, Higgins RF, Reddy DJ (1980) Intimal Hyperplasia. An experimental story. Arch Surg 115:332–335
3. Bolton AE (1977) Radioiodination techniques, Review 18. The Radiochemical Centre, Amersham, pp 45–48
4. Boncheck LI (1980) Prevention of endothelial damage during preparation of saphenous veins for bypass grafting. J Thorac Cardiovasc Surg 79:911–915
5. Boncheck LI, Boerboom LE, Olinger GN, Pepper JR, Munns J, Hutchinson L, Kissebah AH (1982) Prevention of lipid accumulation in experimental vein bypass grafts by antiplatelet therapy. Circulation 66:338–341

6. Brody WR, Kosek JC, Angell WW (1972) Changes in vein grafts following aortocoronary bypass induced by pressure and ischemia. J Thorac Cardiovasc Surg 64:847–854
7. Caro CG, Lever MJ (1983) Effect of vasoconstrictive agents and applied stress on the albumin space of excised rabbit carotid arteries. Atherosclerosis 46:137–146
8. Duncan L, Cornfield J, Buck J (1982) Effect of blood pressure on passage of labelled plasma albumin into canine aortic wall. J Clin Invest 41:1537–1545
9. Falcone DJ, Hajjar DP, Minick CR (1984) Lipoprotein and albumin accumulation in reendothelialized artery wall. Am J Pathol 114:112–120
10. Fry DL (1973) Atherogenesis: initiating factors. Ciba Found Symp 12:93–120
11. Kennedy JH, Wieting DW, Hwang NHC, Anderson MS, Bayardo RJ, Howell JF, De Bakey ME (1974) Hydraulic and morphologic study of fibrous subintimal hyperplasia. J Thorac Cardiovasc Surg 67:805–813
12. Landymore RW, MacAulay M, Sheridan B, Cameron C (1986) Comparison of cod-liver oil and aspirin-dipyridimole for the prevention of intimal hyperplasia in autologous vein grafts. Ann Thorac Surg 41:54–57
13. Meyer FA, Laver-Rudich Z, Tanenbaum R (1983) Evidence for Mechanical coupling of Glycoprotein Microfibrils with collagen fibrils in Wharton's Telly. Biochemica et Biophysica Acta 755:376–387
14. Ramirez CA, Colton CK, Smith KA, Stemerman MB, Lees RS (1984) Transport of ^{125}I albumin across normal and de-endothelialized rabbit aorta in vivo. Arteriosclerosis 4:283–291
15. Wetherhill GB (1967) Elementary statistical methods. Methuen, London

Abstract

Autologous Vein Harvesting Using the Subcutaneous Extraluminal Dissector

W. R. Dimitri, I. E. West, and B. T. Williams

An atraumatic technique for vein procurement has been employed by our team since January 1984 on all patients undergoing myocardial revascularisation, using the subcutaneous vein dissector. To date, 724 long saphenous and 6 cephalic veins were harvested from 672 unselected consecutive patients (568 males and 104 females). Minor early and late leg wound complications were minimized (superficial wound inflammation, 2.6%; small inguinal haematoma, 1.2%; saphenous nerve damage, 1.4%; leg oedema for 3 months, 0.9%). Serious leg problems (wound dehiscence, suppuration and re-exploration) were abolished. This contrasts sharply with a 12% wound complication rate previously reported from this unit. Scanning electron microscope studies of harvested veins reveal a well-preserved vein architecture and lack of damage to the tributaries. The relief of angina in this series compares well with our previous results using the conventional method of open dissection. The simplicity and efficacy of the operative technique is demonstrated, stressing ways of minimising vein handling and trauma. Our results confirm this technique to be of advantage in reducing the early and late morbidity of vein procurement, particularly in high-risk patients, without compromising on vein quality and recommend its wide adoption.

Applications of New Techniques in Saphenous Vein Aortocoronary Bypass Graft Operations

J. E. MOLINA and J. A. ESTRIN

Materials and Methods

Two groups of patients were studied and compared for results. Group I, in which a set of new techniques [1, 2, 3] were implemented, consisted of 80 patients undergoing elective or urgent surgery for coronary obstructive disease and angina. Among this group, seven patients (8.7%) required emergency surgery for unstable angina and four patients (5%) were given reoperations for recurring angina due to occluded previously implanted grafts. Group II consisted of 76 patients operated upon simultaneously but in whom the distal anastomosis of the graft was done first and the proximal end later. In these patients reversed saphenous veins were used in the standard manner. Placement of the grafts was done anteriorly, and standard nonoxygenated clear cardioplegia (St. Thomas II solution) was used in larger amounts than in group I. Although pulmonary pressure monitoring was also used in this group, no esophageal probe for two-dimensional echo monitoring was placed. The mean age in both groups was not significantly different (group I, 61.6 years vs. group II, 65.3 years). The number of graft implanted in group I was 253, with a mean of 3.1 per patient vs. 220 in group II with a mean of 2.8 per patient (Table 1). Among the group who underwent proximal anastomosis first (group I), in 71 patients (89%) partial clamping of the aorta to implant the grafts proximally was well tolerated, and in 9 patients (11%) signs of an increase in pulmonary artery pressure and dilatation of the left ventricle and atrium occurred as detected by the two-dimensional echo probe. Therefore in these patients cardiopulmonary bypass was implemented at

Table 1. Number of grafts

		Group I	Group II
1		5	6
2		12	18
3		36	32
4		21	18
5		4	2
6		2	–
Total	Patients	80	76
	Grafts	253 (average of 3.1/patient)	220 (average of 2.8/patient)

that point, and the proximal anastomosis done first nevertheless. To assess the graft-coronary artery size match, the distal end of the graft was measured directly on the table compared with the diameter measured in the coronary artery. A ratio was established dividing the coronary artery diameter by the vein diameter. A ratio of 1 meant that both diameters were equal; therefore the lower the ratio the more severe was the mismatch. Other parameters monitored were: (a) aorta to coronary artery distance by measuring the length of the vein graft utilized, (b) postcardiac bypass performance assessed by cardiac output measurement with the thermodilution technique using the Swans-Ganz catheter, (c) release of cardiac isoenzymes CK-MB fraction measured to estimate the degree of myocardial damage, and (d) postoperative arrhythmia occurrence.

Results

Cardiopulmonary Bypass Time

Because the cardiopulmonary bypass time was directly related to the number of grafts implanted, each group was subdivided according to the number of grafts received. The more grafts implanted the longer the period of cardiopulmonary bypass. Only patients receiving one to four grafts were analyzed statistically because the number of patients receiving five and six grafts was too small and there was not an equal number of patients in each group. The difference in time of connecting the graft proximally first, before going on cardiopulmonary bypass, was highly significant for patients undergoing two, three, and four grafts (Table 2). This was due to the fact that in group I the proximal anastomosis stage is done off cardiopulmonary (CP) bypass, and after the distal grafts are implanted reperfusion of the myocardium occurs immediately and the patient can be taken off bypass sooner. On the other hand in group II another 30 to 45 min was spent in connecting the grafts proximally to the aorta before the patient could be removed from CP bypass. A few of the patients who were taken off bypass before all grafts had been connected to the ascending aorta needed to be placed on bypass again until the proximal connection was completed. Some tolerated being off bypass even when the proximal anastomoses were not finished but their number was so small (three) that they did not make any difference in the final statistical analysis.

Table 2. Cardiopulmonary bypass time (mean values = minutes)

Grafts	Group I	Group II	*P*	Minutes difference
1	32.6	36.3	NS	–
2	66.8	78.5	<0.05	11.7
3	69.8	97.4	<0.001	27.6
4	78.5	120.0	<0.001	41.5

Ischemia Time

The time of ischemia was measured from the instant the aorta was cross-clamped until all the grafts were connected proximally in group II. Therefore in group I, where the proximal end of the graft had been connected before placing the patient on cardiopulmonary bypass, the patients did not suffer any additional cross-clamp ischemia until these grafts were functioning and ready to be connected distally. As soon as each distal anastomosis was completed, cardioplegia was injected, and those ischemic areas were perfused with the cold solution. At the end of the procedure, as the cross-clamp was removed, instantaneous reperfusion of the entire heart occurs. On the other hand, in group II it was not until all the proximal ends were connected to the ascending aorta that the ischemic areas were reperfused. As expected, the more grafts were implanted, the longer the period of ischemia. Group I patients undergoing one single graft implant did not have a statistically significant difference with patients in group II. But other patients undergoing two, three, and four grafts did show quite a significant difference, thus, group I had shorter periods of ischemia time (Table 3).

Positioning of the Grafts

Connecting a graft going to the left side of the heart approximately somewhat posterior and toward the right side of the ascending aorta was quite easily done without compromising the afterload of the left ventricle as shown by the monitoring done using a two-dimensional echo via an esophageal probe and the pulmonary artery pressure measured by the Swan-Ganz catheter. As the grafts are implanted they should be oriented posteriorly in order to avoid any kinks while the grafts are passed in the transverse sinus to exist between the pulmonary artery and the left atrium. This positioning of the graft is more favorable than placing it anteriorly if sequential grafting is contemplated; thus the first and second diagonal along with the left anterior descending artery are almost in a straight line without any sharp angulations caused to the graft. This is not the case when the graft is implanted anteriorly; thus almost a right angle has to be created connecting any of the diagonal arteries then the left anterior descending artery in the same vein. The graft is also pushed anteriorly by the outflow tract of the right ventricle or the pulmonary artery itself. Reaching the first and second diagonal artery, the left anterior descending system or the circumflex system as a whole required shorter lengths in the graft opposed to placing the

Table 3. Ischemia time (mean values = minutes)

Grafts	Group I	Group II	*P*	Minutes difference
1	13.7	16.6	NS	–
2	36.4	56.7	<0.01	20.3
3	47.3	83.1	<0.001	35.7
4	61.6	108.3	<0.001	46.5

grafts anteriorly. Mean values in the length of the graft shown for group I: left anterior descending artery was 11.5 cm, to the second diagonal artery was 10.8, and to the circumflex artery was 11.3 vs. group II at 13.1, 14.6, and 15.6 cm respectively. The distance between the left anterior descending artery in group I and II was not statistically significantly different. However, the lengths measured for the second diagonals and circumflex system were highly significant. Both of these calculations show a P value <0.05.

Nonreversed Saphenous Vein Grafts [3]

Using the vein in the normal position, having the femoral end of the vein, which is the largest opening, connected to the aorta and having the distal end connected to the coronary artery allowed better matching of the graft to the coronary artery. The vein is always larger but the ratio measured artery-vein was significantly higher (better matched) in group I at 0.6 ± 0.01 vs. group II at 0.4 ± 0.05, P value of this analysis <0.001. The long-term patency rate using valvotomized veins is now in its 2nd year, and the patients who have undergone reangiography have shown them to be patent without any signs of thrombosis or stenosis in the area where the valves were divided.

Oxygenated Cardioplegia [1, 2]

The system we used for oxygenation of clear cardioplegia was the Gish type, where the cardioplegia is contained in a sterile rigid reservoir and oxygen flows over the solution without bubbling through it. The PO_2s measured in the solution during the operative procedure ranged from 500 to 650 Torr. In group I cardioplegia was injected in amounts ranging from 330 ml for patients undergoing single-vessel bypass, to a maximum of 700 ml in patients undergoing five graft implants; compared with group II, where the minimal amount used was 700 ml to a maximum of over 2000 ml in patients undergoing five grafts. The mean value for patients having four graft implants was 1670 ml.

Postoperative Cardiac Performance

Two methods of assessment of cardiac function were used: monitoring of the arrhythmias and measurements of cardiac output. Utilizing a bipolar system for pacing the atrium (surface leads) in group I was compared with group II, where no pacing was used. The number of supraventricular arrhythmias in group I was 3 patients (3.7%) vs. 14 (18.4%) in group II. The pacing of the atrium was made in an asynchronous mode from the time the patient was being weaned off CP bypass up to 30 h after surgery [4]. Comparing group I with group II the statistical analysis was significant to a P value of <0.001. Routinely as the patient is rewarmed and weaned off cardiopulmonary bypass the atrium is paced at 90 beaths/min in an asynchronous mode and cardiac output is measured. At least six measurements were taken each time to have meaningful values compared. Group I had an average of 9.6 ± 1.9 liters/min of cardiac output right off bypass vs. group II with 4.2 ± 0.8 liters/min. The statistical analysis agave a P value <0.001 in favor of group I.

Discussion

Several advantages appeared obvious, utilizing the techniques followed in group I rather than the standard classic approach followed in group II patients. Among the advantages of connecting the saphenous vein proximally first, is that after completing each anastomosis in the distal coronary artery that area of muscle can be immediately perfused with cold cardioplegic solution since the proximal end is already connected [3]. Connecting the distal ends first will not provide such an advantage unless each vein is injected individually with cardioplegic solution. Venting of the air from the graft is also simply done by following the technique used in group I. Injection of cardioplegia expels the air via the distal end before the distal suture line is tightened and tied. Following the routine standard techniques of group II, after the distal anastomosis is completed the patient is routinely rewarmed when the ischemic areas are not yet receiving any perfusion, This, to our way of thinking, risks the occurrence of further myocardial damage in those ischemic areas during the 15, 30, or 45 min that it takes to connect the proximal ends to the aorta.

The monitoring implemented by the anesthesiologist is very useful in two major areas. One is to assess the left ventricular function which cannot be done even under direct vision, with the sternum opened, before and after the patient is placed on cardiopulmonary bypass. If the patient has some difficulties in coming off bypass the two-dimensional echo image will give us a very clear idea which walls of the left ventricular chamber are not moving and whether there is any ischemia, any degree of mitral insufficiency, or simply a hypokinetic ventricle that would require a longer perfusion time to recover from the reperfusion injury. The other useful information that the two-dimensional echo and the Swan-Ganz pressure measurements of the pulmonary artery provide is an assessment of the tolerance of heart to afterload, namely partial clamping of the aorta while the proximal end of the saphenous vein grafts are being connected. If the pulmonary artery pressure rises and the left ventricular chamber becomes dilated or hypokinetic, this can be appreciated immediately by the two-dimensional echo and the Swan-Ganz monitoring line and this facilitates the decision to place the patient on CP bypass and not risk an ischemic event.

Conclusion

Because of the advantages found in following the technique of connecting the saphenous vein grafts proximally first before the patient is placed on cardiopulmonary bypass we strongly recommend following this method whenever possible. Our results show that the total period of CP bypass is shortened, that the period of global ischemia to the myocardium is also shortened, that cooling of ischemic areas is accomplished as soon as the distal anastomosis is performed, and that immediate reperfusion of the entire myocardium occurs upon releasing the cross-clamp from the ascending aorta.

The use of oxygenated cardioplegia is also recommended because it seems to provide better protection of the myocardium at the same temperature levels provided by other methods as has been demonstrated by other investigators [1, 2]. The use of nonreversed valvotomized veins is also recommended to accomplish a better size matching of the graft with the coronary artery as well as the feasibility of using normally natural bifurcation in the veins used for "Y" grafting, and to avoid trapping of air in the veins when reversed saphenous veins are used. The rheology between the graft and the artery seems to be more desirable.

References

1. Guyton RA, Dorsey LMA, Craver JM, Bone DK, Jones EL, Murphy DA, Hatcher CR, Jr (1985) Improved myocardial recovery after cardioplegia arrest with an oxygenated crystalloid solution. J Thorac Cardiovasc Surg 89:877–887
2. Bodenhammer RM, DeBoer LWV, Geffin GA, O'Keefe DD, Fallon JT, Aretz TH, Haas GS, Dagget WM (1983) Enhanced myocardial protection during ischemic arrest. Oxygenation of a crystalloid cardioplegic solution. J Thorac Cardiovasc Surg 85:769–780
3. Molina JE, Gani K, Voss DM (1982) How should clear cardioplegia be administered? J Thorac Cardiovasc Surg 84:762–772
4. Zaidan JR, Waller JL, Lonergan JH (1983) Hemodynamics of pacing after aortic valve replacement and coronary surgery. Ann Thorac Surg 36:69–72

The Mammary Artery as Preferential Conduit in Coronary Artery Bypass Operations

E. Berreklouw, R. de Geest, O. Alfieri, A. Brutel de la Riviere, J. Defauw, P. Knaepen, H. van Swieten, and F. Vermeulen

As cardiac surgeons most of us try to perform a complete revascularization with saphenous veins as conduits. But we should know that after 12 years more than 50% of all vein grafts are narrowed or occluded. In the first postoperative year 10% will occlude, mostly due to poor peripheral runoff or surgical technical reasons.

Most of the other grafts will show diffuse or localized narrowings caused by fibrous intima hyperplasia or atherosclerosis, especially in patients with hyperlipidemia. In contrary to vein grafts, the mammary artery (IMA) does not develop intima hyperplasia and rarely atherosclerosis, and has a patency of about 95% after 12 years [1, 2]. As a result of this superior patency, the survival after 10 years in a large group of patients with an IMA to the left anterior descending artery (LAD) is about 15% better than in a comparable group with only vein grafts [3, 4]. Also, the "event-free" survival is far superior for the IMA group, when an "event" is defined as angina or left heart failure class 3 or 4, myocardial infarction, or death [4]. For other anastomoses than left mammary artery (LIMA) to LAD the patency seems to be as good but the duration of follow-up is sometimes shorter [5–11].

Besides the advantages of better patency and survival, the IMA offers immediate reperfusion and adaptation to flow demand, is always available, and does not require a proximal anastomosis or long-term anticoagulation. Limitations are that it can with great difficulty or not at all reach the diaphragmatic side of the heart and sometimes it is less suitable to perform extensive sequential grafting.

The contraindications for the use of the IMA are stenosis of the subclavian artery or if the IMA itself is not suitable. In situations where there is possible competition of flows between the IMA and vein grafts, like in an isolated mainstem lesion, it seems wise not to use the IMA. Also when the patient is being resuscitated it seems better not to lose time and to proceed with vein conduits.

Patients and Methods

Since January 1984 we have started to use the mammary artery more frequently, which has resulted in its use in almost 700 patients. The decision to use the IMA or not is taken by the surgeon depending on his own experience and the specific circumstances of the patient, as long as its use did not interfere with the principle of complete revascularization.

Three hundred and eighty-two patients, followed at our clinic, were studied. Most were men, who had angina class 3 or 4. There were 38 patients older than 70 years. Thirty-two patients were operated on for an impending infarction. Besides the usual clinical risk factors like smoking (49%), hypertriglyceridemia (39%), hypercholesterolemia (33%), hypertension (23%), and diabetes (9%), there were 32 patients with problems with their venous material; in two patients there was a contraindication for anticoagulation and one patient had a severe calcified ascending aorta. Twenty-one patients had a left ventricular hypertrophy. Most patients had two- or three-vessel disease (92%) with a good or mildly impaired left ventricular function (86%). In almost half of the patients the IMA was implanted in an area of old infarction. In 43 patients the IMA was used in a reoperation. These patients had more frequently hyperlipidemia and in almost all there were problems with the previous venous conduits.

The operative technique used closely resembles that of Mills, Loop, and others [12, 13] (Table 1). Ths single LIMA was almost exclusively anastomosed to the LAD. The LIMA-jump grafts were mostly used to revascularize the anterior wall (Table 2).

For making sequential anastomoses with the left mammary artery we found the ideal case is the patient where the diseased diagonal runs almost parallel to the LAD. In the case of a high diagonal branch or anterolateral branch where there is a large angle with the LAD, there is a chance of kinking of the IMA in two directions. In this situation we prefer to include this anterolateral branch with a venous jump graft. Also if the diagonal branch is only graftable peripherally, it can be difficult to perform a sequential graft with the left mammary artery.

Table 1. Operative variables ($n = 382$)

Mean number of distals	3.59	(SD 1.29)
Number venous anastomoses	897	
IMA single	76%	(292)
IMA jump	21%	(82)
IMA bilateral	2%	(8)
IMA only	8%	(30)

Table 2. Distal anastomoses

IMA-single ($n = 289$)	%	n	IMA-jump ($n = 84$)	%	n
LAD	95	(277)	Diagonal-LAD	92	(77)
Diagonal	2	(6)	LAD (2 ×)	5	(4)
Obtuse marginal	1	(2)	Dia-Dia-LAD	2	(2)
Right (RIMA)	1	(2)	Septal-LAD	1	(1)
Septal	1	(2)			
IMA-bilateral ($n = 8$)					
RIMA-LAD	50	(4)	LIMA-obtuse marginal	50	(4)
RIMA-right	25	(2)	LIMA-posterolateral CX	25	(2)
RIMA-diagonal	25	(2)	LIMA-diagonal-LAD	25	(2)

When both mammary arteries were used, the right one was used more often for the anterior wall and the left one for the circumflex system. The mammary arteries can be used with all kinds of other cardiac and noncardiac procedures.

Results

At an early stage postoperatively a rethoracotomy for bleeding was required in 6% of the patients. In 5% there was a pleural effusion or an elevated diaphragm, which did not require prolonged ventilation. In 2% perioperative infarction occurred, mostly not in the area where the IMA was implanted.

One patient died in the hospital due to a stroke. The remaining 381 patients had a complete follow-up, with a mean duration of about ½ year, the longest almost 5 years. Two patients died later, one probably due to a cardiac death.

During the follow-up period no patient developed a new myocardial infarction in the area where the IMA was implanted. Some patients still had a pleural effusion or complaints about chestwall pain, although most of these pa-

Table 3. Learning[a] vs. late IMA[b]

	Learning IMA ($n = 74$)		Late IMA ($n = 233$)	
	%	n	%	n
Ischemia time	60.2 min	(SD 18.5)	54.9 min	(SD 19.3)
Pump time	91.8 min	(SD 31.1)	86.3 min	(SD 29.7)
Mean blood loss	1553 cc	(SD 638)	1335 cc	(SD 566)
Rethoracotomy	8	(6)	6	(15)
Early complications	18	(13)	18	(42)
Late complications	15	(11)	9	(20)

[a] First 100 patients; [b] Last 282 patients
[a] and [b] both without reoperations and combined procedures

Table 4. Pre- and postoperative clinical variables ($n = 381$)

	Pre		Post	
	%	n	%	n
Angina				
Class 1	1.8	(7)	95.5	(365)
Class 2	25.5	(97)	3.9	(15)
Class 3	41.0	(156)	0.3	(1)
Class 4	23.4	(89)	0.3	(1)
Class 5	8.4	(32)	0	(0)
Positive excercise test				
	90	(181/201)	5	(12/244)
Positive thallium scan				
	91	(30/33)	14	(1/7)

tients were just operated on recently, when they were seen at the clinics. One patient, without a bilateral IMA, was treated for mediastinitis.

If one looks at a "learning" group of the first 100 patients versus the last 282 patients, there was a clear decrease in cross-clamp time, pump time, mean blood loss, rethoracotomies, and late complications (Table 3).

At late follow-up 95% of the patients were free of angina. Fifteen patients had angina class 2, one patient class 3, and one patient class 4. The percentage of positive exercise tests and thallium scans decreased (Table 4).

Table 5. Angina class 1 at follow-up ($n = 365/381 = 95.5\%$)

Patients with	%	n
Impending infarction	94	(32)
Old infarction	96	(157)
Bad ventricle	100	(8)
LV hypertrophy	95	(21)
Reoperation	86	(43)
Combined procedure	96	(24)
Single IMA	93	(289)
Jump IMA	94	(84)
Bilateral IMA	87	(8)
Age > 70 years	100	(38)
Age < 50 years	96	(49)
Follow-up < 1 year	94	(347)
Follow-up > 1 year	91	(35)
LAD > 50 < 70 stenosis	92	(38)
LAD > 70 stenosis	94	(344)
IMA without veins	96	(27)
IMA with veins	94	(355)

Table 6. IMA recatheterization ($n = 15/381 = 3.9\%$)

	%	n
Delay (mean)	6.1 months (SD 4.6)	
Indications:		
Class 1 [a]	67	(10)
Class 2	27	(4)
Class 3	6	(1)
Patency veins		
No veins		(3/15)
All patent	42	(5/12)
Stenosis, one graft	8	(1/12)
Occlusion, one graft	33	(4/12)
Occlusion, more grafts	17	(2/12)
Problems with venous grafts	58	(7/12)
Patency IMA	100	(15/15)

[a] Aspecific pain, syncope, arrhythmia, OTA (operative transluminal angioplasty), septum branch

Equally good results were obtained in different subgroups of patients (Table 5).

In 15 patients a recatheterization was performed, after a mean delay of about ½ year. In a third a recatheterization was performed because of angina, but mostly because of aspecific complaints or other reasons. In about 50% of patients there was a significant narrowing or occlusion of vein grafts, with a perfect functioning mammary artery in all patients (Table 6).

Discussion

We feel that the mammary artery can be used very well as a preferential conduit, with a low morbidity. Although our follow-up is short, the clinical results are excellent in different kinds of patient subgroups.

The choice which conduit should be used depends on the specific pathology of the individual patient. When the mammary artery is quite small and extensive sequential grafting is needed, one rather choses a vein conduit. When there are no veins available or in reoperations, where vein grafts have failed, the choice of the mammary artery is easy. The same is true for a severely calcified ascending aorta or when anticoagulation is contraindicated. Where vein grafts probably perform poorly, due to poor peripheral runoff or hyperlipidemia, the mammary is the conduit of choice.

In the nineties the cardiac surgeon will require much creativity and skill to perform in some cases a complete revascularization with arterial conduits only.

References

1. Campeau L, Enjalbert M, Lesperance J, Vaislic C, Grondin C, Bourassa M (1983) Atherosclerosis and late closure of aortocoronary saphenous vein grafts: sequential angiographic studies at 2 weeks, 1 year, 5 to 7 years, and 10 to 12 years after surgery. Circulation 68 [suppl II]II-1
2. Lytle B, Loop F, Cosgrove D, Ratliff N, Easley K, Taylor P (1985) Long-term (5 to 12 years) serial studies of internal mammary artery and saphenous vein coronary bypass grafts. J Thorac Cardiovasc Surg 89:248
3. Loop F (1985) Cass continued. Circulation 72 [suppl II]:II-1
4. Okies J, Page U, Bigelow J, Krause A, Salomon N (1984) The left internal mammary artery: the graft of choice. Circulation 70 [suppl I]:I-213
5. Barner H (1974) Double internal mammary-coronary artery bypass. Arch Surg 109:626
6. Barner H (1976) Patency of internal mammary-coronary grafts. Circulation [suppl III]:III-70
7. Barner B, Swartz M, Mudd G, Tyras D (1982) Late patency of the internal mammary artery as a coronary bypass conduit. Ann Thorac Surg 34:408
8. Lytle B, Cosgrove D, Saltus G, Taylor P, Loop F (1983) Multivessel coronary revascularisation without saphenous vein: long-term results of bilateral internal mammary artery grafting. Ann Thorac Surg 36:540
9. Harjola P, Frick M, Harjula A, Jarvinen A, Meurala H, Valle M (1984) Sequential internal mammary artery (IMA) grafts in coronary artery bypass surgery. Thorac Cardiovasc Surg 32:288
10. Kamath M, Matysik L, Schmidt D, Smith L (1985) Sequential internal mammary artery grafts, expanded utilization of an ideal conduit. J Thorac Cardiovasc Surg 89:163

11. Galbut D, Traad E, Dorman M, DeWitt P, Larsen P, Weinstein D, Ally J, Gentsch T (1985) Twelve-year experience with bilateral internal mammary artery grafts. Ann Thorac Surg 40:264
12. Mills N (1982) Physiological and technical aspects of internal mammary artery-coronary artery bypass grafts. Modern technics in cardiac/thoracic surgery. Futura Mount Kisco, New York, pp 48-2
13. Tector A, Schmahl T (1984) Techniques for multiple internal mammary artery bypass grafts. Ann Thorac Surg 38:281

Mammary Versus Saphena Grafting to the Left Anterior Descending Artery

M. MASOTTI, P. GUITERAS, C. CREXELLS, J. M. AUGÉ, A. ARÍS, J. M. CARALPS, J. M. PADRÓ, and A. ORIOL

Introduction

Clinical and basic research is presently being applied to ascertain whether left internal mammary artery (LIMA) grafts are superior to saphenous vein (SV) grafts in the surgical treatment of left anterior descending artery (LAD) coronary lesions. Although LIMA grafts have been documented to show better long-term permeability [5, 10, 13], less is known about their behavior in the early and mid-term postoperative period as compared with venous grafts. This study was designed to (1) determine the variables that differentiate the behavior of both types of grafts soon after surgery and at 6 months and (2) discriminate the variables related to occlusion of both types of grafts to LAD, also soon after surgery and at 6 months.

Patients and Methods

From February 1984 to Octover 1985 coronary artery bypass surgery (CABG) was performed in 110 patients, 5 women and 105 men.

The total number of grafts inserted was 256, of which 110 were to LAD. Fifty were of SV, 50 of LIMA, and 10 were sequenial to LAD and a diagonal. Endarterectomy of LAD was performed in 8% of SV grafts and 5.4% of LIMA grafts.

Angiographic control was performed 10 days after operation (0.3 ± 0.07 months) in the 110 patients, and repeated 6 months later (6.3 ± 1 months) in 65 patients of whom 36 received SV grafts (8 with endarterectomy), 23 received LIMA grafts (1 endarterectomy), and 6 sequential bypasses.

Seven patients refused second angiographic control and the rest have not yet been recatheterized. Variables analyzed were 40, of which 15 were clinical, 20 angiographic, and 5 surgical (Table 1).

Angiographic Evaluation

Coronary artery, SV, and LIMA graft segments were drawn manually in end diastole from two orthogonal projections. Diameters were measured with a hand-held sonic pen and a digitizer connected to a Kontron P/M 2.2 computer. Measurements were taken in healthy segments of the coronary artery proximal to the stenosis, the stenotic segment itself, the two distal thirds of the bypass,

Table 1. Variables entering univariate analysis

Clinical	Angiographic	Surgical
Age	Previous ejection fraction	Type of bypass:
Sex	Gensini score (1)	Internal mammary artery
Smoking status	Extent score (1)	Saphenous vein
Serum cholesterol (nmol/liter)	% Stenosis LAD (1)	∅ Distal bed (mm)
Serum tryglycerides (nmol/liter)	Stenosis situation (proximal, mid-distal)	Distal bed morphology
Actual obesity	∅ Distal bed (mm) (1)	Snake
Actual systemic hypertension	∅ Proximal healthy artery (mm)	Endarterectomy
Actual diabetes mellitus	Morphology:	
Family history of CAD	Distal bed (healthy, diseased)	
History of:	Lesion (discrete, tubular, diffuse)	
Prior MI in CABG region	Total No. stenosis 50%	
Prior MI in other regions	Total No. stenosis 70% or LMT 50%	
Prior CHF	Newly formed stenosis (%) (2)	
Prior unstable angina	CAD progression (2)	
Duration of angina	Site of CAD progression (2)	
Actual angina class:	Bypass:	
On effort [a]	Proximal ∅ (2)	
Unstable, excluding variant	Middle ∅ (2)	
Variant	Distal ∅ (end to side) (2)	
	Distal ∅ (side to side) (2)	
	Patency (2)	
	Stenosis (%) (2)	

CAD, coronary artery disease; CHF, congestive heart failure; CABG, coronary artery bypass grafting; LMT, Left main trunk; LAD, left anterior descending artery; ∅, diameter.
[a] Canadian Cardiovascular Society Angina Class.
(1), variables obtained prior to CABG and at first and second controls afterwards
(2), variables obtained only at the first and second controls.

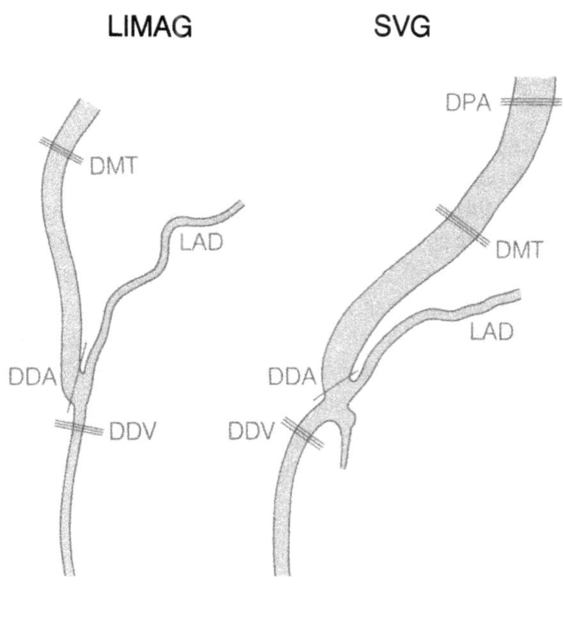

Fig. 1. Drawing from a cineangiogram of a saphenous vein graft (*SVG*) and a left internal mammary artery graft (*LIMAG*) to a left anterior descending artery (*LAD*) in lateral positions. The *thin lines* show where measurements were routinely obtained. *DMT*, diameter of mid-third; *DDA*, diameter of distal anastomosis; *DDV*, diameter of distal vessel; *DPA* diameter of proximal anastomosis

and the distal coronary bed. Three measurements were averaged for each of the above-mentioned segments and corrected for X-ray magnification using the catheter diameter as a reference (Fig. 1). In all cases the chosen radiographic positions were the same before and after surgery.

Left ventriculography was performed in 30° projection. Gensini score [3] was used to assess the severity of coronary artery disease and extent score, defined as the total number of coronary stenoses, to quantify extension of the disease. In the case of progression the location of the stenosis was identified as proximal or distal to the graft or at the level of the preexisting lesion, whether it was bypassed or not.

Significant stenosis was defined as equal to or greater than 70% reduction in lumen except for the left main trunk, where a 50% reduction was considered significant. Variables listed in Table 1 were analyzed comparing SV versus LIMA grafts, and factors related to occlusion of bypass in the early postoperative period and 6 months later were identified.

Statistical Analysis

Univariate analysis was applied to all variables mentioned. Pearson's and maximal likelihood chi squares were complemented with Fisher's exact test to analyze discrete variables. Continuous variables were treated with the t test for nondependent data.

Variables which were significant on univariate analysis were submitted to multivariate analysis using a discriminant function to compare SV and LIMA grafts, and the logistic regression model was used to analyze permeability at 1 week and 6 months after surgery. In all cases a P value of 0.05 was accepted.

Results

Saphenous Vein Grafts Versus LIMA Grafts to the LAD

Table 2a shows the results of the univariate analysis applied to compare SV with LIMA grafts. The discriminant function considers as independent variables those which became significant by the univariate analysis but rearranges the order as shown in Table 2b, according to its degree of significance.

The rate of occlusion of SV grafts at 1 week after surgery was 11.6% (7/60), of which three were nonfunctional. LIMA graft occlusion rate was 8% (4/50) with one nonfunctional. This difference was not statistically significant. Two of the four grafts occluded at 1 week were patent at 6 months. At this date, 4 out of 42 SV grafts (9.5%) were occluded, of which 2 were nonfunctional, and 1 out of 23 LIMA grafts (4.3%) was not functional, and although this difference was not statistically significant a certain tendency toward a greater patency of LIMA grafts appeared evident.

Table 2. Saphenous versus mammary grafting

a) Univariate analysis ($n = 110$)

Variables	SV	LIMA	*P*
∅ Distal bed at 6 months (mm)	1.2± 0.5	1.7± 0.4	0.0025
Lesion before CABG (%)	75.5±19.7	85.9±13.3	0.002
Gensini before CABG	66.3±38.6	53.3±34.6	0.05
Bypass stenosis at 6 months (%)	9.6± 0.5	0	0.05
Bypass middle ∅ at 6 months (mm)	2.8± 0.9	2.3± 0.2	0.05

b) Multivariate analysis

Variables	*F*
Lesion before CABG (%)	14.23
Bypass middle ∅ at 6 months (mm)	10.24
∅ Distal bed at 6 months (mm)	9.77
Bypass stenosis at 6 months (%)	8.18
Gensini before CABG	5.65

CABG, coronary artery bypass graft; ∅, diameter

Table 3. Occluded versus nonoccluded grafts at the first control

a) Univariate analysis ($n = 110$)

Angiographic variables	Occluded ($n = 11$)	Nonoccluded ($n = 99$)	*P*
∅ Distal bed (before CABG)	1.1± 0.1	1.5± 0.4	0.00029
% Stenosis LAD	94.5±10.8	78.7±18.0	0.0054
Stenosis situated distally	10/11 (91%)	54/99 (55%)	0.0125
Surgical variables			
Good distal bed	1/11 (9%)	31/83 (37%)	0.0410
Endarterectomy	4/11 (36%)	11/99 (11%)	0.034

b) Multivariate analysis

Variables	Coefficient	*P*
% Stenosis LAD	−0.145	0.0056
∅ Distal bed (before (CABG)	2.792	0.0071
Constant	11.88	

CABG, coronary artery bypass graft; LAD, left anterior descending artery, ∅ diameter

Graft Occlusion 1 Week After CABG

Occlusion rate at 1 week was 11%. Univariate analysis showed that occlusion was related to poor distal bed (Table 3a), severity of lesion prior to CABG, distal location of the stenosis, and endarterectomy. Multivariate analysis (Table 3b) correlated early occlusion solely to severity of the lesion and poor distal bed.

Table 4. Occluded versus nonoccluded (second control)

a) Univariate analysis ($n = 65$)			
Angiographic variables	Occluded ($n = 5$)	Nonoccluded ($n = 60$)	P
Site of CAD progression (distal)	3/5 (60%)	5/54 (3%)	0.005
Newly formed stenosis (%) (In the first control)	45.8±45	10.9±29	0.0162
Bypass stenosis (%) (In the first control)	19.8±44.3	3.0±14.8	0.051
Surgical variables			
Endarterectomy	4/5 (80%)	5/60 (8.3%)	0.00001
Good distal bed	0/5 (0%)	22/51 (43%)	0.021

b) Multivariate analysis		
Variables	β-coefficient	P
Endarterectomy	−2.058	0.0002
Constant	1.770	–

CAD, coronary artery disease

Graft Occlusion at 6 Months

The rate of occlusion at 6 months was 7.7%. Univariate analysis (Table 4a) showed that endarterectomy, poor quality of distal bed, development of new stenosis, appearance of graft stenosis, and progression of disease in the distal vessel were all related to graft occlusion. Yet, logistic regression analysis (Table 4b) found LAD endarterectomy the only variable to correlate with occlusion at 6 months.

Discussion

A greater diameter of the distal bed at 6 months with LIMA grafts as compared with SV grafts may well be considered a consequence of a higher flow through this type of conduct; yet, results obtained by others [2, 6] who did actually measure flow seem to indicate that this parameter is up to three times greater with SV grafts.

On the other hand, long-term results [10] point toward the advantage of using LIMA. A possible explanation, in an attempt to put everything together, would be that the mammary artery might just adapt its flow to actual necessity through an autoregulatory mechanism [12].

Kay, Sims and Grondin [5, 7, 11] have all shown that atherosclerosis is unusual in LIMA. Our results confirm this point.

When looking for occlusion, our results are not statistically significant but clearly show a tendency toward a better long-term result with the LIMA graft. This has been shown by Grondin at 10 years follow-up.

Our study of the total occlusion rate in the first control shows results similar to those of FitzGibbon or Grondin [1, 4]; yet what might be new and of certain interest is that early occlusion may be predicted through severity of previous stenosis and quality of distal bed.

Finally, occlusion at 6 months seems to be solely related to the performance of endarterectomy. This might possibly point toward a failure in surgery although we consider this technique is controversial. Some authors such as Yacoub [14] find no difference in permeability after endarterectomy, while others such as Miller or Keon [8, 9] relate endarterectomy to myocardial infarction or a greater rate of occlusion.

Our conclusions, although preliminary, might be summarized as follows:

1. There is a better distal bed at 6 months with LIMA than with SV graft.
2. The saphenous vein has a greater tendency to develop new stenosis than LIMA.
3. At both 10 days and 6 months there is a tendency for greater occlusion rate with SV than with LIMA grafts.
4. As a whole, previous stenosis severity and quality of distal bed are good predictors for early occlusion.
5. At the 6-month control only endarterectomy correlates to occlusion.

More cases should be studied, especially the remaining controls at 6 months, to confirm or reject those conclusions. The role of endarterectomy is of special concern.

References

1. FitzGibbon GM, Burton JR, Leach AJ (1978) Coronary bypass graft fate. Angiographic grading of 1400 consecutive grafts early after operation and of 1132 after one year. Circulation 57:1070–1074
2. Flemma RJ, Singh HM, Tector AJ, Lepley D, Frazier BL (1975) Comparative hemodynamic properties of vein and mammary artery in coronary bypass operations. Ann Thorac Surg 20:619–627
3. Gensini GG, Kelly AE (1972) Incidence and progression of coronary artery disease. Arch Intern Med 129:814–827
4. Grondin CM, Lespérance J, Bourassa MG, Pasternac A, Campeau L, Grondin P (1974) Serial angiographic evaluation in 60 consecutive patients with aorto-coronary artery vein grafts 2 weeks, 1 year, and 3 years after operation. J Thorac Cardiovasc Surg 67:1–6
5. Grondin CM, Campeau L, Lespérance J, Enjalbert M, Bourassa MG (1984) Comparison of late changes in internal mammary artery and saphenous vein grafts in two consecutive series of patients 10 years after operation. Circulation 70 (Suppl 1):I-208–212
6. Hamby RI, Aintablian A, Wisoff BG, Hartstein ML (1977) Comparative study of the postoperative flow in the saphenous vein and internal mammary artery bypass grafts. Am Heart J 93:306–315
7. Kay HR, Korns ME, Flemma RJ, Tector AJ, Lepley D (1976) Atherosclerosis of the internal mammary artery. Ann Thorac Surg 21:504–507
8. Keon WJ, Akyurekli Y, Bedard P, Brais MP, Goldstein W, Beanlands DS (1979) Coronary endarterectomy: an adjunct to coronary artery bypass grafting. Surgery 86:859–857
9. Miller DC, Stinson EB, Oyer PE, Jamieson SW, Mitchell RS, Reitz BA, Baumgartner WA, Shumway NE (1983) Discriminant analysis of the changing risks of coronary artery operations: 1971–1979. J Thorac Cardiovasc Surg 85:197–213

10. Okies JE, Page US, Bigelow JC, Krause AH, Salomon NW (1984) The left internal mammary artery: the graft of choice. Circulation 70 (Suppl 1):213–221
11. Sims FH (1983) A comparison of coronary and internal mammary arteries and implications of the results in the etiology of arteriosclerosis. Am Heart J 105:560–566
12. Singh RN, Sosa JA (1984) Internal mammary artery: a livre conduit for coronary bypass. J Thorac Cardiovasc Surg 87:936–938
13. Tector AJ, Schmahl TM, Janson B, Kallies JR, Johnson G (1981) The internal mammary artery graft. Its longevity after coronary bypass. JAMA 246:2181–2183
14. Yacoub MH, Fawzy E, Anyanwu H, Towers M (1975) Combined gas endarterectomy and coronary artery bypass graft. A follow-up study. Circulation 51 (Suppl 1):I-182–187

Abstract

Crossed Double Internal Mammary Artery-Coronary Grafts: 12-Year Follow-up

A. S. GEHA

Crossed double internal mammary artery (IMA)-coronary artery grafts (left IMA to LAD, right IMA to diagonal or obtuse marginal) were used without operative mortality in 44 patients, age 36–70 years, requiring grafts to these vessels during 1973–1977; 32 of them had additional saphenous grafts (SVG) to achieve revascularization. At complete follow-up, 8–12 years after operation, all 44 are alive. Recurrent angina developed at 8 and 9 years postoperatively in two patients because of closed SVGs to other coronaries, and is well controlled medically. One patient developed a uniform narrowing "string sign" of both IMAs 2 years postoperatively, probably because of less than critical coronary lesions, and had an attempt at revascularization. All patients are fully active on late follow-up, and all IMAs studied angiographically are patent.

The direction and location of the LAD and of diagonal and marginal branches allow excellent alignment of these shorter and wider double IMA grafts. The excellent long-term survival and functional results indicate that the left IMA is the graft of choice for the LAD, and the right IMA for a high diagonal or early-arising marginal artery that requires an additional separate graft.

Behaviour of Interstitial Biopolymers in Normal and Stretched Saphenous Vein Excised for Aortocoronary Bypass

J. H. KENNEDY

Introduction

Aortocoronary bypass has become a recognized treatment, and is carried out in cardiac surgical centres worldwide with acceptable mortality and relief of angina. However, some patients develop concentric subintimal fibrous stenosis of the graft and recurrence of symptoms. A number of experimental studies have emphasized the importance of elevated intraluminal pressure (Boncheck 1980), mural ischaemia brought about by interruption of the vasa vasora (Brody et al. 1972), the aortovenous anastomotic angle (Kennedy et al. 1974), endothelial damage (Gunstensen et al. 1982) and reduced flow velocity (Berguer et al. 1980) in the development of venous subintimal hyperplasia. Bonchek et al. (1982) and Landymore et al. (1985) have suggested platelet aggregation as an aetiological factor and reported prevention in experimental animals by anti-activation agents. A number of other technical reasons for graft occlusion exist, e.g. progression of atherosclerosis, poor distal run-off, kinking and suture compromise of the anastomosis; changes in the interstitium of the vessel wall may also be a factor. As in other surgical grafts, the quality of the graft is an essential factor in its success.

Histological findings in reported cases also suggest trauma to the venous endothelium and interstitium. Such changes may be caused by hydraulic overdistension of the vein, which is frequently used during preparation. We describe a preliminary study designed to test the response of the venous interstitium to changes in pressure, in order to measure mechanical properties as a function of applied intraluminal pressure, and correlate these with studies of the colligative properties of the venous interstitium reported elsewhere (Kennedy et al. 1985).

Materials and Method

Fifteen consecutive unselected patients undergoing aortocoronary bypass constituted the study group. Saphenous vein was harvested through linear incisions by a standard technique by the same surgical team. Hydraulic distension with heparinized saline solution to >280 mm Hg for a varying length of time was used to prepare the vein graft. One undistended segment, and one segment after distension, each $1-2$ cm in length, were cut into 3-mm rings and weighed on tared foil onto which a drop of PBS was then decanted to prevent drying, and the breaking strength of each was determined on an Instron material testing machine modified to hold the vein ring between stainless steel hooks at a 20° angle in a bath containing PBS at 4° C. Extension at the rate of 50 mm/min was applied until the tissue fractured. The specimens were removed and dried to a constant weight. For the purposes of the clinical study, as will be discussed below, the deformation was assumed to be tensile, ignoring shear, and monotonic in response. The more complicated treatment of deformation of a thick torus described by Timoshenko (1941) was ignored.

Statistical analysis was based on the method of Weatherill (1967) and was accomplished by a program written for the purpose ("T-test") for both equal and unequal population variance.

Results

Preliminary experiments using hydraulic distension at normal venous pressure (Fig. 1) up to 20 mm Hg showed no difference between moduli of control and distended vein from the same patient. Figure 2 shows the results in a pilot study

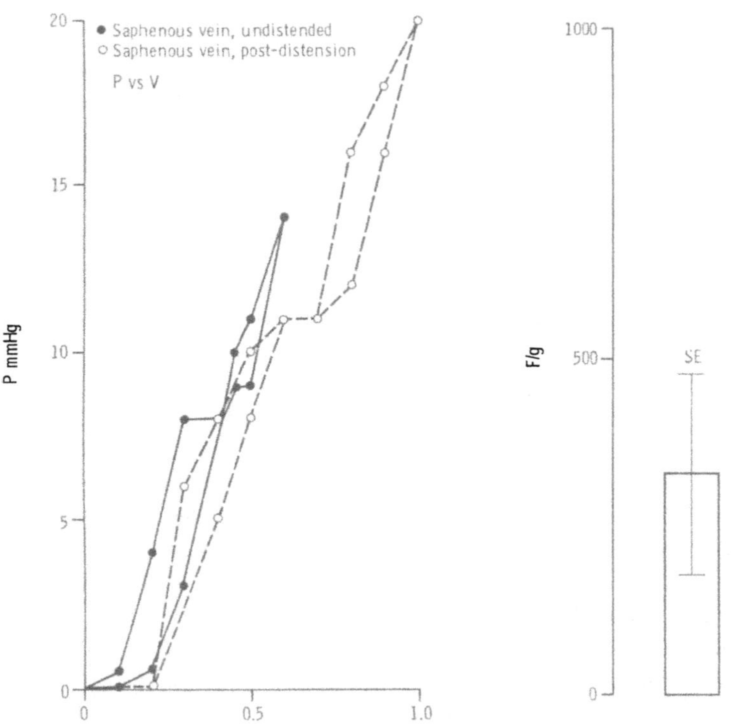

Fig. 1. Pressure–volume relationship in undistended and distended vein from the same patient; at low pressure there is no difference

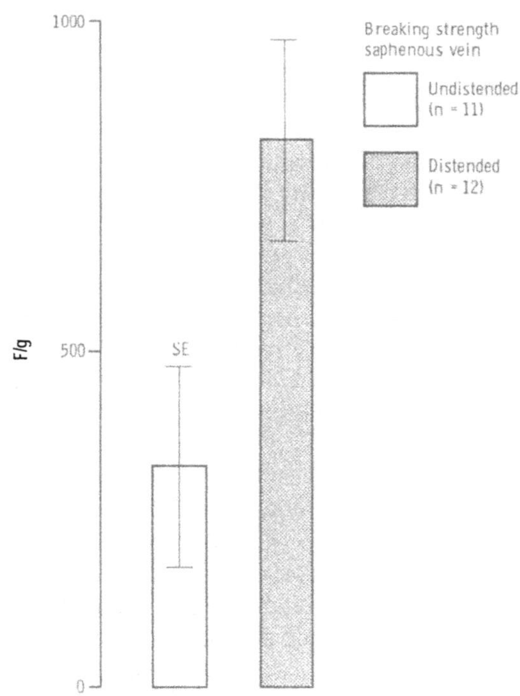

Fig. 2. Average values for breaking strength per gram of dry weight of tissue. The difference is significant ($P < 0.01$)

in which vein rings were extended to the point of failure in an Instron apparatus. The breaking strength in newtons (kg × 9.8 m/s^2) per gram of dry weight was higher in previously distended vein specimens; 863 (SE = 158, n = 11) vs 527 (SE = 158, n = 10) in controls ($P < 0.05$). In the same specimens, weight gain, change in water content, uronic acid eluted and ^{125}I-SA concentration normalized to incubating bath relative to ^{51}Cr-EDTA concentration normalized to incubating bath over a period of 24 h were determined. These two probes were selected because the mobility and distribution of albumin, which has a relatively large molecule, is influenced by the steric exclusion by the extracellular matrix and is therefore affected by the state of hydration of the tissue, while EDTA, which has a small molecule, has access to almost all the extracellular water space and therefore acts as a reference material for the investigation of changes in the interstitium. These results are reported elsewhere (Kennedy et al. 1985) and will only be summarized here. Distended veins swelled less, and desorbed less uronic acid. These findings, together with increase in strength, suggest injury to the interstitial matrix of distended veins not unlike those arising in the ageing process.

Discussion

Connective tissue has been characterized by Scott (1983) as "the natural fibre-reinforced composite material": systems of insoluble fibres which take the stresses of movement and maintenance of shape, and soluble polymers trapped in the mesh, which imbibe water to resist compressive forces. This interstitial matrix also serves as an important link in the transport of proteins and other substances from the plasma to the lymph.

Mechanical properties of macromolecular systems are dependent on the proportions, distribution, and individual characteristics of the constituents. This is particularly true of biomacromolecules in living mammals; for example, structure–property relationships of the connective tissue – the interstitium – vary with age in various tissues (Baer and Torp 1974; Lakatta and Yin 1982) owing, in part, to changes in the modules of the native collagen and elastin; the relative proportions vary from tissue to tissue. In the case of vein from the saphenofemoral system, Yamada (1970) has reported autopsy-derived studies which indicate a gradual deterioration in strength from a maximum at 20–39 years to 60–69 years, the age range of the patients in the present study; the results are similar, allowing for strength measurements normalized to dry weight. Veins greater than 0.2 cm in diameter have three distinct layers – intima, media, and adventitia; the bulk is adventitia, principally made up of collagen fibres (Cliff 1976; Caro et al. 1978). From the bidirectional strength measurements reported by Yamada (1970) a helical configuration would be predictable, as in arteries (Wainwright et al. 1976). While histological proof is not yet available, helic configuration of collagen fibres would also explain why distension increases the strength of the veins in the present study; irrevocable deformation of the coiled collagen fibres so that they are end-bearing, at the same time releasing the enmeshed glycosaminoglycal aggregates so that swelling behaviour and elutable uronic acid are reduced. While not confirmed in the present study, accompanying abnormalities in transport through damaged interstitium, perhaps leading to fibrosis, would be expected.

Reports from other workers suggest that transport through a vessel wall is influenced by intraluminal pressure (Duncan et al. 1962; Fry 1973; Caro and Lever 1983) or by removal of the endothelium (Ramirez et al. 1984; Falcon et - al. 1984; Tedgui and Lever 1984); the latter in turn can be brought about by collapse of the vessel wall (Baldwin et al. 1978). The present mechanical and macromolecular studies have been conducted in a nonuniform population and with whole vein, whereas several of the studies referred to above have been performed in specimens separated from endothelium and adventitia, either of which might obscure changes in transport, as the endothelium is a strong barrier to macromolecular transport (Caro and Lever 1982) and adventitia represents such a large interstitium as to obscure more subtle changes. The mechanical changes observed in distended veins in the present study are probably due to modification of the media, while the chemical observations are the result of alterations in the adventitia.

Conclusions

1. The results of a preliminary study on the effect of distension of saphenous veins removed at aortocoronary bypass on mechanical behaviour and transport have been presented.
2. Within the limitations of the model, there appears to be damage to the interstitial matrix in distended veins.
3. The significance of these findings for development of fibrous intimal hyperplasia in these patients is uncertain; the patients are being followed for evidence of graft failure.

Acknowledgements. The Author wishes to thank Mr. M. Paneth, The Brompton Hospital, London, for permitting this study to be carried out and for providing vein specimens, and Dr. B. O. Weightman, Biomechanics Unit, Department of Mechanical Engineering, Imperial College, London for providing access to the Instron apparatus, and advice about design of this study.

References

1. Baldwin AL, Caro CG, Davis J, Winlove CP (1978) Structural and mechanical aspects of vascular collapse. J Physiol (Lond) 278:14–15P
2. Berguer R, Higgins RF, Reddy DJ (1980) Intimal hyperplasia. An experimental study. Arch Surg 115:332–335
3. Bitter T, Muir HM (1962) A modified uronic acid carbazole reaction. Anal Biochem 4:330–334
4. Bolton AE (1977) Preparation of radioiodinated albumin by a chloramine-I method. Radioiodination techniques. The Radiochemical Centre Review 18:45–48 (Amersham)
5. Boncheck LI (1980) Prevention on endothelial damage during preparation of saphenous veins for bypass grafting. J Thor Cardiovasc Surg 79:911–915

6. Boncheck LI, Boerboom LE, Olinger GN, Pepper JR, Munns J, Hutchinson L, Kissebah AH (1982) Prevention of lipid accumulation in experimental vein bypass grasts by antiplatelet therapy. Circulation 66:338–341
7. Brody WR, Kosek JC, Angell WW (1972) Changes in venigrafts following aortocoronary bypass induced by pressure and ischemia. J Thorac Cardiovasc Surg 64:847–854
8. Caro CG, Lever MJ (1983) Effect of vasoactive agents and applied stress on the albumin space of excised rabbit carotid arteries. Atherosclerosis 46:137–146
9. Caro CG, Pedley TJ, Schroter RC, Seed WA (1978) The mechanics of the circulation. Oxford University Press, London, p 437
10. Cliff WJ (1976) Blood vessels. Cambridge University Press, Cambridge, p 156
11. Duncan L, Cornfield J, Buck K (1962) Effect of blood pressure on passage of labelled plasma albumin into canine aortic wall. J Clin Invest 41:1537–1545
12. Falcone DJ, Hajjar DP, Minick CR (1984) Lipoprotein and albumin accumulation in reendothelialized and de-endothelialized artery wall. Am J Pathol 114:112–120
13. Fry DL (1973) Atherogenesis: Initiating Factors. Ciba Foundation Symposia (new series) 12:93–120
14. Gunstensen J, Smith RC, El-Maraghi N, Julian J, Belbeck L (1982) Intimal hyperplasia in autogenous veins used for arterial replacement. Can J Surg 25:158–160
15. Kennedy JH, Wieting DW, Hwang NHC, Anderson MS, Bayardo RJ, Howell JF, De Bakey ME (1974) Hydraulic and morphologic study of fibrous intimal hyperplasia in autogenous saphenous vein bypass grafts. J Thorac Cardiovasc Surg 67:805–813
16. Kennedy JH, Lever MJ, Paneth M; Addis BJ (1986) Graft stenosis following aortocoronary bypass: state of vein interstitium. Proc European Society for Cardiovasc. Surgery, Brighton, 4 July 1986 (Abstract)
17. Landymore RW, Kinley CE, Cooper JH (1985) Cod liver oil in the prevention of intimal hyperplasia in autogenous vein grafts used for arterial bypass. J Thorac Cardiovasc Surg 89:351–357
18. Ramirez CA, Colton CK, Smith KA, Stemerman MB, Lees RS (1984) Transport of 125-I albumin across normal and de-endothelialized rabbit aorta in vivo. Arteriosclerosis 4:283–291
19. Scott JE (ed) (1983) Connective tissues: The natural fibre-reinforced composite material. J R Soc Med 76:993–994
20. Timoshenko S (1941) Strength of materials. Van Nostrand, New York, pp 80–85
21. Wainwright SA, Biggs WD, Currey JD, Gosline JM (1976) Mechanical design in organisms. Arnold, London, p 137
22. Yamada H (1970) In: Evans FG (ed) Strength of biological materials. Williams and Wilkins, Baltimore, p 106

IV. Coronary Artery Surgery in Acute Myocardial Infarction

Severe Perioperative Cardiogenic Shock in Open Heart Surgery: Benefits of Combined Therapy

M. GOENEN

Introduction

The occurrence of perioperative myocardial ischemia, with various degrees of severity, is not uncommon during heart surgery despite adequate measures of myocardial protection by cardioplegia and hypothermia.

Consequently, if cardiac function is inefficient to maintain adequate circulation, isolated or combined treatment involving intraaortic counterpulsation, positive inotropic drugs, and vasodilators very often enhances myocardial performance in order to ensure adequate tissue perfusion.

Nevertheless, postischemic myocardial depression may require several days of treatment before normal function is restored, provided that the myocardial damage is not irreversible [1].

The number of patients requiring such treatment is likely to increase because of surgical indication in patients with seriously altered ventricular function by acute myocardial infarction, postinfarction complications, recurrent postinfarction angina, acute endocarditis, and advanced cardiopathies. Positive inotropic adrenergic drugs and vasodilators suffice in most cases, but fail in others. Our attention was therefore attracted by a new positive inotropic and vasodilating drug, amrinone, with a different nonadrenergic mechanism of action, suitable for combination to lower doses of beta$_1$-agonists, without causing any major side effects.

Patient Material

Fourty patients, 26 males and 14 females, aged from 4 to 74 years, developed severe perioperative cardiogenic shock, 15 of them after single- or multiple-valve replacements, 3 after correction of complex congenital cardiopathies, and finally 22 patients after aortocoronary bypass. Twenty-eight patients had emergency operations, 11 with the intraaortic balloon pump. The wean off bypass was difficult in all patients and needed combined adrenergic drugs and vasodilators. The intraaortic balloon pump was inserted 23 times: 11 preoperatively, 11 during the operation and 2 additional times in the ICU. The catheter could not be inserted in two other patients.

Criteria of cardiogenic shock, refractory to combined adrenergic and vasodilating drugs and intraaortic balloon pumping, were the following: cardiac index < 2 liters/min/m^2 and pulmonary capillary wedge pressure > 20 mm Hg,

Table 1. Management of perioperative cardiogenic shock prior to administration of amrinone

	n
1. Dopamine and dobutamine up to 15 μg/kg/min	39
2. Isoprenaline up to 1 μg/min	6
3. Nitroglycerine 1 – 2 μg/kg/min	28
4. Noradrenaline, when SBP < 85 mm Hg, SVR = 10 units	5
5. IABP (11 preoperatively)	23
6. Amrinone IV up to 20 μg/kg/min (12 h to 7 days)	40

systolic blood pressure < 100 mm Hg, poor tissue perfusion, cold extremities, oliguria, and metabolic acidosis.

Management of cardiogenic shock is presented in Table 1. Amrinone, a nonglycoside, noncatecholamine cardiotonic agent, possesses significant positive inotropic effects [2] and vasodilatory properties [3] and potentiates the effects of adrenergic drugs [4].

The drug was administered in addition to the former therapy, in doses up to 20 mcg/kg/min. Duration of therapy ranged from 12 h to 7 days.

Complete hemodynamic data, including cardiac output measurements by thermodilution, could only be obtained in some cases, because of emergency administration of the drug during or early after operation.

Results

Clinical and hemodynamic conditions improved markedly in 34 patients, in whom the intraaortic balloon pump and inotropic therapy was progressively

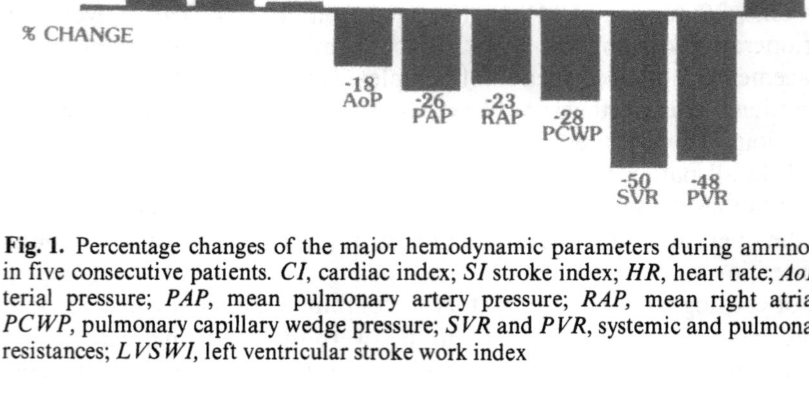

Fig. 1. Percentage changes of the major hemodynamic parameters during amrinone infusion in five consecutive patients. *CI*, cardiac index; *SI* stroke index; *HR*, heart rate; *AoP*, mean arterial pressure; *PAP*, mean pulmonary artery pressure; *RAP*, mean right atrial pressure; *PCWP*, pulmonary capillary wedge pressure; *SVR* and *PVR*, systemic and pulmonary vascular resistances; *LVSWI*, left ventricular stroke work index

withdrawn. The six other patients died of refractory cardiogenic shock. Autopsy findings demonstrated extensive subendocardial necrosis in four patients and major myocardial infarction in two.

Two additional patients died later of noncardiac causes.

Percentage changes of most hemodynamic parameters in five consecutive patients are shown in Fig. 1 and their left ventricular function curve in Fig. 2, while Fig. 3 describes a case of severe cardiogenic shock after emergency aortic valve replacement, despite intraaortic balloon pump, dopamine, and dobutamine 10, mcg/kg/min each.

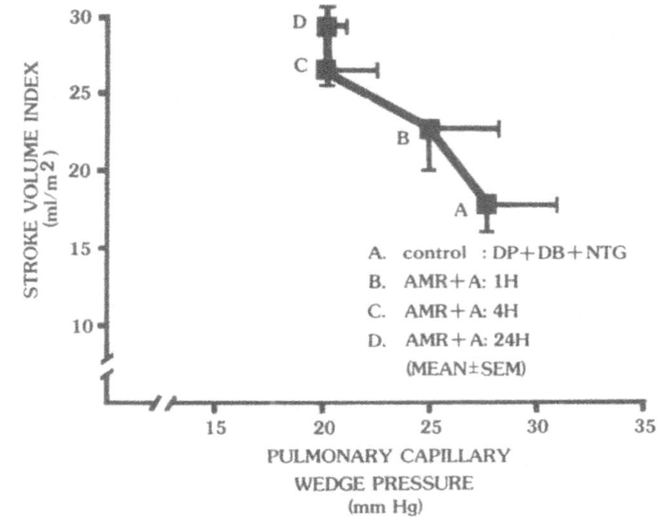

Fig. 2. Left ventricular function curve, as a relationship between pulmonary capillary wedge pressure and stroke volume index. *DP*, dopamine; *DB*, dobutamine; *NTG*, nitroglycerine; *AMR*, amrinone

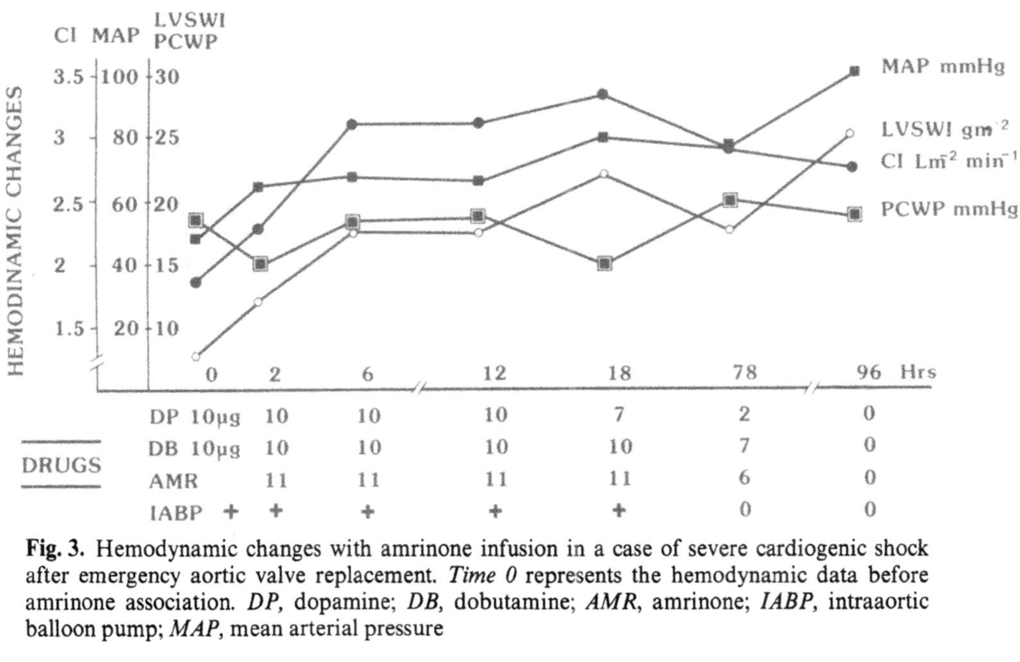

DRUGS	0	2	6	12	18	78	96 Hrs
DP 10μg		10	10	10	7	2	0
DB 10μg		10	10	10	10	7	0
AMR		11	11	11	11	6	0
IABP	+	+	+	+	+	0	0

Fig. 3. Hemodynamic changes with amrinone infusion in a case of severe cardiogenic shock after emergency aortic valve replacement. *Time 0* represents the hemodynamic data before amrinone association. *DP*, dopamine; *DB*, dobutamine; *AMR*, amrinone; *IABP*, intraaortic balloon pump; *MAP*, mean arterial pressure

Discussion

Low cardiac output after open heart surgery remains one of the major postoperative problems. Intraaortic balloon pump, catecholamines, and vasodilators constitute the basis of current therapy [5]. In some patients, this therapy fails to restore adequate hemodynamic function.

Amrinone, a nonglycoside, noncatecholamine, inotropic, and vasodilating drug, has shown significant hemodynamic improvement in moderate postoperative heart failure [6], but the potentiation of amrinone of the effect of adrenergic drugs in severe cardiogenic shock may be one of its most attractive features [7, 8]. This new therapeutic approach may be based on the presumption that cyclic-AMP is increased by two different pathways : adenylcyclase activation by beta-agonists and inhibition of cyclic-AMP breakdown by phosphodiesterase III inhibitors such as amrinone.

The major advantage of amrinone consists in its direct inotropic and vasodilating activity, which decreases pre- and afterload and increases cardiac index and left ventricular stroke work index without major side effects [7]. The drug was well tolerated in most cases. Nevertheless, arrhythmias may occur and transitory hypoxemia is common; the paO_2 decreased by nearly 10% after initiation of the infusion, especially after a bolus. Undesirable reduction of mean arterial pressure may also occur, but can be easily reversed by volume loading in the case of inadequate filling pressure or by low dosis of norepinephrine.

In summary, the additional administration of amrinone to adrenergic inotropic drugs may actually be considered as a major step in the treatment of postoperative cardiogenic shock. Used alone, this new drug may have at least similar hemodynamic benefits to adrenergic drugs and only minor side effects in intravenous administration.

References

1. Braunwald E, Kloner RA (1982) The stunned myocardium prolonged postischemic ventricular dysfunction. Circulation 66:1146–1149
2. Farah AE, Alousi AA (1978) New cardiotonic agents: a search for digitalis substitute. Life Sci 22:1139–1148
3. Millard RW, Dube G, Grupp I, Alousi AA, Schwartz A (1980) Direct vasodilator and positive inotropic actions of Amrinone. J Mol Cell Cardiol 12:647–652
4. Honerjäger P, Schafer-Korting M, Reiter M (1981) Involvement of cyclic AMP in the direct inotropic action of Amrinone. Biochemical and functional evidence. Naunyn Schmiedebergs Arch Pharmacol 318:112–120
5. Miller CD (1980) Postoperative enhancement of left ventricular performance by combined inotropic-vasodilator therapy with preload control. Surgery 88:108–117
6. Goenen M, Pedemonte O, Paele Ph, Jaumin P, Trémouroux J (1985) Effets hémodynamiques de l'Amrinone sur le bas débit cardiaque après chirurgie à cœur ouvert. Réanimation, Soins Intensifs, Médecine d'Urgence 3:151–156
7. Goenen M, Pedemonte O, Baele Ph, Amrinone T (1985) in the management of low cardiac output after open heart surgery. Am J Cardiol 22:33–38 B
8. Caradonna E, Driel H Van, Alfieri O, Hemel NH, Swieten HA, Vermeulen F (1983) Preliminary experience with Amrinone in patients with low cardiac output states after open heart surgery. RBM 7:29–31

Improved Detection of Perioperative Myocardial Infarction After Cardiac Surgery Using CK-MB Mass Measurements

J.-P. CHAPELLE, M. EL ALLAF, R. LARBUISSON, R. LIMET, M. LAMY, and C. HEUSGHEM

Introduction

After coronary bypass surgery (CBS), late survival is reduced in patients who develop perioperative myocardial infarction (PMI) as compared with the uncomplicated cases [4, 8]. Therefore the improvement of individual therapy in these patients depends on our capacity reliably to select high-risk cases during the early postoperative period.

From a biochemical point of view, the MB isoenzyme of creatine kinase (CK-MB) and myoglobin can be considered as the most useful indicators of myocardial injury after CBS [1, 5, 11, 12]. Although these two tissue markers can regularly be detected in the blood following the intervention, the analysis of their liberation patterns enables normal intraoperative trauma to be differentiated from myocardial necrosis. In this study, CK-MB and serum myoglobin (SMb) were serially measured per- and postoperatively in 41 patients who underwent CBS. SMb was determined by radioimmunoassay (RIA) and CK-MB by five different techniques : immunoinhibition, immunoinhibition-immunoprecipitation, column chromatography, and electrophoresis, all methods measuring the activity of the isoenzyme, and a new immunoenzymetric assay (IEMA) designed for measuring its concentration. Our purpose was twofold: (a) to compare the relative merits of SMb and CK-MB for identifying the patients suffering from PMI and (b) to select the most sensitive assay for CK-MB, and particularly to determine whether this isoenzyme should be measured by mass or by means of its catalytic activity.

Material and Methods

Patient Population

CK-MB and SMb measurements were performed in an initial population of 92 patients who underwent elective coronary bypass grafting as an isolated surgical procedure; definite information about the clinical factors and complete biochemical data (CK-MB could not be measured by immunoinhibition in hemolyzed samples) was, however, available in only 41 patients (30 men and 11 women, mean age 57 years). In this series, 33 cases followed a completely uneventful postoperative course; eight cases showed electrocardiographic evidence of PMI (new Q waves on the ECG).

Peripheral blood samples were taken before operation, at 1-h intervals during the intervention, upon the patient arrival in the intensive care room immediately after surgery, every 4 h during the first postoperative day, and finally 36 and 48 h after the intervention was started. Serum was separated promptly, kept at 4° C, and analyzed within 24 h.

Thirty-two patients (20 men and 12 women, mean age 58 years) with documented acute myocardial infarction (AMI) served as reference to determine the time course of the investigated constituents in the blood following myocardial necrosis. The mean time elapsed from onset of chest pain to hospital admission was 2.8 ± 1.4 h. The initial blood sample was taken upon admission; the others at 4-h intervals during the first 36 h and every 12 h until day 3.

Biochemical Measurements

Total CK (2.7.3.2) was measured according to Rosalki [10] and SMb by means of a commercially available RIA kit (MYOK, No. 1135, International CIS, United States). Our reference values for total CK and SMb were 0–100 U/liter and 5 – 80 µg/liter, respectively.

The *mass* concentration of CK-MB was determined using a solid-phase, two-site IEMA method (Tandem-E CKMB, Hybritech Inc., San Diego, United States) [7], without modifying the manufacturer's current protocol. CK-MB *activity* was determined using four different techniques: (a) immunoinhibition (CK-MB UV test, No. 15600, Merck, Darmstadt, FRG) [9]; (b) immunoinhibition-immunoprecipitation (Isomune-CK, No. 43173, Roche Diagnostics, Nutley, NJ 07110, United States) [13]; (c) ion-exchange chromatography on minicolumns containing DEAE-Sephadex (Boehringer-Mannheim, FRG) [6]; and (d) electrophoresis on polyacrylamide gel [3].

Results

Serum CK-MB Mass and Activity Measurements After CBS

The CK-MB concentrations (IEMA) obtained after CBS in the 33 uncomplicated cases were compared with the CK-MB activities determined at the same measurement times by immunoinhibition, immunoinhibition-immunoprecipitation, column chromatography, and electrophoresis (Fig. 1).

CK-MB was detected in each patient by the five techniques and there was an excellent agreement between mass and activity curves. Maximum levels occurred after 7 h and the increase above preoperative levels was observed during 24 – 36 h. At peak, CK-MB concentrations averaged 36 µg/liter and maximum activities ranged from 11 U/liter (electrophoresis) to 23 U/liter (immunoinhibition). In order to compare the methods measuring mass and activity in standard conditions, we divided the individual CK-MB values obtained at peak by the value recorded at the 24th postoperative hour using the corresponding technique. The range of the ratios obtained in this calculation reflected, to some extent, the relative sensitivity of the methods (Table 1).

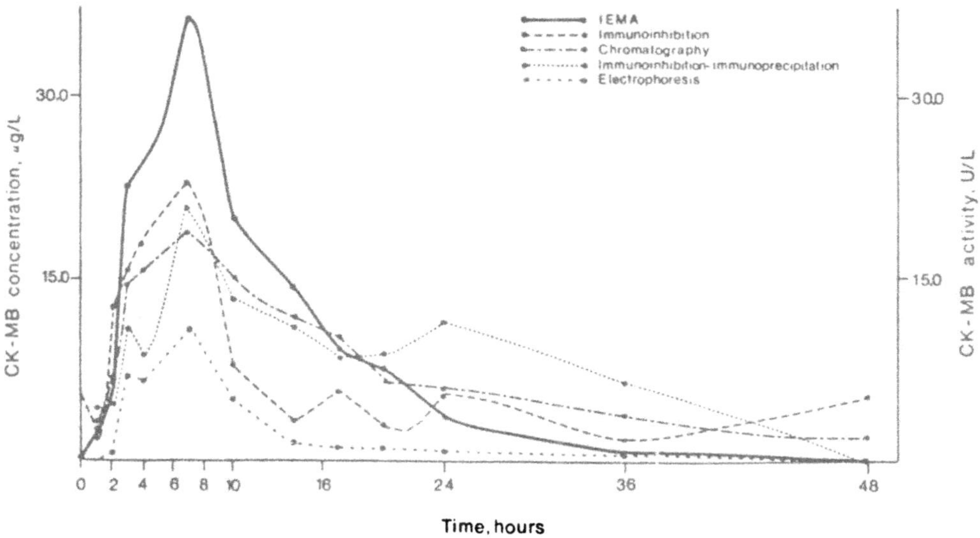

Fig. 1. Comparison of the postoperative CK-MB concentration (IEMA) and catalytic activity curves in the 33 patients without PMI complication

Table 1. Mean ratio between the serum CK-MB levels recorded at peak and at the 24th postoperative hour using the five techniques investigated

Methods	CK-MB ratio
Immunoenzymetric assay	12.5
Electrophoresis	9.0
Immunoinhibition	4.3
Column chromatography	3.1
Immunoinhibition-immunoprecipitation	1.9

Serum CK-MB Concentration After CBS and AMI

CK-MB concentrations peaked earlier in the uncomplicated patients after CBS than in the AMI patients (6.4±2.6 vs. 16.2±7.6 h, $P<0.01$) and returned to normal within shorter periods (22.0±6.0 vs. 59.7±16.1 h, $P<0.01$). Peak levels were 7.5 times more elevated after AMI (Fig. 2a). Earlier SMb peak levels were also recorded after CBS than following AMI (3.3±0.5 vs. 5.5±3.9, $P<0.01$), but there were no significant differences for the magnitude of the changes and delays in normalization. In the CBS patients, sustained elevations of SMb were recorded 24–36 h after surgery (Fig. 2b).

Serum CK-MB Concentration in the Patients with ECG Abnormalities

In the eight patients with ECG abnormalities, we found three different patterns of CK-MB liberation (Fig. 3): the pattern of type I (three patients) was similar

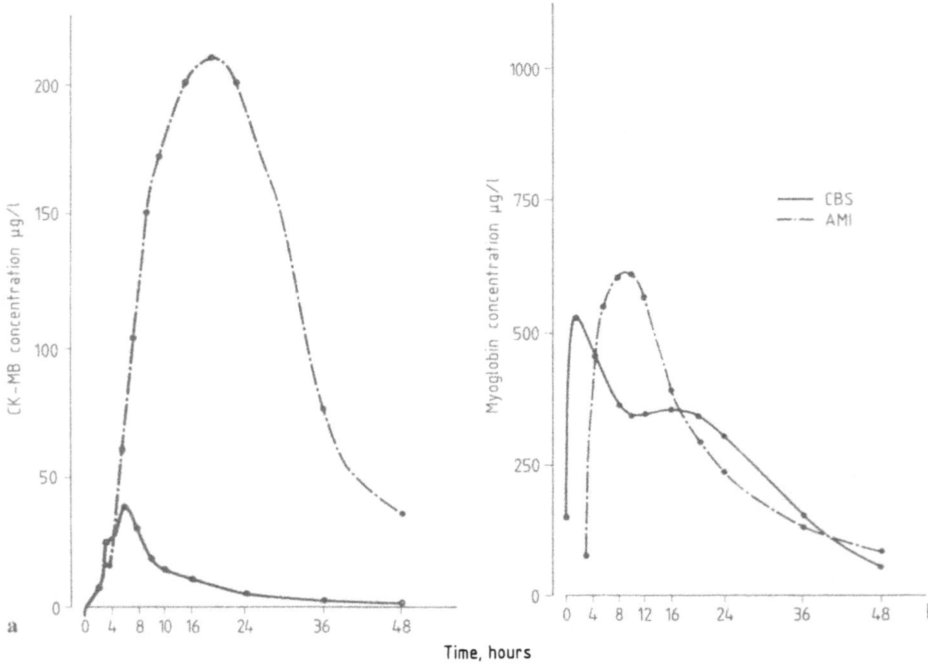

Fig. 2a, b. Mean serum CK-MB (**a**) and SMb (**b**) concentrations after CBS ($n = 33$, no PMI complication) and AMI ($n = 32$)

Table 2. Mean (±SD) serum total CK, CK-MB, and SMb levels recorded 10 h (A) and 24 h (B) after CBS in the patients with ($n = 8$) and without PMI ($n = 33$). Discriminant power of the methods at the two measurement times (*F* test with 1 and 39 degrees of freedom)

	A			B		
	Patients without PMI	Patients with PMI	*F* test	Patients without PMI	Patients with PMI	*F* test
CK-MB (IEMA) (µg/liter)	18±9	121±51	114.2	3±2	70±80	24.5
CK-MB (electrophoresis) (U/liter)	5±8	30±7	64.5	1±1	27±36	18.2
CK-MB (immunoinhibition-immunoprecipitation) (U/liter)	13±3	29±6	57.7	11±8	29±24	18.7
CK-MB (immunoinhibition) (U/liter)	7±7	38±22	47.1	5±5	31±43	12.7
CK-MB (chromatography) (U/liter)	15±6	46±27	37.9	6±5	26±28	16.6
Total CK (U/liter)	409±162	619±260	8.3	603±232	1014±295	18.1
Myoglobin (RIA), (µg/liter)	334±101	458±217	5.9	298±177	695±417	17.8

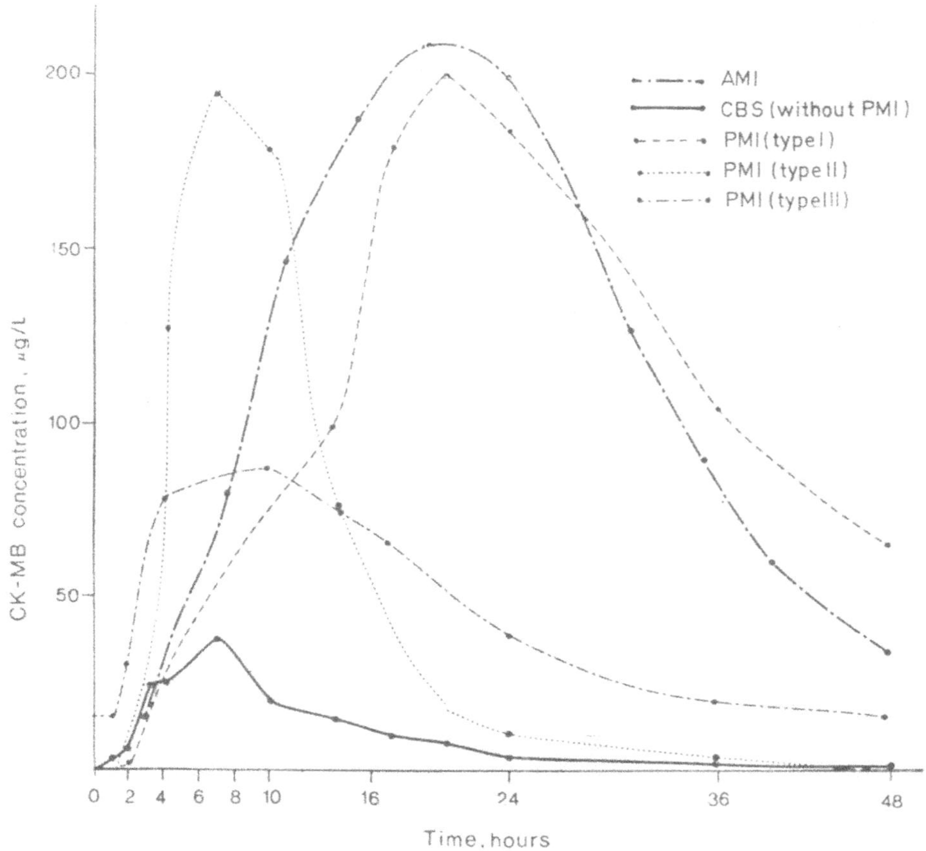

Fig. 3. Patterns of CK-MB release in the patients who developed PMI (type I, $n = 3$; type II, $n = 2$; type III, $n = 3$). Comparison with the CK-MB concentration curves obtained in the uncomplicated cases ($n = 33$) and in the patients with AMI ($n = 32$)

to that recorded in the AMI patients; the initial rise was followed by a second increase of CK-MB, and the maximum concentration (> 150 μg/liter) was reached 20 h after the beginning of the intervention. In the two other patterns, peak concentrations occurred much sooner (6–8 h). For the two patients of type II, fast CK-MB disappearance rates, leading to the normalization of the levels of the cardiac isoenzyme within 36 h, suggested a severe intraoperative damage without secondary extension of the lesion. The low disappearance rates observed in the three patients of type III were responsible for sustained CK-MB elevation after 24 h (25–50 μg/liter). Such concentration curves are consistent with a continuous CK-MB release at least during the first postoperative day.

Ability of the Investigated Analytical Methods to Detect Abnormal Myocardial Damage After CBS

It appeared from Fig. 3 that the 8–12 h and 20–24 h postoperative periods, corresponding to the beginning of the descending slope and to the normalization of the CK concentrations in the uncomplicated cases, are particularly appropriate for the detection of myocardial damage. The serum levels recorded for the investigated parameters at the 10th and 24th postoperative hours were therefore selected for comparing the performances of CK-MB and SMb for differentiating the patients with PMI. Table 2 gave the mean serum values obtained for these constituents in the patients with and without complication of PMI, at these two measurement times. The differences between the two groups were evaluated by an F test. The statistical treatment indicated that the best discrimination was obtained by means of CK-MB concentrations determined by IEMA; among the methods measuring CK-MB activity, the electrophoretic and the immunoinhibition-immunoprecipitation techniques yielded the highest F values. The immunoinhibition method, very sensitive to the interference of adenylate kinase [2], had the poorest performances. All CK-MB assays were superior to the determination of SMb by RIA for detecting PMI.

Conclusion

Although there were no fundamental differences between CK-MB concentration and activity curves after cardiac surgery, the comparison of five of the most widely used techniques in the routine laboratory demonstrated that the IEMA had the highest sensitivity and was superior to the other methods for discriminating the patients at high risk of PMI. The good performances of SMb, recently reported by others [9], could not be confirmed in this study. It also appeared, from a practical point of view, that serum CK-MB concentrations > 50 µg/liter 10 h after the intervention are indicative of abnormal intraoperative damage. At the 24th postoperative hour, CK-MB levels > 25 µg/liter suggest persistent enzyme liberation from the myocardium and concentrations > 100 µg/liter indicate severe myocardial necrosis.

References

1. Bendz R, Ström S, Olin C (1980) CK-MB in serum and in heart and skeletal muscles in patients subjected to mitral valve replacement. Eur J Cardiol 12:25–39
2. Chapelle JP, Heusghem C (1978) Intérêt de l'adénylate kinase comme marqueur de la nécrose myocardique. In: Siest G, Galteau MM (eds) Biologie prospective. Masson, Paris, 597–601
3. Chapelle JP, Heusghem C (1980) Further heterogeneity demonstrated for serum creatine kinase isoenzyme MM. Clin Chem 26:457–462
4. Hammermeister KE (1983) Myocardial infarction during coronary artery bypass surgery – not a benign event. Int J Cardiol 2:516–518
5. Johnson RN, Neutze JM, Kerr AR, Gillain B (1983) Serum myoglobin concentration as an index of myocardial damage after cardiac surgery. Int J Cardiol 4:33–37

6. Mercer DW (1974) Separation of tissue and serum creatine kinase isoenzymes by ion-exchange column chromatography. Clin Chem 20:36–40
7. Myrtle JF, Shimizu I, Varga M, Kotler H, Bartholomew RM (1983) Creatine kinase MB quantitation in serum by simultaneous immunoenzymetric assay. Clin Chem 20:1232–1233 (Abstract)
8. Namay DL, Hammermeister KE, Zia MS, Derouen TA, Dodge HT, Nomay K (1982) The effect of perioperative myocardial infarction on late survival in patients undergoing coronary bypass surgery. Circulation 65:1066–1071
9. Neumeier D, Knedel M, Würzburg U, Hennrich N, Lang H (1975) Immunologischer Nachweis von Creatinkinase-MB in Serum beim Myokardinfarkt. Klin Wochenschr 53:329–333
10. Rosalki SB (1967) An improved procedure for serum creatine phosphokinase determination. J Lab Clin Med 69:696–705
11. Sylvén JCH, Bomfin V, Ivert T, Olin C (1982) Myocardial and non-myocardial release of myoglobin and creatine-kinase MB following cardiac operations with hypothermic potassium cardioplegia. Cardiovasc Res 16:151–157
12. Val PG, Pelletier LC, Hernandez MG, Jais JM, Chaitman BR, Dupras G, Solymoss BC (1983) Diagnostic criteria and prognosis of perioperative myocardial infarction following coronary bypass. J Thorac Cardiovasc Surg 86:878–886
13. Wicks R, Usategui-Gomez M, Miller M, Warshaw M (1982) Immunochemical determination of CK-MB isoenzyme in human serum. II. An enzymic approach. Clin Chem 28:54–58

Advantages of Revascularization in Patients After Myocardial Infarction

A. MARKEWITZ, N. SCHAD, W. HEMMER, B. REICHART, and E. KREUZER

Introduction

The aim of our study was to verify and quantify the benefit of revascularization with regard to regional left ventricular function at rest and during exercise in patients after myocardial infarction.

Patients and Methods

Fifty patients who had undergone coronary artery bypass grafting (CABG) at our hospital were matched with 50 nonoperated on patients. They were comparable in age (57.6±5.7 years vs 56.7±6.4 years), sex, findings of coronary angiography, global left ventricular ejection fraction (EF), and increase of heart rate during exercise (34.1±16.2 bpm vs. 27.1±16.7 bpm). The patients were investigated with first-pass radionuclide angiography at rest and during exercise after a mean follow-up of 50 months after CABG or catheterization. Statistical evaluation was performed with Student's *t*-test. According to coronary angiography the three major coronary arteries were associated individually with three corresponding vascular territories. Table 1 shows the number of vascular territories compromised by myocardial infarction. Altogether 123 anastomoses were performed, resulting in a revascularization rate of 85% (LAD territory), 60% (CX territory), and 41% (RCA territory) with a total rate of 56%. The low percentage in RCA territories was caused by the fact that only those coronary arteries were bypassed in which an increase in blood supply promised benefit with regard to the area of intact myocardium seen intraoperatively.

Table 1. Number of vascular territories compromised by myocardial infarction

Vascular territory	Operated on patients	Not operated on patients	Total
LAD	13 (29%)	17 (36%)	30 (33%)
CX	5 (11%)	9 (19%)	14 (15%)
RCA	27 (60%)	21 (45%)	48 (52%)
Total	45	47	92

Results

Table 2 shows the average results in regional EF of revascularized versus nonrevascularized vascular territories at rest and under exercise conditions. There is a marked difference in regional EF between bypassed and nonbypassed coronary territories. In addition regional EF increases in operated territories under exercise while it decreases in nonoperated territories. However, the mean difference in regional EF at rest and during exercise within each group is not significant. The results gain statistical significance by calculating the average difference in regional EF at rest and under exercise conditions between revascularized and nonrevascularized areas (see Table 3). Both differences are highly significant. Related to the basic regional EF at rest we found some further interesting results (see Table 4). Vascular territories with poor function benefit the most by CABG. The effect of revascularization decreases with increasing EF.

Table 2. Regional ejection fraction at rest and during exercise in revascularized vs. nonrevascularized coronary territories

	Operated on patients	Not operated on patients
Rest	38.2±17.3%	29.2±14.3%
Exercise	41.3±16.4%	28.7±14.8%
Mean difference	+ 3.1 (NS)	−0.5 (NS)

Table 3. Mean difference in regional EF of revascularized vs. nonrevascularized coronary territories

	Δ EF in %	Significance
Rest	+ 9.4±3.56	$P<0.01$
Exercise	+ 12.6±3.57	$P<0.001$

Table 4. Mean difference in regional EF at rest and during exercise related to regional ventricular function: operated on patients versus nonoperated on patients

Basic EF	Δ EF in %		Significance
30%	OP	+ 7.3	$P<0.005$
	NOP	+ 1.5	
30% to 50%	OP	+ 3.7	$P<0.05$
	NOP	− 2.5	
50%	OP	+ 0.5	$P<0.25$
	NOP	− 4.2	

Discussion

Patients after CABG normally experience an improvement in clinical findings. Global hemodynamic parameters on the other hand do not change or show only minor improvement under exercise compared with preoperative findings [1, 4]. The discrepancy of these findings can be explained by the extent of the coronary heart disease and its secondary damages.

A coronary heart disease which requires operative treatment has often resulted in fibrotic, dys-, or akinetic zones nearly occupying a total vascular territory, or one of the three major coronary arteries is not suitable for grafting due to peripheral stenosis or occlusion. Additionally it is impossible to bypass smaller side branches because of technical reasons. This implies that revascularization is only rarely complete. Regional ventricular function of these vascular territories cannot improve while regional EF of revascularized areas shows a marked increase especially under exercise.

This increase, however, only rarely influences global EF to an extent that it gains statistical significance. On the other hand, it is sufficient that patients experience an improved exercise capacity and report an improvement in general wellbeing. In addition, our results confirm, similar to other studies [2, 3, 5], that the benefit of CABG increases with decreasing EF of a vascular territory. This means that regional left ventricular function can improve by revascularization even if major parts of a vascular territory are compromised by myocardial infarction.

Conclusions

1. Global EF is not a suitable parameter to quantify the benefits of CABG.
2. Revascularization should be performed as completely as possible especially in vascular territories showing poor left ventricular function due to serious myocardial damage by myocardial infarction.
3. This also applies for smaller coronary arteries and their side branches.

References

1. Austin EH, Oldham HN, Sabiston DC et al. (1981) Early assessment of rest and exercise left ventricular function following coronary artery surgery. Ann Thorac Surg 35:159
2. CASS Principal Investigators and Their Associates (1983) Coronary Artery Surgery Study (CASS): a randomized trial of coronary artery bypass surgery. Survival data. Circulation 68:939
3. European Coronary Surgery Study Group (1982) Prospective randomized study of coronary artery bypass surgery in stable angina pectoris: a progress report on survival. Circulation 65:II-67
4. Lim YI, Kalff V, Kelly MJ et al. (1982) Radionuclide angiographic assessment of global and segmental left ventricular function at rest and during exercise after coronary artery bypass grafting. Circulation 66:972
5. Takaro T, Huldgren HN, Detre KM et al. (1982) The Veterans Administration Study: current status. Circulation 65:II-60

V. Reoperation

Coronary Artery Reoperations: A 6-Year Experience

A. Schütz, Ch. Weinhold, B. M. Kemkes, E. Kreuzer, and J. Beenisch

Introduction

Since 1974 aortocoronary bypass operation has been a common method in the surgical treatment of coronary heart disease in Germany. Consequently the increasing number of these operations causes more reoperations. We review our experience of coronary artery reoperations carried out at the Department of Cardiac Surgery of the University of Munich.

Methods and Results

From April 1979 to August 1985 3798 aortocoronary bypass operations were performed including 74 reoperations, an incidence of 1.8%. Sixty-seven male and 7 female patients had to be reoperated on at an interval of 24.9 ± 25.4 months after initial surgery. The mean age was 53.7 ± 7.2 years at the time of primary revascularization.

All patients developed recurrent angina caused by graft closure or graft stenosis with still patent distal vessels in 42 patients. Five patients showed progression of disease in previously unbypassed vessels and 27 patients suffered from a combination of graft closure and progression of disease. However, angiographic findings demonstrated vessel modifications consisting of wall irregularities and obstructive lesions in the proximal and distal part of the main 3 coronary arteries in 43 patients (58.4%). This progressive atherosclerosis represents the most malignant form of coronary heart disease. The elevated serum lipid concentration divided into increased triglyceride and cholesterol levels was the outstanding risk factor which occurred in 82% of these patients (Fig. 1).

Complete revascularization should be achieved at initial surgery and 1.7 distal anastomoses were performed at the time of reoperation. Early mortality was 5.3% (4/74) and late mortality was 4.1% (3/74), but decreased significantly during the last 3 years (2.4% each) (Table 1).

The postoperative examination of our patients was carried out after the NYHA classification: 70% of those patients who showed graft failure or significant proximal stenoses of previously unbypassed vessels but still had patent distal vessels had no further symptoms of angina pectoris (Table 2). In contrast only 24.3% of those patients with progressive atherosclerosis became asymptomatic after second surgery (Table 3).

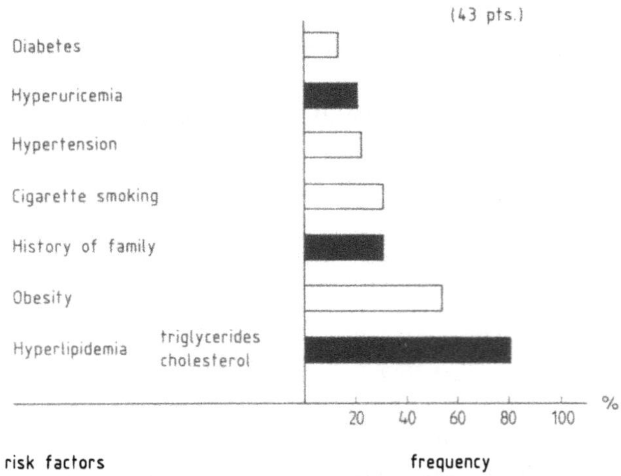

Fig. 1. Risk factors of patients with progressive atherosclerosis

Table 1. Mortalities of 74 reoperated on patients

	Group I (33 patients) (4.79–12.82)	Group II (41 patients) (1.83–7.85)
Early death	3 patients (9.1%)	1 patient (2.4%)
Late death	2 patients (6.1%)	1 patient (2.4%)

Table 2. Follow-up of 37 patients with progressive atherosclerosis

General state		Angina	
Better	26 patients (70.3%)	None	9 patients (24.3%)
Unchanged	9 patients (24.3%)	During exercise – Mild	7 patients (17.9%)
Worse	2 patients (5.4%)	– Severe	10 patients (25.6%)
		At rest	11 patients (29.7%)

Table 3. Follow-up of 30 patients with nonprogressive atherosclerosis

General state		Angina	
Better	28 patients (90.0%)	None	21 patients (70.0%)
Unchanged	1 patient (6.7%)	During exercise – Mild	2 patients (6.7%)
Worse	1 patient (3.3%)	– Severe	1 patient (3.3%)
		At rest	6 patients (20.0%)

Discussion

The incidence of coronary artery reoperations can be compared with the results of other authors [4, 5]. The average time interval of 24.9 ± 25.4 (range 1 – 144 months) between the two operations was lower than those documented in other studies [3, 5]. An important reason for this is the high number of patients with progressive atherosclerosis, which is a very malignant form of coronary heart disease. In addition 82% of these patients suffered from hyperlipidemia with an especially high cholesterol fraction. It is known that the elevated serum lipid concentration forces the development of atherosclerosis even in the saphenous vein grafts after the first postoperative year [1]. Six of seven patients who died suffered from progressive atherosclerosis. In our opinion an accurate indication for aortocoronary reoperation is extremely necessary. Increasing experience has led to better results in the last 3 years. From January 1983 to August 1985 we lost only 2 patients (1 early death, 1 late death) out of a total of 41, an early and late mortality of 2.4%, which approaches the results of initial surgery.

References

1. Campeau C, Enjalbert M, Lesperance J, Vaislic C et al. (1983) Atherosclerosis and late closure of aortocoronary saphenous vein grafts: sequential angiographic studies at 2 weeks, 1 year, 5 to 7 years, and 10 to 12 years after surgery. Circulation 69 (Suppl 2):1
2. Campeau C, Enjalbert M, Lesperance J, Bourassa MG et al. (1984) The relation of risk factors to the development of atherosclerosis in saphenous vein bypass grafts and the progression of disease in the native circulation. A study 10 years after aortocoronary bypass surgery. N Engl J Med 311:1329
3. Gorny P, Deloche A, Fabiani JN, Chauvaud S et al. (1985) Reintervention après pontage saphene aorto-coronaire. Arch Mal Cœur 78:31
4. Hanna ES, Ellerton DG, Jones RJ, Crew JR (1982) Coronary artery revascularisation: reoperations performed on 124 consecutive patients. Texas Heart Inst J 9:293
5. Loop FD, Lytle BW, Goll CC, Golding LAR et al. (1983) Trends in selection and results of coronary artery reoperations. Ann Thorac Surg 36:380
6. Lytle BW, Kramer JR, Golding LR, Cosgrove DM et al. (1984) Young adults with coronary atherosclerosis: 10 year results of surgical myocardial revascularisation. J Am Coll Cardiol 4:445
7. Pidgeon J, Brooks N, Magee P, Pepper JR et al. (1985) Reoperation for angina after previous aortocoronary bypass surgery. Br Heart J 53:269
8. Wukasch DC, Toscano M, Cooley DA, Reul GJ et al. (1977) Reoperation following direct myocardial revascularisation. Circulation 56 [Suppl 2]:3

Late Results in Coronary Reoperations and Investigations Concerning Their Cause, Mortality, and Morbidity

J. M. HABICHT, PH. BETTENDORFF, H. P. WIJNEN, and E. HAUF

Introduction

Worldwide, coronary reoperations are carried out more and more frequently in centers dealing with cardiovascular operations. According to Loop et al. of the Cleveland Clinic Foundation [2], reoperations in the 1970s were mainly performed for early graft failure and insufficient first revascularization. Now, in the 1980s, a second wave of reoperations is expected. These patients often had a successful first operation 5–10 years ago, and angina has recurred because of progressive coronary atherosclerosis or because of late graft thrombosis due to atherosclerosis. *Figure 1* illustrates the increase of reoperations at our institution in the 10-year period from 1974 to 1984.

It is important to realize that the percentages described do not reflect patients needing reoperation after unsuccessful first revascularization, but merely show the relationship between coronary reoperations and first operations independently of the cause of reoperation or of whether the first operation was carried out at our institution or elsewhere. The purpose of this review was a long-term follow-up of patients reoperated on at our institution in the 5-year period between 1974 and 1979. We also investigated this series of patients in relation to mortality, morbidity, and cause of reoperation.

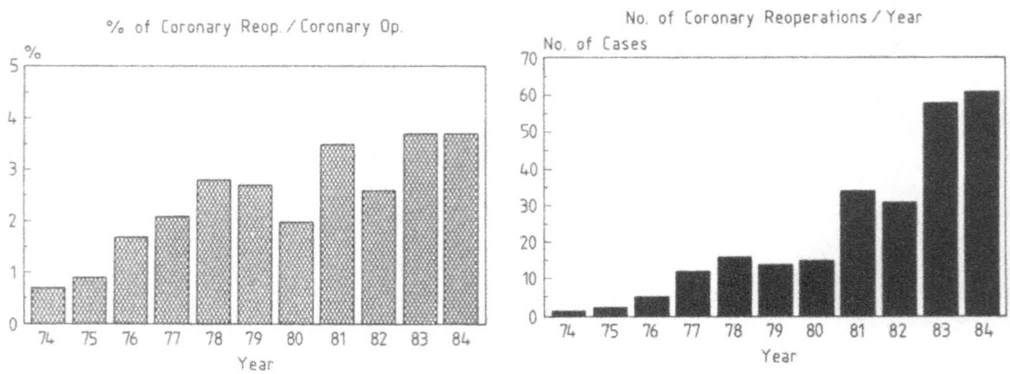

Fig. 1. Coronary surgery reoperations (CABG only)

Patients and Methods

This series includes 49 patients reoperated on consecutively between 1974 and 1979 for coronary disease only. Mean age at revascularization was 50.7 years, at reoperation 52.7 years, and mean interval between the two interventions was 24.3 months. There were 7 women and 42 men, and 77.5% (38) of these patients did *not* have their first revascularization at our institution. All 49 patients had angina pectoris before reoperation, 96% (47) of them in NYHA class III or IV. Three-vessel disease was found in 67.3% (33), two-vessel disease in 30.6% (15), and one-vessel disease in 2.0% (1) at the time of reoperation. Fifty-five percent (27) had myocardial infarction either before (41%) or during and after (14.3%) the first procedure. To determine the cause of reoperation, angiographic and operative reports were reviewed. Data for long-term follow-up were obtained by distributing questionnaires. Follow-up data concerning the year 1985 were complete for 30 of 43 operative survivors (67.4%). Mean follow-up time was 7.2 years (86.8 months), with a range of 5.6–8.7 years (67.2–104.4 months).

Results

General Results

In total, 110 bypasses (2.2/patient) had been carried out at the first revascularization. Graft patency at the time of reoperation is seen in Tables 1 and 2.

At reoperation, a total of 83 bypasses were carried out (1.7/patient). This means that generally all of the occluded and failing grafts (74) were replaced, and that others were additionally carried out to previously nonbypassed vessels.

Table 3 shows a classification of the causes of reoperation.

Table 1. Bypass patency after first revascularization

	No.	%
Total bypasses	110	100
Patent	36	32.7
Failing (significant stenosis)	13	11.8
Occluded	61	55.5

Table 2. Distribution of occlusions

	No.	% of occlusions related to total bypasses	% of occlusions related to territory
LAD	22/46	36.1	47.8
RCA	17/31	27.9	54.8
Cx	16/26	26.2	61.5
Diagonal	6/7	9.8	85.7

Table 3. Causes of reoperation ($n = 49$)

	No.	%	Mean operation/ reoperation interval (months)
Group I	24	49.0	14.0 (2–39)
Group II	7	14.3	32.0 (12–62)
Group III	18	36.7	34.9 (5–97)

Group I	Graft failure and occlusion + insufficient first revascularization
Group II	Progressive atherosclerosis
Group III	Combination of Groups I and II

Forty-nine percent of the patients were reoperated on for graft failure and occlusion as well as insufficient first revascularization. Mean interval in this group was shorter than in groups II and III.

According to operative reports, mistakes in surgical technique were assumed to be the cause of bypass occlusion in a total of ten grafts (involving seven patients). Three were probably too short, two showed mistakes in the suture of distal anastomoses, two were implanted too distally, two were implanted proximally to the stenosis which was intended to be bypassed, and one showed proximal anastomosis on the wrong side of the aorta.

Mortality

Operative mortality (first 30 postoperative days) was 12.2% (6 of 49 in this series). A summary of operative mortality is seen in Table 4.

Impaired left ventricular function was the only significant risk factor relating to mortality ($P < 0.01$). Age and frequency of three-vessel disease was slightly but not significantly higher in patients who did not survive reoperation. Five of six had only systemic hypothermia as a means of myocardial protection; one had chemical cardioplegia at normothermia. This is not statistically significant as most cases (84%) in this series were reoperated on under systemic hypothermia only. Insulin-dependent diabetes or other coronary risk factors were of no importance with regard to mortality in this series.

Table 4. Operative mortality 1974–1979: total operative mortality (within 30 days) = 6/49 (12.2%)

Cardiac: 4		Noncardiac: 2	
Perioperative infarction/operative ischemia:	3	Massive hemolysis: (with acute renal failure)	1
Refractory ventricular arrhythmia:	1	Mesenteric embolization: (with intestinal necrosis)	1
Preoperative EF $\leqq$ 25% in three cases			

Cardiac operative mortality in patients with normal EF = 1/44 (2.3%).

Table 5. Operative morbidity 1974–1979 ($n = 43$)

	No.	%
Hypotensive episodes (drug therapy required)	4	9.3
Perioperative infarctions	3	7.0
Ventricular arrhythmias (drug therapy required)	2	4.7
Postoperative bleeding (reexploration required)	1	
Pneumonia	1	
Sternal infection (successfully treated)	1	
Transient hemisyndrome	1	

Morbidity

Table 5 lists all major complications having occurred in the postoperative phase of reoperation. These complications concern only operative survivors. On the whole, the operative morbidity was not significantly higher than the usual operative morbidity of first revascularization operations.

Complications at reentry of the thorax were the following: in one case the right ventricle was opened unintentionally without serious damage; in another case, dissection of the heart was impossible because of severely calcified adhesions; in a third case, manipulation of a still patent mammary bypass may have been the cause of death due to embolization in LAD territory.

Long-term Results

Development of NYHA (angina) classification for operative survivors for whom data of long-term follow-up were complete for 1985 is seen in Fig. 2.

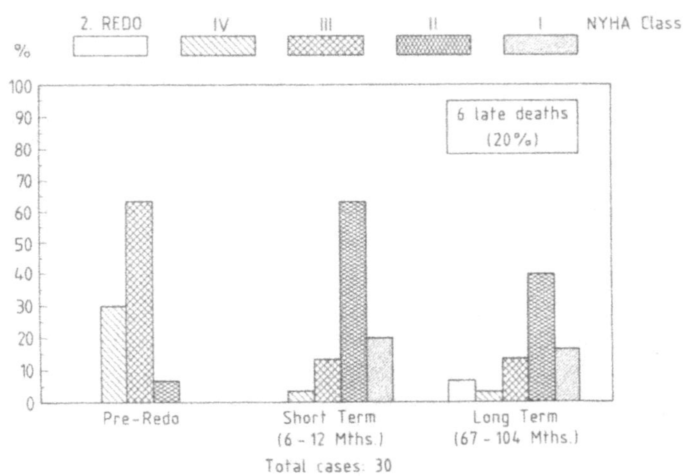

Fig. 2. Coronary surgery reoperations: long-term follow-up (mean = 7.2 years)

Three stages are shown: before reoperation, shortly after reoperation (6 – 12 months), and late results, a mean 7.2 years after reoperation (67 – 104 months). Seventy-nine percent (19 of 24) of late survivors were in NYHA class I or II in 1985, but it must be considered that 8% (2) of these patients had been reoperated on a second time in between. Of all operative survivors 12.4% (3 of 24) had late infarction. An additional 8% (2) were suffering from manifest cardiac insufficiency. No percutaneous transluminal coronary angioplasty (PTCA) had been done after reoperation in this series. The cause of the six late deaths was cardiac in five cases and unknown in one case. Five of six had three-vessel disease at the time of reoperation. Age or coronary risk factors were not significantly higher in these patients.

Conclusions

In summary, a group of candidates for reoperation with severe coronary artery disease was reviewed: more than 90% had angina pectoris NYHA class III or IV before reoperation, and around two-thirds of the patients had three-vessel disease at that time. Only one patient of 49 had one-vessel disease. Over 55% had infarction prior to reoperation. This group of reoperated on patients was not part of a consecutive series of primary revascularizations, and more than 77% of the patients had their first procedure done at other institutions and were transferred to us for reoperation only. We, therefore, believe that this group is not necessarily representative for evaluating general results concerning *primary* coronary artery bypass graft (CABG).

Mortality was rather high, with 12.2% deaths in the perioperative period, for several reasons: half of the deceased had an ejection fraction ≦ 25%. Myocardial protection in these years (1974 – 1979) was mainly done with hypothermia only (84%) at our institution, without associating chemical cardioplegia. Two of six perioperative deaths were noncardiac. This is a rather accidentally high proportion. Foster et al. had not found one case of noncardiac death in the perioperative period of 283 coronary reoperations investigated by them (mortality had been 15 of 283) [1].

On the whole, however, the late results of the reoperations investigated by us can be considered good if taking into account the severe disease of this group. An event-free interval (as defined by Schaff et al. of the Mayo Clinic in 1982) was seen in 50% (15 of 30) of the operative survivors followed up over a mean of 7.2 years. An event-free interval [3] means a postoperative interval free of: cardiac death, late myocardial infarction, cardiac insufficiency, reoperation, and recurrence of NYHA III or IV. A percentage can be thus calculated for patients free of angina pectoris (NYHA I) or for patients in NYHA I and II. Schaff et al. found an event-free interval for patients in NYHA I and II in 63% over a period of 7 years after reoperation. Their estimation, however, was calculated in the actuarial mode.

To what extent PTCA will replace reoperation remains to be seen. We do not know of any long-term results on PTCA after CABG for 5 years or more, but PTCA will surely assert itself for certain indications. We believe that recurrent angina caused by early segmental and anastomotic stenosis of grafts or local progression of ATS (Atherosclerotic disease) in coronary vessels will be a good indication for PTCA in the future. Possibly, patients with poor left ventricular function should have PTCA as well, as the operative risk in these patients is still high (although less high since the general introduction of cold chemical cardioplegia). However, graft failure due to late stenosis caused by ATS of the graft may be theoretically too dangerous for PTCA since bypasses are brittle and risk of atheromatous embolization is high. Diffuse lesions in grafts and arteries as well as total occlusions will most probably always remain surgical indications.

References

1. Eric D, Foster MD, Lloyd D, Fisher PD et al. (1984) Comparison of operative mortality and morbidity for initial and repeat coronary artery bypass grafting: the Coronary Artery Surgery Study Registry experience. Ann Thorac Surg 38 (6):563–570
2. Floyd D, Loop MD, Bruce W, Lytle MD et al. (1983) Trends in selection and results of coronary artery reoperations. Ann Thorac Surg 36(4):380–388
3. Hartzell V, Schaff MD, Thomas A, Orszulak MD et al. (1983) The morbidity and mortality of reoperation for coronary artery disease and analysis of late results with use of actuarial estimate of event-free interval. J Thorac Cardiovasc Surg 85:508–515

Outcome of Re-interventions After Aorto-Coronary Bypass Operations

K. LAIRD-MEETER, R. VAN DOMBURG, M. J. B. M. VAN DEN BRAND, E. BOS, and P. G. HUGENHOLTZ

Introduction

As more time passes since the introduction of the aorto-coronary bypass graft operation, it is becoming increasingly obvious that this form of treatment of angina pectoris is not a definitive one. After a revascularization procedure the atherosclerotic process is not quiescent, nor do the venous grafts remain unaltered by their new role as coronary arterial channel [1]. Many patients therefore come back after a bypass graft operation with unrelieved or recurring angina pectoris [2–4]. A second intervention, either a repeat bypass operation or a percutaneous transluminal angioplasty, is necessary in an increasing number of cases [5–7]. This study was undertaken to enhance our insight into the frequency and outcome of re-intervention procedures.

Methods

Patient Selection and Characteristics

All 1041 patients undergoing single aorto-coronary bypass surgery at our institution prior to July 1980 were included in the study. The clinical characteristics

Table 1. Clinical profile of patients in this study ($n = 1041$)

Sex		
Males	915	88%
Females	126	12%
Age (mean)		
Men	52.6	(SD 7.7)
Women	55.5	(SD 8.2)
Disease affecting		
1 vessel	192	19%
2 vessels	320	31%
3 vessels	444	42%
Left main vessel	85	8%
Ejection fraction		
$\geqq 0.55$	600	57%
0.31–0.55	248	24%
$\leqq 0.30$	27	3%
Unknown	166	16%

of these patients are presented in Table 1. All re-interventions performed in this group of patients up to July 1985 are included. Until 1982 a re-intervention always took the form of a repeat bypass operation, while after 1982 either angioplasty or a repeat bypass operation was performed.

Catheterization Data

Selective coronary angiography was performed in all patients before the primary operation and before the re-intervention. A vessel was considered diseased when in more than one projection a luminal narrowing by more than 50% was seen in a main coronary artery. A classification into one-, two-, three-vessel disease and left main vessel disease. At recatheterization selective injection into the bypass graft was performed whenever possible. If the bypass graft could not be opacified, was found at surgery to be closed, or could be opacified but was narrowed by more than 90%, the graft was considered a failure.

Angioplasty

The technique of Grüntzig was used for angioplasty [8], which was performed in 34 of the patients. A steerable balloon catheter was inserted via the femoral route. Dilatation of a narrowed or occluded bypass graft was performed in 14 patients, dilatation of native vessel(s) in 19, and dilatation of both a native vessel and a graft in 1.

Surgical Technique

Complete revascularization was attempted in all cases. At the original surgical procedure a mean of 2.6 distal anastomoses were placed, with a range of 1 – 7. At the repeat operation, vascularization was improved in all patients but two, one of whom received an aortic valve prosthesis while the other underwent aneurysmectomy and mitral valve replacement.

Statistical Data Analysis

Where appropriate, the Chi-square contingency test was used for statistical testing. The probability of survival was calculated by the Kaplan-Meier method [9].

Results

After a mean follow-up period of 7.5 years (range 5 – 14.5), 143 patients had died (14%). The probability of survival for the total population is 95% at 3 years, 90% ± 2% at 6 years and 83% ± 3% at 9 years.

At the reference date, re-interventions had been performed in 123 patients, or 12% of the studied group. More patients had re-interventions in the first year after the primary surgical procedure than in later years: 23 in the first year, as against 10 per year up to the 9th postoperative year subsequently (Fig. 1). The

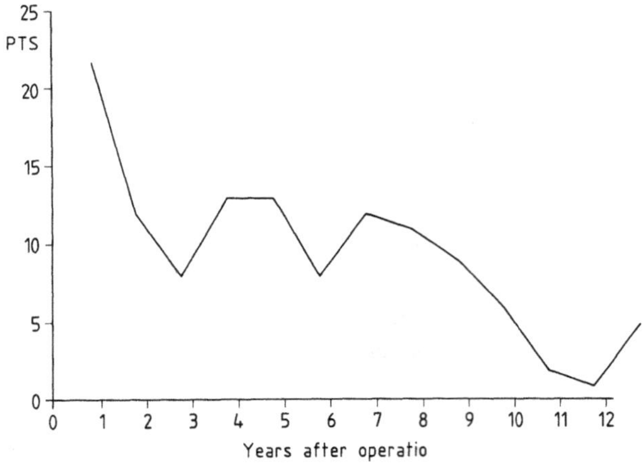

Fig. 1. On the vertical axis is shown the number of patients which underwent a re-intervention in that particular post-operative year, on the horizontal axis the years after surgery. In the first year the number was 23 of 1041 operated upon (2.3%), thereafter up to the 9th postoperative year it was around 10 per year (1%)

Table 2. Anatomical lesion at the time of re-intervention

Findings	No. of patients (%)
Graft failure alone	32 (26%)
Graft failure and disease progression in grafted artery	24 (20%)
Graft failure and disease progression in nongrafted arteries ± disease progression grafted artery	42 (34%)
Progression in nongrafted artery	15 (12%)
Technical inadequacy at first operation	5 (4%)
Aortic valve stenosis	5 (4%)
Total	123

mean interval between the qualifying operation and the re-intervention was 4.5 years (range 1.5 months to 12.5 years).

The indication for re-intervention was severe angina pectoris unrelieved by drug treatment. The symptoms were generally worse than before the first operation: only 1 patient (1%) fell in class II of the NYHA classification, while 46 (37%) had been in this class before the original operation. At recatheterization graft failure with or without disease progression was found in 80% of the patients. In 53% at least one graft was still patent. Table 2 shows the anatomical lesions found at the time of re-intervention. Graft failure as the sole reason for re-intervention is relatively uncommon and was the case in only 32 patients (26%). In most cases progression of atherosclerotic lesions in the native coronary arteries was found in addition.

The lethality of repeat bypass operation was 6% (6 in 101 procedures). In three cases the cause of death was a myocardial infarction sustained at a repeat operation performed 7.8, 9.3 or 12.6 years after the original surgery. Most probably the cause of death in these cases was embolization of atherosclerotic material, as described by Keon in 1983 [10]. One patient died of pump failure after left ventricular aneurysmectomy and mitral valve replacement; he had sustained a massive myocardial infarction in the interval since the first operation.

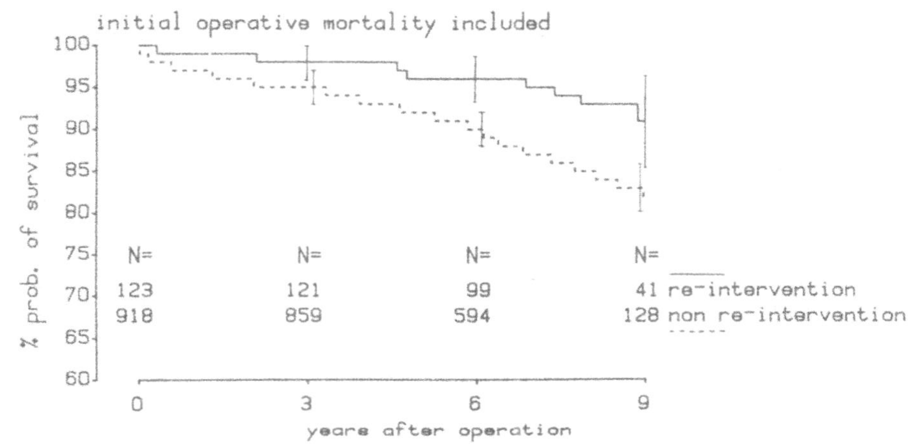

Fig. 2. Survival probability of patients with a later re-intervention (n = 123) and without (n = 918), the initial operative mortality (n = 12) included. The vertical bars denote the 95% confidence limits. The patients with a re-intervention have a higher survival probability, at 9 years 91% versus 82%

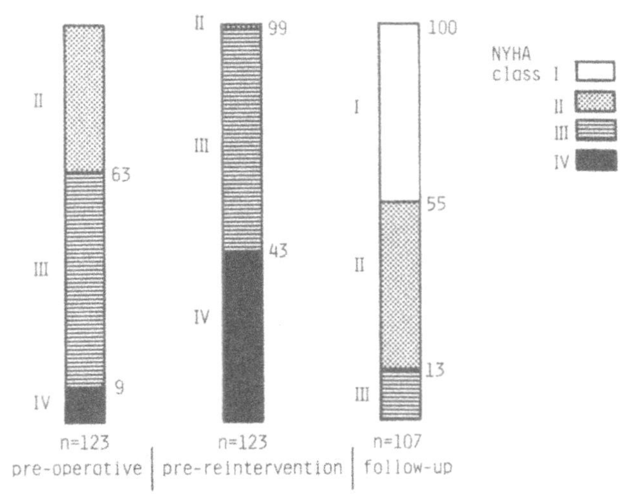

Fig. 3. The vertical bars represent in percentages the angina pectoris classifications of the patients prior to the first operation, prior to the re-intervention and at follow-up. Note the absence of patients in class IV at follow-up, while 43% were in that class before the re-intervention

The two other patients died of infections. Deaths related to angioplasty numbered 2, among 41 procedures (4.9%). These deaths were caused by acute myocardial infarctions and pump failure. The total number of 8 deaths in 142 procedures gave an overall mortality rate of 5.6%, significantly higher than the 1.2% perioperative mortality rate found after the primary procedures ($P < 0.005$).

Survival in the group of patients with a re-intervention is quite good. Figure 2 shows the probability of survival for the patients with a later re-intervention and those without. The probability of survival for the patients with a re-intervention, intervention-related mortality included, is 98% ± 2% at 3 years, 96% ± 3% at 6 years, and 91% ± 6% at 9 years. For those without a later re-intervention the corresponding figures are 96% ± 2%, 91% ± 2%, 82% ± 3%.

Symptomatic condition for the group of patients with a re-intervention is depicted in Figure 3. At follow-up, 49% of the 107 survivors still had anginal complaints, but 89% felt better than before either procedure.

Conclusions

1. Re-interventions are not only necessary immediately after initial aorto-coronary bypass surgery, but also much later. In this study of 1041 patients, after a mean follow-up time of 7.5 years the number who had needed a re-intervention was 123 (12%).
2. The procedure-related mortality is higher at re-intervention than at the primary operation: 5.6% versus 1.2%, but probability of survival at 5–10 years is not worse for the group with a re-intervention than for the group without. This is probably caused by a selection bias. Selection for a re-intervention means that the patient is symptomatic, reaches the hospital alive, does not have a massive acute infarction at that time and has a coronary anatomy amenable to bypass grafting.
3. Angioplasty procedure as an alternative to repeat bypass operation was equally effective as regrafting in the relief of angina pectoris; procedure-related mortality was also similar.
4. Symptomatic improvement after a re-intervention occurred in 89% of the surviving patients, and 51% became pain free. This is not significantly different from the results 3–5 years after a first aorto-coronary bypass operation [2, 4].

References

1. Bourassa MG, Campeau L, Lespérance J, Grondin CM (1982) Changes in grafts and coronary arteries after saphenous vein aorto-coronary bypass surgery. Results at repeat angiography. Circulation 65 [Suppl II]:90–97
2. Campeau L, Lespérance J, Hermann J, et al. (1979) Loss of improvement of angina between 1 and 7 years after coronary bypass surgery. Circulation 60 [Suppl I]:1–5
3. Cameron A, Kemp HG, Shimomura S, et al. (1979) Aorto-coronary bypass surgery. A 7-year follow-up. Circulation 60 [Suppl I]:9–13
4. Laird-Meeter K, ten Katen HJ, Brower RW, et al. (1983) Angina pectoris 1 to 10 years after aortocoronary bypass surgery. Eur Heart J 4:678–686

5. Foster ED (1985) Reoperation for coronary artery disease. Circulation 72 [Suppl V]:59–64
6. Jones EL, Douglas JS, Grüntzig AR, et al. (1983) Percutaneous saphenous vein angioplasty to avoid re-operative bypass surgery. Ann Thorac Surg 36:389–395
7. Block PC, Cowley MJ, Kaltenbach M, et al. (1984) Treatment of coronary artery bypass graft stenosis with percutaneous angioplasty: an alternative to repeat surgery. Am J Cardiol 53:666–668
8. Grüntzig AR, Senning A, Siegenthaler WE (1979) Nonoperative dilatation of coronary artery stenosis: percutaneous transluminal coronary angioplasty. N Engl J Med 301:61–67
9. Kaplan EL, Meier P (1958) Nonparametric estimation from incomplete observation. J Am Stat Assoc 43:457–481
10. Keon WJ, Heggtveit HA (1983) Coronary atheroembolism causes peri-operative myocardial infarction. A hazard at reoperation. Cardiovasc Surg 24:287

Coronary Artery Regrafting in 64 Cases: Results and Experience

J. Ramström, T. Åberg, S.-O. Nyström, A. Hallén, S. Brunnkvist, L. Nordgren, and E. Enghoff

After coronary bypass operations some patients will have persistent pain or recurrence of symptoms. A proportion of these patients will be candidates for reoperation.

The aim of this study is to give a short review of our experience with reoperations, especially as regards the selection of patients for the procedure.

Material and Methods

From 1970 until the end of 1984, 1678 patients with stable and unstable angina pectoris were revascularized at the Department of Thoracic Surgery, University Hospital, Uppsala, Sweden. Patients with severe recurrent angina pectoris refractory to medical treatment with a desire for a second operation were investigated with coronary and graft angiogram and left ventriculogram. During the same time interval, 64 of these patients (3.8%) had a second operation.

At the *primary operation*, the mean age in these 64 patients was 52 years (range 37 – 62 years). Three of the patients had left main disease, 26 three-vessel, 21 two-vessel, and 14 one-vessel disease. Twenty patients had ejection fraction of more than 50%, 32 between 30% and 50%, and 12 below 30%. The number of grafts placed per patient was 2.3. Fourteen of the patients were subsequently judged to be incompletely revascularized.

Mean age at regrafting was 55 years (range 39 – 68 years). Eight patients were female. Four had diabetes mellitus and 14 hypertension. Fourteen smoked more than ten cigarettes a day at the time of regrafting.

Mean interval between primary operation and regrafting was 36 months (range 1 – 130 months). A mean of 3.1 new peripheral anastomoses on an average of 1.8 grafts were placed, giving the patients a mean of 2.9 patent grafts at the end of the operation. Follow-up was made after a mean of about 1.5 years. Information about the patient was obtained either by personal contact via telephone or via letter. Among other things information was sought about the symptom level and the physical activity level before and after the second operation. Symptom level was graded as 1 = no angina, 2 = much improved, 3 = slightly improved, 4 = unchanged, and 5 = worse. Physical activity was graded as 1 = no angina, 2 = much improved, 3 = slightly improved, 4 = unchanged, and 5 = worse.

The material was divided into two groups, the first being operated upon from 1975 to April 1983. After this period we analyzed our material of cases and found the results to be mediocre. Indications for reoperation were greater. Between June 1983 and December 1985, we regrafted a further 23 cases.

Results

In a majority of the patients (64%), the return of symptoms occurred early after the primary operation. Probable causes of the recurrence are given in Table 1. The most common cause was graft failure and progressive disease. In a given case, several causative factors were often involved.

Two patients died at the reoperation. In one case, glutaraldehyde-treated homograft veins had been used at the primary operation because of lack of the patients own veins 10 months earlier. She suddenly occluded all her grafts and developed an unstable angina. She could not be weaned from the heart-lung machine and autopsy revealed a preoperative infarction. The second case died 2 weeks postoperatively because of left ventricular failure. Autopsy showed signs of perioperative myocardial infarction. The aortic balloon pump had to be used in four cases. In two surviving cases, there were signs of a definite perioperative infarction (Q-wave and high enzymes). Eight cases were classified as probable myocardial infarctions due to a CK-MB level of more than 2.0 µmol/ml 20 h after operation. Neurological complications occurred in three cases. Two of them had temporary partial hemiplegia, and the third patient had a frank stroke with permanent hemiplegia. CT examination showed signs of brain infarction.

Follow-up in group I was done in June 1983 after the first 41 cases. Mean observation time was 18 months (range 2–65 months). Results are given in Table 2. Only three patients were free of pain and one-third of the patients were

Table 1. Putative causes of recurrent angina after the first operations

Graft failure only	19
Graft failure + progressive disease	16
Graft failure + incomplete revascularization	3
Progressive disease only	15
Progressive disease + incomplete revascularization	5
Incomplete revascularization only	3
All three factors	3

Table 2. Angina status after reoperation: the first 41 cases

Without pain	3	8%	69%
Much improved	13	33%	
Slightly improved	11	28%	
Not improved	8	21%	
Worse	4	10%	
Follow-up time, 18 months (4–65 months)			

Table 3. Angina status after reoperation: the last 23 patients (1 death, June 1983 – January 1985)

Without pain	4	18%	82%
Much improved	11	50%	
Slightly improved	3	14%	
Not improved	3	14%	
Worse	1	4%	
Follow-up time, 14 months (8–26 months)			

either not improved or worse. Patients in whom the cause of recurrence was progressive disease had somewhat worse results than other groups. Especially if the progressive disease was diffuse and situated in peripheral arteries, results of regrafting were poor.

After changing indications for operation, avoiding patients with progressive diffuse, small-vessel disease, another 23 patients were operated upon, group II. Follow-up of these patients was done in July 1985. Observation time was 14 months (range 8–26 months). Eighteen percent of the patients were free of angina and 82% had had at least slight improvement (Table 3). No patient in either group had died late after operation.

Discussion

A majority of the patients that are subsequently reoperated upon have their recurrence of angina during the 1st year after operation [4, 9]. In most of these cases graft occlusion is a major reason [2, 4, 9, 10, 12]. Technical failure is probably the reason in many cases [4]. Other reasons may be poor runoff in the grafted vessels [13] and thrombogenic factors in the vessel wall and the blood. Arteriosclerosis in the vein grafts is not a major reason a short time after the operation [3]. Fourteen patients were incompletely revascularized at the first operation. Most of these were at the beginning of our experience before the importance of complete revascularization was realized. In three cases this was the only reason for recurrent pain after the first operation. All these patients were completely relieved of angina after the reoperation. In 58% progressive disease was the only or a contributing factor for recurrence. In most cases progressive disease was found in the ungrafted vessels. Progressive disease distal in the grafted vessel was not so common [13]. The mortality of 3.1% is higher than 1.4% mortality for the last 600 patients at the primary operation, but of the same magnitude as found in several materials [8, 10, 13]. No death was caused by an intraoperative complication specific for reoperation. In two cases (3.1%) we had a proven perioperative infarction with positive Q-waves on ECG and high enzymes, which is similar to the infarction rate for primary operations [5].

At the first follow-up of the first 41 cases 69% were improved but only 8% were free of angina.

This can be compared with 85% improvement and 40% free of angina after the primary operation. Most series published during the later years have results better than this at least for patients free of angina [1, 7, 8, 10, 13, 14]. The worst result was seen in patients with progressive distal disease. In almost all these cases the graft had also occluded. It is easy to understand that a new attempt with a vein graft to a vessel with a compromised runoff will have a great tendency for a new occlusion. During the past 2 years we have not operated on patients with distal small vessel disease or patients with massive diffuse progressive arteriosclerosis. We attribute our improved results to this factor. In most cases it is probably possible to avoid patients unsuitable for regrafting by the combined information obtained from the first operation (operative report) and the angiography before the contemplated reoperation. A good description of the quality of the coronary pathology in the operative report is of utmost importance when judging the prognosis of a reoperation or indeed the need for a repeat coronary angiography.

References

1. Allen RA, Stinson EB, Oyer PE, Shumway NE (1978) Predictive variables in reoperation for coronary artery disease. J Thorac Cardiovasc Surg 78:186–192
2. Barboriak J, Barboriak D, Andersson A, Rimm A, Tristani F, Flemma R (1978) Risk factors in patients undergoing a second aortocoronary bypass procedure. J Thorac Cardiovasc Surg 76:111–114
3. Campean L, Lespérance J, Herman J, Corbora F, Grandin CM, Bourassa MG (1979) Loss of improvement of angina 1 and 7 years after aortocoronary bypass surgery. Correlations with changes in vein grafts and in coronary arteries. Circulation 60 [Suppl 1]: 1
4. Culliford AT, Girdwood RW, Isom OW, Krauss KR, Spencer FC (1979) Angina following myocardial revascularization. Does time of recurrence predict etiology and influence results of operation? J Thorac Cardiovasc Surg 77:889–895
5. Foster F, Fisher LD, Kaiser GC, Myers WO (1984) Comparison of operative mortality and morbidity for initial and repeat coronary artery bypass grafting: the coronary artery surgery study (CASS) registry experience. Ann Thorac Surg 38:563–570
6. Hanna E, Ellertson DG, Jones RJ, Crew JR (1982) Coronary artery revascularization: reoperations performed on 124 consecutive patients. Texas Heart Inst J 9:293–297
7. Kobayashi T, Mendez AM, Zubiate P, Vanstrom NR, Yokoyama T, Kay JH (1978) Repeat aortocoronary bypass grafting. Chest 73:446–449
8. Krause AH jr, Page VS, Bigelow JC, Okies JE, Dunlop SF (1978) Reoperation in symptomatic patients after direct coronary artery revascularization. J Thorac Cardiovasc Surg 75:448–504
9. Laird-Meeter K, van den Brand MJBM, Serruys PM et al. (1983) Reoperation after aortocoronary bypass procedure. Results in 53 patients in a group of 1041 with consecutive first operations. Br Heart J 50:157–162
10. Loop FD, Cosgrave PM, Kramer JR et al. (1981) Late clinical and arteriographic results in 500 coronary artery reoperations. J Thorac Cardiovasc Surg 81:675–685
11. Pidgeon J, Brooks N, Magee P, Pepper JR, Sturridge MF, Wright JEC (1985) Reoperation for angina after previous aortocoronary bypass surgery. Br Heart J 53:269–275
12. Pucci JJ, Walesby RK, Smith EEJ et al. (1982) Reoperation for failed aortocoronary bypass grafts. J Cardiovasc Surg 23:453–457
13. Reul GJ Jr, Cooley DA, Ott DA, Coelho A, Chapa L, Eterovic I (1979) Reoperations for recurrent coronary artery disease. Arch Surg 114:1269–1275
14. Schaff HV, Orszulak TA, Gersh BJ et al. (1983) The morbidity and mortality of reoperations for coronary artery disease and analysis of late results with use of actuarial estimate of event-free interval. J Thorac Cardiovasc Surg 85:508–515

Reopertion After Coronary Bypass Surgery: Technical Aspects and Long-term Follow-up

R. A. E. DION, G. JAMBROES, B. JAMBROES, B. J. AMSEL, R. VAN HAASE, P. WALTER, and J. F. HITCHCOCK

Introduction

Angina pectoris has been reported to recur after initial revascularization at rates of 3.5%–7.2%/year [1, 3, 4, 9, 13, 14, 16, 19]. Fortunately the reported results from repeat coronary artery bypass grafting have been encouraging: mortality ranged from 0% to 12.5% [2, 5, 7, 8, 10, 12, 13, 16, 21] and less than 3% in a few reported series [10, 14]; perioperative myocardial infarction has been reported, depending on definition, in 5%–15% of cases [1, 5, 7–9, 12–14, 16, 19]; at 5 years 30%–55% of patients remained markedly improved [1, 2, 7, 10, 13, 14, 16, 21].

Material and Methods

One hundred and nineteen consecutive patients reoperated on between September 1978 and June 1985 with a maximum follow-up (100%) of 82 months were analyzed. One of them had a third operation. Ninety-nine patients were treated at the University Hospital of Utrecht and 20 at the University Hospital of Antwerp. There were 95 males (80%). The mean age at reoperation was 56 years (35–75 years).

Thirteen percent of the patients were 45 years old or less. Seventy-one patients (60%) had undergone their first operation at another institution. Sixty-three (53%) patients had sustained at least one myocardial infarction before the first operation, 82 (70%) before reoperation. At the first operation, 45 patients (38%) had three-vessel disease, and a mean of 2.7 distal anastomoses per patient were performed, with a perioperative infarction rate of 15.1%.

The symptom-free period ranged from 0 to 132 months, mean 25 months, median 6 months. The initial operation-reoperation interval ranged from 1 to 180 months, mean 42 months, median 36 months. Graft failure was emerging as the most frequent cause of recurrence (38%) (see Fig. 1). There was a clear correlation between symptom-free interval and cause of recurrence: less than 6 months in the case of graft failure, 3 years in the case of progression of the disease (Table 1).

Hyperlipidemia, diabetes, obesity, and peripheral vascular disease could not be correlated significantly with any of the causes of recurrence, although there were more graft failures among diabetic (9% vs. 0%) and obese (15% vs. 4%) patients as compared with progression of the disease among patients presenting

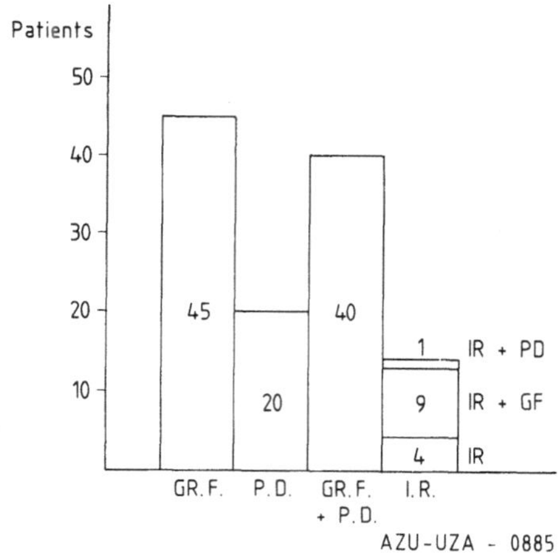

Fig. 1. Cause of recurrent angina. *GR.F.*, graft failure; *P.D.*, progression of the disease; *I.R.*, incomplete revascularization

Table 1. Reoperations for recurrent angina. Relationship between causes of recurrence and symptom-free interval (months)

Graft failure	Med 3 Mean 12	(0–102)
Progressive disease	Med 36 Mean 43.2	(5–120)
Graft failure + progressive disease	Med 18 Mean 34	(0–132)
Incomplete revascularization	0-2-26-108	
Incomplete revascularization + graft failure	Med 3	(1–10)
Incomplete revascularization + progressive disease	2	

MED = median

with peripheral vascular disease (12% vs. 6%). Male patients presenting more frequently with the combination graft failure progression of the disease than female patients (38% vs 16%, $P = 0.005$). Before reoperation, 118 patients were in class III or IV NYHA, and 1 was asymptomatic but had a strongly positive thallium scan with ECG-monitored stress study. Twenty-six patients underwent emergency repeat operation for unstable angina. Ninety-three patients (78%) had three-vessel disease. Thirty patients (25.3%) had a poor left ventricular (LV) function as defined by ejection fraction (EF) equal to or less than 0.4, left ventricular end-diastolic pressure (LVEDP) equal to or higher than 20 mm Hg, and/or diffuse hypokinesia with LV dilatation (Table 2): in this group, there were more female patients, a higher incidence of graft failure, of hyperlipidemia and of diabetes ($P = 0.001$), and a lower incidence of progression of the disease. At reoperation, resternotomy was used in all cases. Injuries of the innominate vein (two patients), of a previous graft (two patients), of the pulmonary artery (two patients), and of the right ventricle (RV) (two patients) could not be avoided: in these cases, the pericardium had not been closed at first operation. Cannulation of the ascending aorta was feasible in all but five cases

Table 2. Reoperations for recurrent angina: influence of LV function

	EF < 0.4[a]	EF > 0.4[a]
Females	8 (27%)	16 (18%)
Graft failure	14 (47%)	31 (35%)
Progressive disease	1 (3.3%)	19 (21.3%)
Graft failure + progressive disease	11 (37%)	30 (34%)
Hyperlipidemia	11 (37%)	20 (22.5%)
Diabetes	5 (17%)	2 (2.2%)
Corrections/patient	3.0	3.0
Hospital deaths	5 (17%)	2 (2.2%)
PMI	6 (20%)	7 (7.8%)

[a] EF < 0.4: 30 patients; EF > 0.4: 89 patients
PMI, perioperative myocardial infarction

Table 3. Reoperations for recurrent angina

Corrections/patient, 3.0 (Mean, 2.2 VD)	
New grafts	309
LIMA	5
Patches	28
TEA	11
Interposition	8
Dilation + exploration	8
LAD not found	3
CX not found	2
LV aneurysm resection	1

LAD, left anterior descending artery; CX, circumflex artery: LV, left ventricle; VD, vessel disease; LIMA, left internal mammary artery; TEA, thrombo-endarterectomy.

(4.2%). Moderate hypothermia (25° – 28° C) and cold crystalloid cardioplegia were used systematically. Surgical corrections are detailed in Table 3. Distal correction per patient averaged 3.0. Aortic cross-clamping time averaged 64 min (11 – 135 min).

Results

Perioperative myocardial infarction was diagnosed in 13 patients (11%). Inotropic agents were used in 27 patients (23%) and insertion of an intraaortic balloon pump catheter was necessary in 12 patients (10%). Ten patients (8.4%) underwent rethoracotomy for postoperative bleeding. Other complications were mediastinitis (one patient), adult respiratory distress syndrome (two patients), pulmonary embolus (one patient), acute liver failure (coma) (one patient), rewiring of the sternum (one patient), superficial wound infection (three patients), and neurologic transient disorder (one patient).

The mean follow-up was 27 months (2 – 82 months). There were seven deaths (5.8%) within 30 days after reoperation: the cause of recurrence in every case was a combination of graft failure and progression of the disease, with a mean symptom-free interval of 38 months (median 36 months, 5 – 65 months) and an operation-reoperation interval of 68 months (median 71, 18 – 119 months); four patients were emergencies (unstable angina in three patients, evolving infarction in one); another had angina at rest, and all but one were denied reoperation elsewhere; perioperative myocardial infarction occurred in four patients, twice as a result of incomplete revascularization (vessels not found); one patient died of acute tamponade on the ninth day postoperatively due to the bleeding of a side branch of a saphenous graft (dislodgement of a hemostatic clip); two

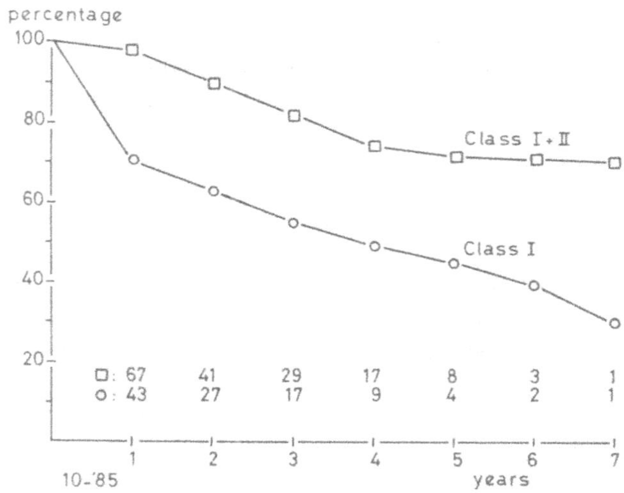

Fig. 2. Actuarial curve of NYHA class after reoperation over 5 years

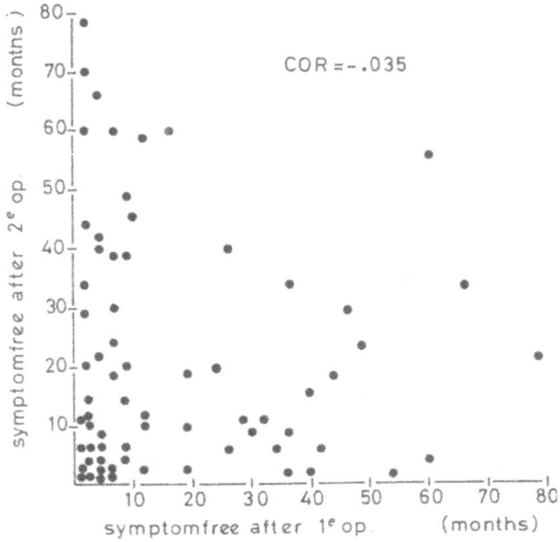

Fig. 3. Improvement (NYHA I and II) after first operation versus reoperation. *Abcissa,* symptom-free period after first operation; *ordinate,* symptom-free period after reoperation

patients died in spite of successful revascularization (four grafts): postmortem examination revealed patent grafts and extensive subendocardial fibrosis of the LV; five patients had a poor LV function. Hospital mortality when the LV EF exceeded 0.4 was 2.2% (two patients) (see Table 2).

Actuarial follow-up showed that nearly 50% of the patients remained symptom free while 75% remained markedly improved after 5 years (Fig. 2). When EF exceeded 0.4, 80% of the patients remained symptom free after 5 years. There was no correlation between the symptom-free intervals after the initial and after the repeat operation (Fig. 3).

Discussion

Progress in coronary angiography, in perioperative medical treatment, and in surgical technique have made repeat coronary operations a viable therapeutic tool: this should be used not only to try and equal the results of an initial revascularization, rather to decrease the cohort of patients who are denied a reoperation for a number of reasons.

Data regarding the number of patients turned down for reoperation along with reasons for avoiding reoperations are scarce: yet appreciation and comparison of the post-operation results would only gain in adequacy if they were displayed [17, 18]. In our opinion, no patient presenting with unstable angina should be turned down for reoperation. Estimation of caliber and runoff of a proximally occluded and collaterally filled coronary artery is hazardous. Systematic patient refusal based on these generally proposed criteria [10, 14, 16, 21] can lead, in our experience, to unjustified elimination of acceptable candidates.

Poor LV function alone (25% in our series) is not a reason to decline reoperation in the presence of severe angina pectoris: relief of angina rather than improvement of LV function is then in prospect. At our institute, six patients (5%) were denied reoperation: all had a poor LV function, none had unstable angina, and all had ungraftable arteries as described by the surgeon at first operation (previous endarterectomy, vessels not found, poor anatomy).

Technical aspects of reoperation have been widely described [1, 6, 9, 11]. An oscillating saw was used at resternotomy after careful examination of a lateral chest X-ray: when there was no retrosternal free space, only the outer table of the sternum was divided using the saw; strong scissors were used carefully to divide the inner table. Once the ascending aorta and right atrium had been freed, cardiopulmonary bypass was instituted and half an empty heart was more easily dissected free all around. When a previous mammary artery graft was still patent, the patient was cooled down to 20 °C to achieve optimal myocardial protection. Complete revascularization was always attempted, small coronary branches being anastomosed to a sequential graft. More recently, the internal mammary artery has been used whenever possible. A combination of prolonged aortic cross-clamping time and of suboptimal revascularization certainly accounts for the higher rate of perioperative myocardial infarction at reoperation [22].

The excellent results in terms of survival (Table 2) and functional status (80% asymptomatic at 5 years) achieved in patients with fair LV function and favorable coronary anatomy, and the incidence of myocardial infarctions occurring between the two operations (13%), lead us to propose a percutaneous angioplasty [18, 19] or a reoperation in order to salvage threatened but not infarcted myocardium, even in the absence of angina pectoris: thallium scan with ECG-monitored stress and stress technetium multiple-gated wall motion studies have their place in determining these situations on time! [21].

Graft failure alone is the cause of recurrence in 38% of the cases, while it is found in combination with another factor in 41% (Fig. 1). Harvesting of the saphenous vein should be handled with extreme care and the mammary artery should be used whenever possible.

According to Loop [10], the incidence of late graft failure due to atherosclerosis is still due to increase, while progression of the disease as the cause of recurrence is expected to decrease [10, 13, 18] even further if surgeons grafting at the first operation all the diseased major vessels, even those with less than 50% stenosis. As observed by others [1, 15], 11% of the reoperated on patients had suffered from a postcardiotomy syndrome after their first operation.

Conclusions

- Early recurrence of angina pectoris does not preclude successful reoperation.
- Mortality and morbidity of reoperations are higher than those of initial revascularization, but remain acceptable.
- Seventy-five percent of the patients remain markedly improved at 5 years.
- No patient with unstable angina should be turned down for repeat coronary operation, and poor LV function alone is no contraindication.
- In the case of fair LV function and of favorable coronary anatomy, angioplasty and/or reoperation may be proposed to salvage threatened myocardium, even in the absence of angina pectoris.
- "Overcomplete" revascularization of all the diseased major vessels at the first operation may be advocated, even more in young patients, and in the presence of hyperlipidemia and peripheral vascular disease.
- Use of the mammary artery should be extended in view of the high (and probably still growing) incidence of venous graft failure.
- Pericardium should be at least approximated whenever possible at the first operation.
- It is the duty of the surgeon to describe minutely the lesions and the quality of the coronary vessels grafted at the first operation.

References

1. Allen RH, Stinson EB, Oyer PE, Shumway NE (1978) Prediction variables in reoperation for coronary artery disease. J Thorac Cardiovasc Surg 75:186–192
2. Brooks N, Honey M, Cattell M, Wright JEC, Sturridge HF, Balcon R, Layton C (1979) Reoperation for recurrent angina. Br Heart J 42:333–338

3. Cameron A, Kemp HG Jr, Shimorura S, Santilli E, Green GE, Hutchinson JE III, Mekhjian HA (1979) Aortocoronary bypass surgery, a 7 years follow-up. Circulation 60 [Suppl 1]:9–13
4. Campeau L, Lesperance J, Hermann J, Corbara F, Grondin CM, Bourassa MG (1979) Loss of improvement of angina between 1 and 7 years after aortocoronary bypass surgery. Correlations with changes in vein grafts and in coronary arteries. Circulation 60 [Suppl 1]: 1–5
5. Culliford AT, Girdwood RW, Isom OW, Krauss KR, Spencer FC (1979) Angina following myocardial revascularization. Does time of recurrence predict etiology and influence results of operation? J Thorac Cardiovasc Surg 77:889–895
6. Dobell ARC, Jain AK (1984) Catastrophic hemorrhage during redo sternotomy. Ann Thorac Surg 37:273–278
7. Gandjbakhch I, Pavie A, Cabrol C, Bachet J, Musat T, Goudot B, Guilmet D (1982) Chirurgie coronarienne itérative, techniques et indications. Ann Chir 36:607–609
8. Krause AH, Scott Page V, Bigelow JC, Okies JE, Duncap SF (1978) Reoperations in symptomatic patient after direct coronary artery revascularization. J Thorac Cardiovasc Surg 75:499–504
9. Loop FD, Cosgrove DM, Kramer JR, Lytle BW, Taylor PC, Golding LAR, Groves LK (1981) Late clinical and arteriographic results in 500 coronary artery reoperations. J Thorac Cardiovasc Surg 81:675–685
10. Loop FD, Lytle BW, Gill CC, Golding LAR, Cosgrove DM, Taylor PC (1983) Trends in selection and results of coronary artery reoperations. Ann Thorac Surg 36:380–388
11. Loop FD (1984) Catastrophic hemorrhage during sternal re-entry. Ann Thorac Surg 37:271
12. Qazi A, Garcia JM, Mispiretta LA, Corso PJ (1981) Reoperation for coronary artery disease. Ann Thorac Surg 32:16–18
13. Reul GJ Jr, Cooley DA, Ott DA, Coelho A, Chapa L, Eterovic I (1979) Reoperation for recurrent coronary artery disease, causes, indications, and results in 168 patients. Arch Surg 114:1269–1275
14. Schaff HV, Orszulak TA, Gersh BJ, Piehler JH, Puga FJ, Danielson GK, Pluth JR (1983) The morbidity and mortality of reoperation for coronary artery disease and analysis of late results with use of actuarial estimate of event free interval. J Thorac Cardiovasc Surg 85:508–515
15. Urschel HC Jr, Razzuk MA, Gardner M (1976) Coronary artery bypass occlusion secondary to postcardiotomy syndrome. Ann Thorac Surg 22:528–531
16. Foster ED, Fischer LD, Kaiser GC, Myers WO (1984) Comparison of operative mortality for initial and repeat coronary artery bypass grafting: the coronary artery surgery study (CASS) registry experience. Ann Thorac Surg 38:563–570
17. Pluth JR (1984) Operative mortality and morbidity for initial and repeat coronary artery bypass grafting. Ann Thorac Surg 38:552–553
18. Mills NL (1983) Trends in selection and results of coronary artery operations. Ann Thorac Surg 36:373–374
19. Jones EL, Douglas JJ, Gruentzig AR, Crauer JM, King SB, Guyton RA, Hatcher CR (1983) Percutaneous saphenous vein angioplasty to avoid reoperative bypass surgery. Ann Thorac Surg 36:389–395
20. Mills NL (1983) Reop. or not. Ann Thorac Surg 36:375–376
21. Shark WM, Kass RM (1981) Repeat myocardial revascularization in coronary disease therapy: consideration of primary bypass failures and success of second graft surgery. Am Heart J 102:303–306
22. Assad-Morell JL, Frye RL, Connolly DC, Gau GT, Pluth JR, Barnhorst DA, Wallace RB, Davis GD, Elveback LR, Danielson GK (1975) Relation of intraoperative or early postoperative transmural myocardial infarction to patency of aortocoronary bypass grafts and to diseased ungrafted coronary arteries. Am J Cardiol 35:767–773

Redo Surgery for Coronary Heart Disease: Do the Operative Problems Determine the Postoperative Results?

A. SCHIESSLER, J. PALENKER, B. HEMPEL, A. JOHN, and E. S. BÜCHERL

Of the 1400 patients who were operated on for coronary artery disease in Berlin during 1984/1985, 13 had previously undergone bypass operations and had come back with recurrent symptoms. Fifty percent of these revision patients were previously operated on in our own center.

At the outset we divided the patients into *two groups:*

1. Those patients who returned within months (in one case only 2 months) after the first operation with significant symptoms and severe restriction of physical activity. The average age of this group was 46 years and one was a 39-year-old woman (Table 1).

   The first group of patients as a rule had stable angina pectoris although exercise tolerance was limited. One case was unstable and three had infarctions with blocked bypasses.

2. The second group had had their first operation several years ago, the longest interval being 11 years and the shortest 6 years. Average age was 53 years (Table 2).

This group had suffered no new myocardial infarctions but had an unstable type of angina pectoris which was not responsive to medical treatment.

Table 1. Preoperative status of the patients and indication for surgery

Group A: redo surgery within 2–23 months ($n = 7$)		No. of patients
Myocardial infarction		3
Angina pectoris	stable	6
	unstable	1

Table 2. Preoperative status of the patients and indication for surgery

Group B: redo surgery within 6–11 years ($n = 6$)		No. of patients
Myocardial infarction		–
Angina pectoris	stable	1
	unstable	5

Table 3. Vascular status at an interval of 2–23 months in group A

Patients	Initial grafts	Graft-occlusions	Additional stenoses/ occlusions	New grafts
7	3.1	2.3	1.7	2.2

Table 4. Vascular status at an interval of 6–11 years in group B

Patients	Initial grafts	Graft-occlusions	Additional stenoses/ occlusions	New grafts
6	1.4	0.3	2.6	2.6

Tables 3 and 4 show the status of the coronaries. The first group initially received an average of three grafts. Repeat catheter and angiography show occlusion of two or three of them. About two additional stenoses of other vessels were seen per patient. On average two new bypasses were placed at the second operation.

The other group had mostly only one bypass. Bypass occlusion was rarer and involvement and extension of disease to the other coronaries was the main problem. This group received two to six new bypasses at the second session.

We are all familiar with the problems of dense adhesions between the heart and pericardium and sometimes the chest wall, especially when the pericardium was left open. Our impression is that this problem is much more difficult in the group who came early for their reoperations. Extensive inflammatory adhesions make the dissection very difficult. Often one enters both pleural cavities.

Sternotomy is carried out using the oscillating saw, which at first is used to divide the outer table. The inner table is split with strong scissors. Separation of the sternal halves is another problem, especially when the right ventricular myocardium is fixed to its posterior surface. With care and patience one can usually overcome this.

Cannulation was done into the ascending aorta and the right atrium using a two-stage venous cannula. Often one cannot fully separate the right atrium from the pericardium. Myocardial protection consisted of internal cooling and a combination of Kirsch and hydroxy-ethyl-starch solutions injected into the aortic root. Only membrane oxygenators were used and flow rate was 2.4 liters/m^2/min. Moderate systemic hypothermia (28 °C) and venting of the left ventricle were also used.

In the group who were admitted early for reoperations, although only two grafts on average were placed, the aortic occlusion time was still an average of 74 min. The other group in spite of receiving an average of three grafts had an average cross-clamp time of 53 min (Table 5). The reperfusion time to achieve a rectal temperature of around 34 °C and good cardiac activity was 60 min in the first group (Table 5).

Table 5. Operative procedure

Preoperation after	2–23 months	6–11 years
Mean aortic cross-clamp time (min)	74	53
Mean reperfusion time (min)	60	51
Mean systemic hypothermia (°C)	26	25
Mean grafts (vein, a. mam. int.)* (No.)	2.1	2.7

* arteria mammaria interna

Table 6. Postoperative complications

Reoperation after	2–23 months	6–11 years
Bleeding, ml/24 h/patient (mean)	970	960
	No. of patients	
Reopening for bleeding	1	1
Catecholamines (> 12 h postoperatively)	2	2
Postoperative infarction	1	–
Prolonged ventilation	2	3
Sternal wound dehiscence	–	1

Table 6 shows the postoperative complications. Four patients required catecholamines (dopamine, dobutamine) for longer than 12 h postoperatively. Twenty-four-hour blood loss was less than 1000 ml in both groups. Two required reopening for persistent bleeding. One patient suffered an infarction probably due to a drop in pressure resulting from excessive bleeding. He was opened up again and a thrombus removed from the bypass. Subsequently he was stable and had normal ECGs. Five patients required prolonged ventilation, that is longer than 6–8 h.

One was ventilated for 14 days as he developed a necrotizing pneumonitis. This patient had massive pulmonary embolism after a month and died in spite of operative intervention. One patient had sternal dehiscence and had to be operated on again to fix the sternum.

In spite of the small number of patients we observed a striking difference between the two groups, as far as symptomatology and operative findings are concerned. Recently operated on patients presented greater difficulty with the dissection and preparation of the heart. Obtaining vein grafts was a problem only in one patient in whom we took an arm vein and mobilized the mammary artery. Postoperative problems were similar in both groups. Excessive bleeding requiring reopening, which is otherwise quite rare in our center, occurred in two patients. Five required prolonged ventilation and four prolonged application of catecholamines.

There is a basic difference between these and those who are operated on for the first time. The early recovery and clinical improvement are certainly good. (Late follow-up is yet to be seen.) In spite of difficulties in the operations and the postoperative care we are encouraged by the results.

Repeat Coronary Revascularization Procedures After Primary Direct Coronary Surgery

P. SERGEANT, W. FLAMENG, M. SCHETZ, L. DEKEYZER, and R. SUY

Coronary redo surgery forms an increasing segment of the coronary revascularization procedures. The "failure" of the primary procedure can be caused by graft failure due to intimal hyperplasia or technical imperfections, caused by progression of atherosclerosis on grafted or nongrafted vessels or caused by incomplete initial surgery.

The total experience in coronary redo surgery of the K. U. Leuven cardiovascular surgery department is presented with special emphasis on the early graft failure group and on the use of the mammarian artery bypass. The Anderson [1] actuarial method is used for the analysis of the follow-up.

Ninety-three consecutive patients were reoperated on for recurrent angina pectoris from January 1973 until December 1984 with exclusion of aneurysmal resections and valvular replacements in primary or secondary procedures. Forty-nine percent of the patients were in anginal class 3 or 4 (range 0−4) and 58 in NYHA functional class III and IV. Two patients were reoperated on during the acute phase of an infarction with both in cardiogenic shock. Forty-one patients had angiographic findings of only graft failure without progression of the disease. In 27 patients these findings of only graft failure were present in the first 6 months after the initial operation, this is the pure early graft failure group.

The mean left ventricular end-diastolic pressure at reoperation was 12.8±6 mm Hg and the left ventricular ejection fraction was 59.5±14%. At the first operation a mean of 2.7±1.3 distal anastomoses were constructed per patient (1−7 distals); 18 distals were mammarian artery anastomoses. Before reoperation a mean of 0.9 ± 0.9 distals were still permeable (0−5) with 11 patent mammarian artery anastomoses. At reoperation 2.2 ± 1.3 new distals were constructed (1−5) with venous material and 46 new mammarian artery grafts, the left and/or right artery in single or jump graft fashion. Fifty-one patients entered the follow-up with at least one mammarian artery anastomosis patent.

The operative mortality was 3.2% (0.7%−9.1%, 95% confidence limits). The mean intensive care stay of the operative survivors was 3.5±2.7 days and the mean total hospital stay was 14.5±8.8 days. The revascularization was complete in 61%, most frequently because the vessel was too calcified or because of a full-thickness scar; in only few patients was there insufficient graft material.

The mean follow-up of the 90 operative survivors was 33±29 months. The mean follow-up of the 27 patients in the pure early graft failure group was 41±33 months. The total actuarial survival of the 93 patients (operative death

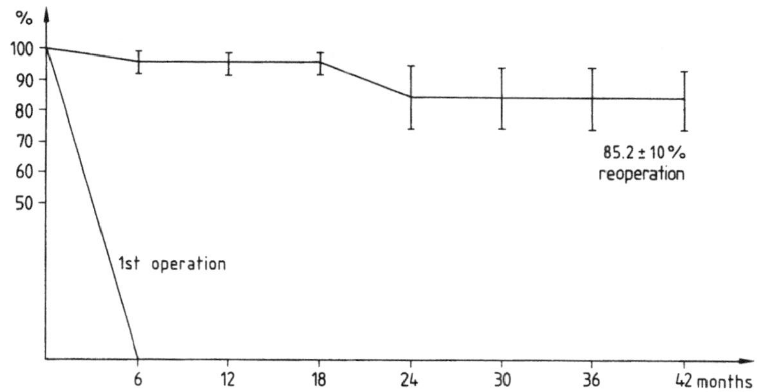

Fig. 1. Actuarial results of the pure early graft failure group, event-free analysis after the first and second procedures

included) was 95.4±2.2% at 42 months after surgery. Their cardiac survival was 97.8±1.5% at 42 months. The event-free group of the operative survivors at 42 months was 79.7 ± 5.2%. An event was defined as the onset of new even minimal angina pectoris, unannounced myocardial infarction, or sudden cardiac death. The event-free group of the operative survivors in the pure early graft failure group was 85.2 ± 10% at 42 months (Fig. 1).

Coronary reoperations can be performed with similar morbidity and mortality as in primary procedures even in the presence of unstable angina pectoris. The use of the left and right mammarian artery as a single or jump graft is essential if this graft material was not used in the primary procedure. The late results are very good, even in the presence of early graft failure. These patients should be reoperated on if there is a recurrence of symptoms, with at least one good size vessel graftable, in the presence of veins, or the possibility of a mammarian artery graft and of course with the full cooperation of the patient.

Reference

1. Anderson R, Bonchek L, Grunkemeier G, Lambert L, Starr A (1974) The analysis and presentation of surgical results by actuarial methods. J Surg Res 16:224–230

Coronary Artery Bypass Reoperation: Indication and Results

P. Spreafico, G. Minzioni, A. Graffigna, E. Arbustini, and M. Vigano'

Introduction

At present, for most patients with coronary artery disease (CAD), coronary artery bypass grafting (CABG) is the therapy which offers the best control of symptoms and, in many cases, longer survival. Although an improvement in clinical status can be achieved in most patients treated with CABG, angina may persist in operated on patients or may appear later in the postoperative course.

In prospective randomized studies [1, 6, 8] it has been reported that 76%–90% of the patients show a definite improvement in symptoms; 33%–55% of these are asymptomatic whereas 5% deteriorate. This latter group of patients must be considered as potential candidates for a new surgical approach. On the basis of the increasing number of patients who yearly undergo CABG, more grafted patients are expected to need reoperation [5].

Patients and Methods

From November 1976 to June 1985, 29 patients who had had CABG were reoperated upon owing to recurrence of angina. There were 26 males and 3 females: mean age was 54 years (range 35–73 years).

In 21 cases angina was unstable, while it was stable in the remaining 8 cases. Time elapsed from the first operation to the recurrence of symptoms ranged from 1 to 129 months (mean free interval, 34 months). Coronarographic studies showed occlusion or stenosis in 35 out of 61 CABGs performed at the first operation (57%) and new coronary lesions in 15 patients (51%).

Indications for surgery were: occlusion or stenosis of the graft in 13 patients, progressive atherosclerosis in previously ungrafted vessels in 4 patients, and a combination of graft occlusion and progressive atherosclerosis in 11 cases; one patient was reoperated on because of a steal from the left anterior descending artery through a collateral of the left internal mammary artery used at the first operation. The interval between operations varied from 1 to 140 months (mean, 44 months).

The surgical technique was the same employed in elective CABG operations with the only precaution of isolating the femoral vessels before opening the chest. Fifty-one new CABGs were performed at the second operation [using the homologous saphenous vein in all patients but one, in whom the left internal mammary artery (LIMA) was used], together with ten new anastomoses to the previously grafted veins, with a CABG/patient ratio of 2.1 at reoperation. Since 26 patent and functioning grafts (out of 61 performed at the first operation) were left in place, the final CABG/patient ratio increased to 3.0. In addition, four endarterectomies, one ligature of a collateral of a LIMA previously anastomized to the left anterior descending artery (LAD), which was responsible for the steal from the LAD artery, one thromboembolectomy according to Fogarty, and one intraluminal dilatation with Grunzig's technique were performed. All grafts removed at operation underwent pathologic studies. Multiple serial sections were stained according to H & E, Masson trichrome, and Weigert methods.

Results

There was one in-hospital death owing to low-output syndrome on day 35 (hospital mortality, 3.4%). There was no perioperative myocardial infarction as detected by new Q-waves on the electrocardiogram. Postoperative course was complicated in one case by sternal dehiscence.

The follow-up of all the discharged patients (range 1–101 months, mean 26 months) shows only one late death due to central nervous system damage following a cardiac arrest 7 months after reoperation. Twenty-five patients have improved their condition (18 are now asymptomatic, 7 have less severe angina), while 2 are unchanged.

Discussion

Indication for reoperation is angina in a patient with graftable vessels and good runoff, as well as for the first operation. Coronarographic study may show: progressive atherosclerosis of the native arteries, graft occlusion, or a combination of both. Thrombosis, inadequate runoff, intimal hyperplasia, progression of arterial disease, and technical faults may be the reason for graft stenosis or occlusion in the first 3 years, responsible for early angina after operation. "Atherosclerosis" of the graft usually occurs later on, usually after 5 years. It has been reported [4] that 10%–25% of the vein grafts become occluded within the 1st year; thereafter the average vein graft occlusion rate is 2%/year. Recent reports [2, 5] have also showed that between 5 and 10 years the graft occlusion rate doubled. Sequential angiographic studies [2] demonstrated that 46% of the vein grafts open 6–18 months postoperatively had evidence of atherosclerotic changes 10–12 years after surgery. In our experience atherosclerotic-like changes were observed in 22% of patients after a mean interval of 70 months (range 32–140 months) after the first operation.

On the basis of an incidence of 7% after 10 years with a linear increment of 10% for each following decade, Loop [5] extrapolates 13700 CABG reoperations at the beginning of the nineties.

With increasing experience in this field, operations can today be performed with acceptable risk: hospital mortality declined from 5% to 2% in Loop's series and similar rates are reported by other well-experienced groups [7, 9–11]. Adhesions may cause accidents during reentry, diffuse bleeding, and longer pump time and may obscure the coronary anatomy [3], but probably at present a diffuse atherosclerosis involving the grafts and a depressed myocardial function play a more important role in determining the operative risk. While some reports gave evidence of the importance of hyperlipidemia as risk factor in the group of patients having reoperation, Loop's large series of 1000 reoperated on patients showed no correlation with the usual risk factor, except for diabetes, the frequency of which was double in the reoperation series. Our experience confirms that when the reoperation is performed by surgeons who have experience of these more complicated procedures, coronary artery reoperation can today be performed with acceptable hospital mortality and symptomatic improvement.

References

1. Anderson RP, Rahimtoola SH, Bonchek LI, Starr A (1974) The prognosis of patients with coronary artery disease after coronary bypass operation. Time-related progress of 532 patients with disabling angina pectoris. Circulation 50:274
2. Grondin CM, Pomar JL, Hebert Y, Bosch X, Santos JM, Enjalbert M, Campeau L (1984) Reoperation in patients with patent atherosclerotic coronary vein grafts. A different approach to a different disease. J Thorac Cardiovasc Surg 87:379
3. Jones EL, Douglas JS, Gruetzig AR, Craver JM, King SV, Guyton RA, Hatcher CR (1983) Percutaneous vein angioplasty to avoid reoperative bypass surgery. Ann Thorac Surg 36:389
4. Lawrie GM, Morris GC, Chapman DW, Winters WL, Lie JT (1977) Pattern of patency of 596 vein grafts up to 7 years after aorta coronary bypass. J Thorac Cardiovasc Surgery 73:433
5. Loop FD, Lytle BW, Gill CC, Golding LAR, Cosgrow DM, Taylor PC (1983) Trends in selection and results of coronary artery operations. Ann Thorac Surg 36:380
6. Mathur VS, Guinn GA (1979) Chronic stable angina: prospective randomized study with 4–7 year follow-up to evaluate surgical vs medical treatment. Chest 76:359
7. Mills NL (1983) Reop or not. Ann Thorac Surg 36:375
8. Read RC, Murphy ML, Hultgren HN, Detre K, Thomsen J, Takaro T (1978) Treatment of chronic stable angina. A preliminary report on survival data of the randomized Veteran Administration Cooperative Study. J Thorac Cardiovasc Surg 75:1
9. Reul GJ, Cooley DA, Oh DA, Coelho A, Chapa L, Eterovic I (1979) Reoperation for recurrent coronary artery disease. Causes, indications and results in 168 patients. Arch Surg 114:1269
10. Schaff HV, Onszulak TA, Gersh BJ, Piehler JM, Puga FJ, Danielson GK, Pluth JR (1983) The morbidity and mortality of reoperation for coronary artery disease and analysis of late results with the use of actuarial estimate of even free interval. J Thorac Cardiovasc Surgery 85:508
11. Vouhé P, Grondin CM (1979) Reoperation for coronary graft failure. Clinical and angiographic result in 43 patients. Ann Thorac Surg 27:328

Subject Index

www.ingramcontent.com/pod-product-compliance
Lightning Source LLC
Chambersburg PA
CBHW061203240926
51846CB00006B/1096
* 9 7 8 3 6 4 2 4 5 6 2 4 4 *